Unconventional Optical Imaging for Biology

SCIENCES

Image, Field Director – Laure Blanc-Féraud

Imagery in Life Sciences, Subject Head – Françoise Peyrin

Unconventional Optical Imaging for Biology

Coordinated by
Corinne Fournier
Olivier Haeberlé

ISTE

WILEY

First published 2024 in Great Britain and the United States by ISTE Ltd and John Wiley & Sons, Inc.

ISTE Ltd
27-37 St George's Road
London SW19 4EU
UK

www.iste.co.uk

John Wiley & Sons, Inc.
111 River Street
Hoboken, NJ 07030
USA

www.wiley.com

Library of Congress Control Number: 2023940645

British Library Cataloguing-in-Publication Data
A CIP record for this book is available from the British Library
ISBN 978-1-78945-132-0

ERC code:
LS2 Genetics, 'Omics', Bioinformatics and Systems Biology
LS2_13 Computational biology
PE1 Mathematics
PE1_20 Application of mathematics in sciences

Contents

Introduction

Corinne FOURNIER[1] **and Olivier HAEBERLÉ**[2]
[1] *Laboratoire Hubert Curien, CNRS, IOGS, Télécom Saint-Étienne, Université Jean Monnet, Saint-Étienne, France*
[2] *IRIMAS, Université de Haute-Alsace, Mulhouse, France*

I.1. Context

Optical imaging in biological systems has undergone spectacular developments in recent years, which have resulted in providing a quantity and a quality of information that, until about 20 years ago, was merely a dream for physicists, biologists or physicians.

The extraordinary progress that has been made can be explained through a combination of contributions in the field of the physics of image formation, in instrumentation with the arrival of new sensors with remarkable performance, and finally by the extraordinary computing power and memory capacity of current computers. To illustrate these remarks, we can refer to two spectacular examples (not addressed in this book).

In fluorescence microscopy, the diffraction barrier has been "broken" in a spectacular way thanks to the developments of STED (Stimulated Emission Depletion) microscopy first, and followed by the invention of pointillist microscopies. STED microscopy utilizes the temporal properties of the fluorescence phenomenon, which is not instantaneous, to cause a stimulated emission. The latter is controlled by the system, being spatially, temporally, spectrally and directionally dissociable from the spontaneous fluorescence emission. Proposed as early as 1994,

Unconventional Optical Imaging for Biology,
coordinated by Corinne FOURNIER and Olivier HAEBERLÉ.

this technique has only recently become widespread, with the emergence of inexpensive and high-performance lasers and detectors. Pointillist microscopies make use of the statistical properties of fluorescence emission, which exhibits a random nature. By processing large quantities of individual images, with few fluorescent spots, it is possible to detect and locate them individually, and thus to reconstruct an image with improved resolution. These techniques have now even made imaging of living specimens possible; this is mainly due to the quality of fluorescence labelings, the right photon yield of fluorophores, but especially the extreme sensitivity of modern cameras, and the speed of image processing allowed by current computers.

Another field that has undergone remarkable development is imaging through scattering media. A large body of techniques has been developed or improved in recent years. The most astounding is perhaps the one that makes use of scattering matrices. It is based on the fact that, in an imaging system, the Green's matrix (set of Green's functions linking each source emitting light to each detector pixel) contains the information accessible in linear scattering processes. Modern experimental means (sensors of large dimension and sensitivity, spatial light modulators with many degrees of freedom, and powerful computers) now contribute to experimentally characterize scattering media by accurately measuring the scattering matrix. Impressive operations until recently unimaginable can now be performed; these include the characterization of surface or volume scattering, separation of the contributions of single and multiple scattering and even focusing through a scattering medium, which paves the way to both transmission and reflection imaging.

This book is concerned with other areas of biological imaging that have also been driven, like these two examples, by advances in instrumentation and computer science, and that have led to making possible concepts that were until recently purely theoretical.

I.2. Unconventional imaging

Unconventional imaging, as opposed to conventional imaging, allows us to access physical quantities (such as the opacity, the refractive index, the property of wave polarization, the chemical composition of an object and so on) not directly accessible by optical systems, in which sensors can only measure information in terms of intensity.

The use of particular optical setups and computer processing for the captured images/signals has enabled the reconstruction of physical quantities. This is also referred to as *computational imaging*. Typical unconventional imaging modalities are: polarimetry, interferometry, holography and phase imaging, as well as hyperspectral imaging. Unconventional imaging can also be used for the purposes of miniaturizing, reducing the costs or improving the quantitativity of conventional imaging systems. This type of imaging requires the co-design of the optical system, sensors and signal and image processing algorithms. A large variety of information obtained through unconventional imaging allows for improved detection, quantitative characterization and classification of imaged objects. These systems are used in many fields of biological imaging, namely endoscopy, microscopy, skin or through-skin imaging and fast phenomena imaging.

I.3. Book contents

In this book, we focus on various unconventional imaging modalities developed for the biomedical field; these include wavefront analysis imaging, digital holography, optical nanoscopy, endoscopy and single-pixel imaging. The first six chapters are complementary and address phase-imaging.

Chapter 1 presents quantitative phase microscopy using a wavefront analyzer. Wavefront analyzers are particular devices that are capable of measuring a wave without making use of holography (more details in the following chapters). In this chapter, the notion of wave phase is first recalled, followed by an introduction to the notion of phase object in the field of biology. The particular modality of quadriwave lateral shearing interferometry is described in detail and applied to solve major problems in biological imaging, such as dry mass measurements, the study of fast biological phenomena and birefringence measurements.

Chapter 2 presents digital holography through a detailed presentation of the principle of interferometry used in holography, based on superposing a reference wave onto the wave diffracted by the object. Introduced by Gabor in electron microscopy, holography is in fact known in particular for its applications in optics. The most commonly used holographic configurations are described. Finally, the digital processing of the obtained data, in order to extract the characteristics of the measured wavefront, in amplitude and phase, is detailed. This chapter serves as an introduction to Chapter 4, which deals with digital holography, in the configuration known as in-line holography, as well as to Chapter 5, which presents tomographic diffractive microscopy.

Chapter 3 is concerned with a general methodology for numerical reconstruction using an approach based on "inverse problems". This approach leads to estimating the parameters of interest of imaged objects from unconventional images. It is presented in a very general way and thus can be applied to different modalities of unconventional imaging. This chapter presents the simple case of likelihood maximization between data and linear imaging models, and then addresses the problem of the nonlinear phase reconstruction (*phase retrieval*) with or without taking into account the a priori on the reconstructed objects. This chapter contains examples of in-line digital holography in connection with the next chapter.

Chapter 4 is dedicated to in-line holographic microscopy. It presents the experimental configurations of holographic microscopy used in the biomedical field along with their specificities. The problem of numerical reconstruction is addressed by comparing different historical and state-of-the-art approaches with experimental images. As a follow-up to Chapter 3, approaches based on "inverse problems" are used and their potential for holographic microscopy is discussed.

Chapter 5 gives an extension of holography, with application to transmission microscopy. Tomographic diffractive microscopy is a technique coupling holography with scanning light illumination on the specimen or with a rotation thereof. This technique allows for much more information to be acquired, which results in a 3D reconstruction of the distribution of optical indices in the observed specimen. The refractive index (in refraction and absorption) has become a contrast allowing for many applications on specimens without preparation (no coloring, no fluorescent tagging), which now finds applications in many fields (such as the study of stem cells, yeasts, bacterial growth and so on).

Chapter 6 describes another phase microscopy technique, known as white light interferometric microscopy. Based on a particular configuration (Linnick interferometer), it differs from the techniques described in the previous chapters in that it is a reflection technique. The demodulation of the reflected signal leads to unequaled precision of measurement, namely in the nanometric range. However, the lateral resolution remains that of a conventional optical microscope. A recent extension involves combining microsphere-assisted microscopy with interferometry, paving the way for surface nanometrology. These techniques are now also used for biological imaging, in particular cellular or tissue imaging.

Chapter 7 addresses white light and endoscopic fluorescence imaging. Following a presentation of the principles of endoscopy, particular emphasis is given to the problem of the 3D reconstruction of hollow organs observed through this technique. Endoscopic images have specific characteristics, requiring dedicated approaches, namely the low contrast of the structures to be observed, delicate fluorescent tagging, strong distortions of the obtained images, and induced by the characteristics of the optical system utilized and the hollow geometry of the organs. This results in specific difficulties in performing the 3D image registration.

Finally, *Chapter 8* is dedicated to single-pixel imaging. Thanks to the optical modulation of scenes by known patterns and advanced digital reconstruction algorithms, it is possible to reconstruct an image from a series of point measurements (on a single pixel). This type of imaging has been developed considerably over the last 15 years and makes it possible to design efficient and low-cost systems for different modalities such as infrared, terahertz or fluorescence imaging. This chapter presents the instrumental aspects and the mathematical foundations of single-pixel computational imaging. In addition, it addresses conventional numerical reconstruction techniques and also the latest approaches that use deep learning.

The purpose of this book is thus to introduce the reader to these new unconventional imaging techniques through a detailed presentation of their principles and implementations, supported by illustrations of application examples drawn mainly from the studies of the various research groups involved in their development.

1

Quantitative Phase Microscopy Using Wavefront Analysis

Serge MONNERET[1], Julien SAVATIER[1] and Pierre BON[2]

[1]*Aix-Marseille Université, CNRS, Centrale Marseille, Institut Fresnel, France*

[2]*Université de Limoges, CNRS, XLIM, France*

1.1. Introduction

The observation of transparent samples using optical techniques may seem by definition not very obvious, since these samples have very little influence on the transmission of light that travels therethrough. Consequently, it is necessary to employ more complex solutions than simple imaging in order to reveal the structures of such samples. Interest in such techniques is particularly heightened in biological imaging, for which the observation of living biological cells placed in an aqueous medium leads to very low contrasts, whereas the observation of subcellular structures is of major relevance for the understanding of living organisms. The first techniques developed were based on the use of interferometry to create contrast, but at the cost of relatively complex systems and/or not allowing measurements (contrast increase only). We will present here a technique based on a wavefront measurement, producing a map of the

For a color version of all the figures in this chapter, see www.iste.co.uk/fournier/unconventional.zip.

Unconventional Optical Imaging for Biology,

optical thickness of the imaged sample resulting in inferring a set of measurements of interest.

1.2. Description of the principles used in phase imaging

We consider an infinite translucent medium (e.g. glass with a refractive index n_0 = 1.5) when a sinusoidal monochromatic light wave of wavelength λ_0 passes through, as shown in Figure 1.1. Consider that this block of glass possesses two internal zones. The first one, in green in the figure, is absorbing and has the same index n_0. The second one, in blue, is transparent but of index $n = n_0 + \Delta n$. If this object is imaged, the green zone that made photons disappear by absorption will create a darker zone than the rest of the image and will consequently be detectable by creating an absorption contrast. On the other hand, the blue zone will not be visible because the photons that traveled through will all reach the detector. Nevertheless, since the index of refraction is different in the blue zone from that of the surrounding medium, these photons will not have taken the same time to reach this detector and will arrive later or earlier than the others according to the sign of Δn.

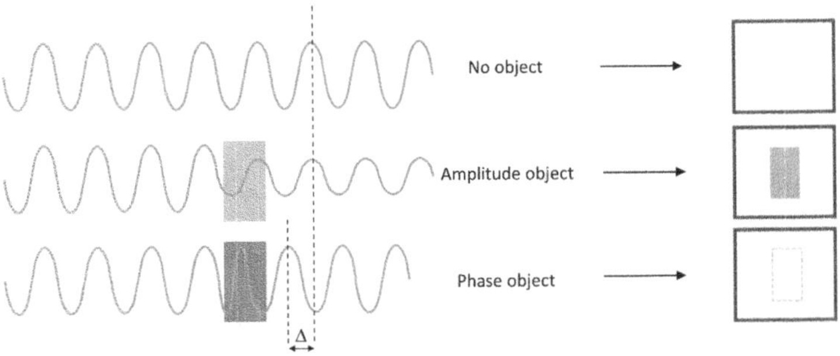

Figure 1.1. *Amplitude and phase in optical imaging*[1]

Let us call Δ the spatial shift of the wave due to passing through the entire blue zone (Figure 1.1). In this simple one-dimensional case, the wave incident on the sample can be written as A cos $(k_0 x)$ exp(-iωt) where $k_0 = 2\pi/\lambda_0$ is the wavenumber and ω is the angular frequency. The output wave will then take the form:

$$A(x,t) = A\ cos(k_0 x - \Phi)\ exp(-i\omega t)\ with\ \Phi = 2\pi\Delta/\lambda_0 \quad [1.1]$$

1 Figure developed from: www.microscopyu.com.

The value of Φ is called the phase of the wave, hence imaging techniques that generate contrast from the spatial distribution of the parameter Δ are called phase imaging. It should be noted that the value of Δ can be identical for a low index and large thickness zone, or another zone of higher refractive index but smaller thickness. Consequently, it is the optical thickness (product of the refractive index and the geometrical thickness) which defines Δ, and which will thus be the contrast parameter in phase imaging. Figure 1.2 illustrates the importance, but also the limitations, of phase imaging: it is impossible to decorrelate the optical index from the thickness. Furthermore, a thinner object with a higher refractive index than another can ultimately produce the same phase shift.

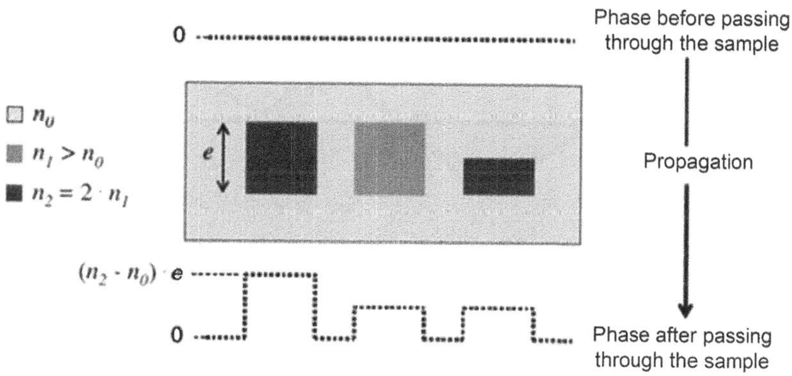

Figure 1.2. *Wave surface deformation when traversing an inhomogeneous object (source: Bon 2011)*

The value of the time shift associated with Δ is tiny (3 fs for every 10 μm crossed for a relative refractive index variation of 0.1) and no current conventional detector can take this time shift into account. Consequently, if they are completely translucent, the red and orange inserts of the sample of Figure 1.2 will be totally undetectable in an imaging system such as a microscope equipped with a conventional camera. On the other hand, making the wave from the sample interfere with another reference wave leads to the creation of an interference contrast that is this time sensitive not to local absorption, but to the parameter Δ and thus to the local optical thickness. Zernike's phase contrast techniques (Zernike 1935), now conventional, as well as Nomarski's contrast techniques (Nomarski 1955), also called *differential interferential contrast* (DIC), are all based on this general principle. Holographic microscopy is probably the most successful version of this principle: it allows access to quantitative information, but requires dedicated microscopes (Cuche et al. 1999).

Consider now a monochromatic plane wave of wavelength λ_0 passing through a phase object considered here as non-diffracting. Its scalar electromagnetic field can be written, after traversal of the object and in a reference plane perpendicular to its mean wave vector:

$$E(x,y) = a(x,y)\ exp(i\ k_0\ W(x,y)) \tag{1.2}$$

with $a(x,y)$ the amplitude of the field and $W(x,y)$ the distance between the wavefront perturbed by the object and the reference plane wave. Figure 1.3 gives a representation of this surface.

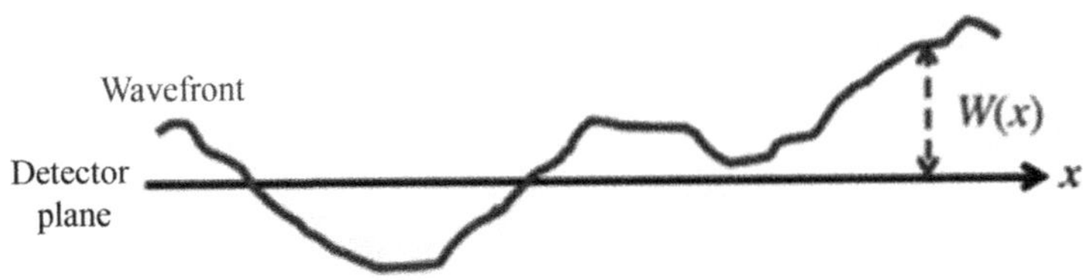

Figure 1.3. *Representation of the W function in a one-dimensional example (source: Bon 2011)*

When illuminating a phased object with an incident plane wave (pictured in Figure 1.2), the wavefront W after traversing the object is directly related to the optical path difference distribution that characterizes this object:

$$W(x,y) = \Delta(x,y) = \int_0^h [n(x,y,z) - n_{med}]\, dz \tag{1.3}$$

where h is the height of the sample, $n(x,y,z)$ is the refractive index distribution and n_{med} is the refractive index of the surrounding medium.

$W(x,y) = Delta(x,y) = OPD(x,y)$ is called the *optical path difference* in the literature. From now on, we will systematically use this notation in the rest of this chapter.

The knowledge of the distribution $OPD(x,y)$ thus provides us with a complete understanding of the constitution of the object traversed by an incident plane wave. In other words, if we consider that the inhomogeneities within the sample introduce local photon delays with respect to one another, sending a plane wave on this sample will result in producing a distorted wavefront as a result of propagating within these inhomogeneities. The technique we propose here consists of simply measuring the wavefront after the sample perturbation, using a wavefront sensor, and then deducing the optical thickness mapping of this sample knowing beforehand the shape of the incident wavefront. This technique has been made possible by the emergence of wavefront sensors with sufficient resolution to produce useful information for biologists.

1.3. Quadriwave lateral shearing interferometry for high spatial resolution wavefront analysis

Wavefront analysis using *quadriwave lateral shearing interferometry* (QLSI) is a technique that can be used to meet the objectives presented above.

It is based on the measurement of the gradient of the wavefront simultaneously in two orthogonal directions. To this end, four replicas of the electromagnetic field shifted from each other in the two directions of the analysis plane (Figure 1.4) will be generated by a specific diffraction mask. The interference between these replicas will create an intensity modulation (interference fringes forming what will be called an interferogram, recorded by the sensor of a digital camera) carrying the information of the phase gradients. Post-acquisition analysis of the recorded interferograms then allows for the calculation of the shape of the incident wavefront on the diffractive mask.

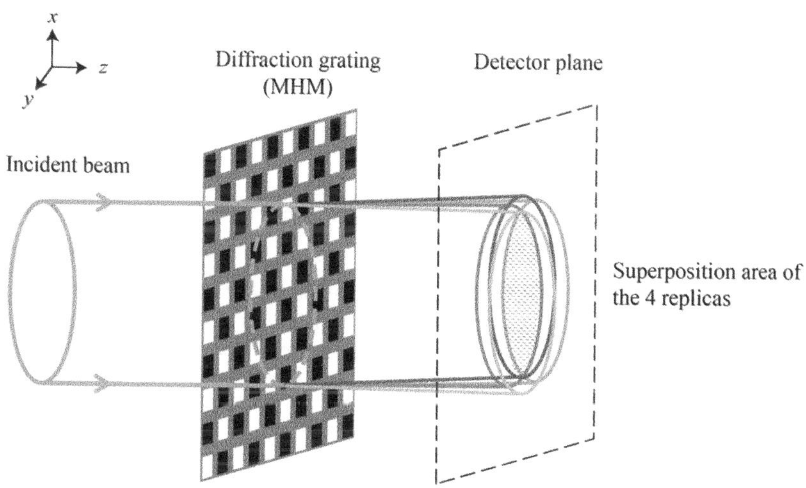

Figure 1.4. *Separation of the incident wavefront into four symmetric replicas along two perpendicular axes by diffraction on a modified Hartmann mask (MHM) (source: Aknoun 2014)*

1.3.1. *Generation of incident field replicas*

As we have just stated, quadriwave lateral shearing interferometry is based on a measurement of wavefront gradients along two perpendicular directions, from the analysis of the interference pattern produced on the sensor of a camera by four replicas of this wavefront slightly inclined along these two directions.

The optical element making possible the generation of these four diffraction orders is a sinusoidal phase grating of transmittance $t(x, y)$ in the two spatial directions. Equation [1.4] describes this transmittance for a grating of period p along x and y; Figure 1.5 presents this theoretical phase grating (Figure 1.5(a)) as well as its diffraction orders (Figure 1.5(c)):

$$t(x, y) = cos(\frac{2\pi}{p}x)\ cos(\frac{2\pi}{p}y) \qquad [1.4]$$

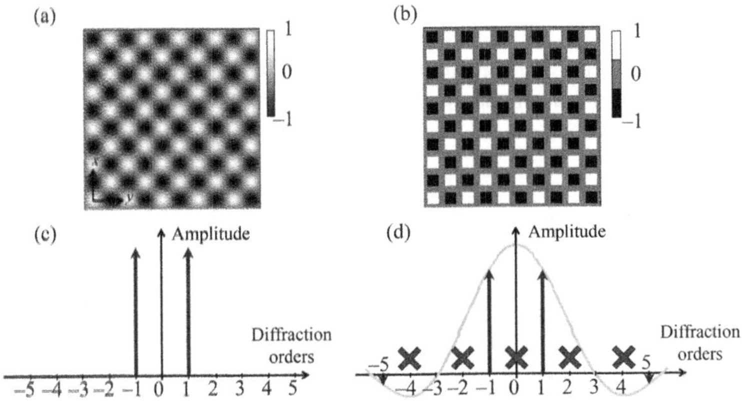

Figure 1.5. *Bisinusoidal phase grating (a) and modified Hartmann grating (b). Graphs (c) and (d) represent the diffracted amplitude distribution in the different orders of these two gratings, respectively (source: Bon 2011)*

Building such a grating is nevertheless difficult. The chosen solution is based on a three-level approximation (+1; 0; 1) of the transmittance function (Figure 1.5(b)). This grating is called a modified Hartmann mask (MHM); it can be seen as the combination of a matrix of square apertures (called the Hartmann mask) and a phase checkerboard dephasing one hole out of two of π. Figure 1.5(d) shows the orders diffracted by an MHM. The choice of a duty cycle of 2/3 results in suppressing orders 3 and –3. The addition of the pure phase grating enables, by destructive interference, the suppression of all even orders, including the zeroth order representing the field not diffracted by the grating. Therefore, an MHM is a good and practical model of the optimal bisinusoidal phase grating. It enables 90% of the diffracted energy in the four desired orders to be distributed, the rest being distributed in odd orders higher than 3. Nevertheless, its main drawback is that it does not provide as much transparency as the optimal two-dimensional phase grating.

The π phase shift of the checkerboard is obtained by increasing the optical path traveled, that is, the grating is locally thicker to introduce the desired delay. Relation [1.5] links the difference in thickness e to the optical index n of the material used to create this π phase shift:

$$e = \frac{\lambda_0}{2(n-1)} \qquad [1.5]$$

This relation shows the obvious dependence of the etching thickness on the usage wavelength of the grating. When the phase shift is not exactly π, a reoccurrence of the even orders is observed, and in particular of zeroth order. These orders will interfere with the useful orders and will create additional frequencies in the interferogram, degrading the signal-to-noise ratio. It is however possible to find distances between the mask and the plane of the detector, minimizing the influence of the parasitic orders (Primot and Guérineau 2000): in these planes, the interferogram is similar to that which would be obtained for a phase shift of π. In practice, when light is not monochromatic, e should be chosen so as to create a phase shift of pi for the central wavelength of the source and a mask/detector distance close to the Talbot distance of the Hartmann mask for this central wavelength (Velghe 2006).

This operating point makes it possible to obtain an achromatic assembly operating regardless of the wavelength spectrum of the source, including white light. This is a major advantage of the technique applied to microscopy, since it enables us to use the conventional illumination of the microscope to perform the measurement (halogen source sufficiently spatially coherent to generate the interferograms, used in a Köhler assembly with a reduced aperture diaphragm).

1.3.2. *Determination of the incident wavefront*

As we have seen above, after a few millimeters of propagation, the beams are slightly separated and then form interference fringes whose pitch is determined by the angle between the propagation directions. If the incident beam is a perfectly plane wave, the interferogram recorded by a camera is a regular two-dimensional array of light points. If the wavefront presents local modulations, this regular mesh is locally deformed. The study of these distortions using spectral analysis methods allows us to find the phase spatial gradients.

More precisely, the intensity distribution at the level of the interferogram, after propagation along a distance z after passing through the mask (placed in the plane z = 0), is given by (Bon 2009):

$$I(x,y,z) = I_0 \left[1 + cos\left(\frac{2\pi}{p}x + \frac{2\pi}{p}z\frac{\partial OPD}{\partial x}\right) + cos\left(\frac{2\pi}{p}y + \frac{2\pi}{p}z\frac{\partial OPD}{\partial y}\right)\right]$$
$$+ \frac{I_0}{2}\left[cos\left(\frac{2\pi}{p}(x+y) + \frac{2\pi}{p}z\frac{\partial OPD}{\partial(x+y)}\right)\right] \qquad [1.6]$$
$$+ \frac{I_0}{2}\left[cos\left(\frac{2\pi}{p}(x-y) + \frac{2\pi}{p}z\frac{\partial OPD}{\partial(x-y)}\right)\right]$$

where I_0 corresponds to the maximum intensity on the diffraction mask output. This equation corresponds to a perfect mask generating only the four desired diffraction orders.

This equation shows that various wavefront gradients are encoded in the form of frequency modulation around characteristic interferogram spatial frequencies, that is, the eigen spatial frequencies of the MHM.

Let us now consider an arbitrary wave arriving at the MHM at normal average incidence. If we merely consider a single dimension to simplify the equations, the intensity recorded at the detector can be written as:

$$I(x) \approx i_0(x) + i_x(x)\, cos\left(\frac{2\pi}{p}\left[x - L\,\frac{\partial W(x)}{\partial x}\right]\right) \qquad [1.7]$$

where L is the distance between the MHM and the camera sensor. This coefficient, placed in front of the wavefront gradient term, is important: it can be used to modulate the sensitivity to gradients (the larger L is, the more sensitive the sensor, however it provides less dynamics).

The gradient along the x-direction of the wavefront can be extracted by demodulation in the Fourier space of the interferogram. We call $|\nu_{int}|$ the maximum spatial frequency of the intensity information i_0. We call $|\nu_{mod}|$ the support in Fourier space of the information modulated around the carrier frequency and 1/p the fundamental frequency of the interferogram. T_{pix} refers to the sampling period of the matrix detector (it is assumed that the pixels are square), θ refers to the orientation of the interferogram with respect to the sensor pixel matrix and $\Delta\nu = 2/\alpha p$ refers to the bandwidth for the extraction of the phase information, α being a parameter used to simplify the computations. All of these notations are represented in Figure 1.6.

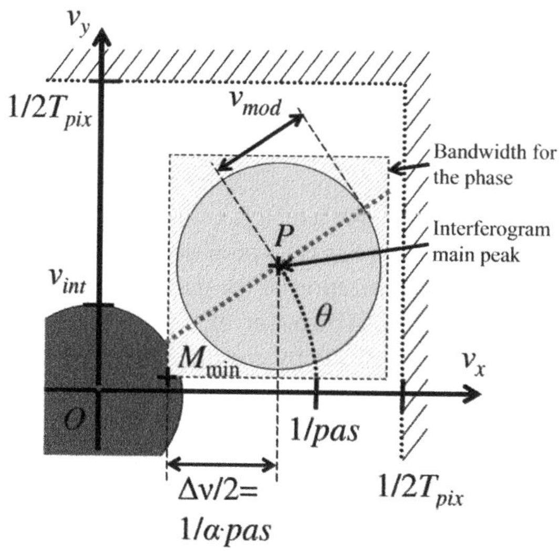

Figure 1.6. *Definition of the various supports in Fourier space (source: Bon 2011)*

Various conditions must be met to ensure that the bandwidth is sufficient, without spectrum aliasing, to accurately reconstruct the phase and intensity signal. First, the main frequency of the grating $cos(\theta)/p$ must be lower than the Nyquist frequency $1/2T_{pix}$ in order to sample the signal correctly; it is also necessary that all the frequencies of the bandwidth around the main frequency satisfy this same Nyquist criterion. Finally, the last condition comes from the necessary non-overlap between the intensity information and the modulated phase information; this must be reflected by a non-overlapping of the red and orange domains of Figure 1.6. It should be noted that for essentially transparent samples, such as those usually employed in the field of cell biology, the energy values (especially for high spatial frequencies) will be lower in intensity than in phase.

In the end, a choice of $\alpha = 2$ is often made at the level of the reconstruction algorithms to best separate the bandwidth of the frequency support from the intensity distribution of the samples. This choice requires that the phase and intensity images resulting from the reconstruction processes have a number of pixels 16 times lower than the images initially produced on the sensor plane. More precisely, with such a value of α a sensor area of 4 x 4 pixels is used to produce a local phase measurement. The lower limit that would just satisfy the Nyquist criterion would be to use 2.73 x 2.73 pixels to sample the interferogram. Some recent commercial systems utilize a reconstruction algorithm based on 3 x 3 pixel sampling (SID4 SC8, Phasics, France). Finally, equation [1.6] shows that we also have access, through the interferogram, to the gradients in the (x + y) and (x – y) directions. This redundant information can be used to increase the signal-to-noise ratio of the wavefront measurement (Velghe et al. 2005).

The most commonly used method to quantitatively reconstruct the wavefront employs the discrete Fourier transform, which leads to artifacts when the phase objects overlap the edges of the image, which is common in cell biology. To address this shortcoming, a simple approach has been proposed to avoid these artifacts, based on the duplication and antisymmetrization of the derivative data, in the direction of the derivative, before integration (Volkov et al. 2002; Bon et al. 2012a). This approach completely erases edge effects by creating continuity and a mathematical differentiability condition at the edge of the image.

It is thus possible to extract the OPD gradients from the Fourier analysis of an interferogram recorded on a CCD or CMOS sensor. The gradients are finally integrated to obtain a two-dimensional OPD map. However, since the phase information is encoded in the interferogram by a frequency modulation, the phase and intensity are independently determined. The intensity image is effectively simply extracted from the application of a low-pass filter on the interferogram (fringe descreen operation). This property offers an advantage over conventional phase contrast methods such as Nomarski/DIC or Zernike contrast, where it is very difficult to attribute the intensity modulations visible in the images either to a spatial variation of the sample absorption or to OPD gradients.

1.3.3. *Wavefront sensor implementation*

The technology of wavefront measurement using quadriwave lateral shearing interferometry until now has been exclusively commercialized by Phasics (Saint-Aubin, France), a company that holds the exploitation rights. The various products developed over the last 20 years have followed some of the technological evolutions of cameras (including the shift from CCD cameras to sCMOS cameras, the development of sensors for specific spectral domains such as infrared), making it possible to address ever wider application fields. Nonetheless, some applications still require very specific cameras (EMCCD in very low light, ultrafast cameras for the measurement of dynamic samples, etc.) to acquire interferograms. The now commercialized (SID4Element, Phasics, France) proposed solution (Berto et al. 2012) consists of using an imaging optical system as a relay to project the image of an MHM, at the appropriate location and magnification, inside the camera optimized for the targeted application. Consequently, it is possible to acquire interferograms under very low light to achieve phase images in full-field coherent Raman microscopy, or to use a fast camera to follow fast-evolving samples (see section 1.5.3).

1.4. Using a wavefront sensor in microscopy

Most non-tissue biological objects (isolated biological cells in culture) appear very faintly in intensity-based imaging (otherwise known as absorption imaging). In this case, when the incident light exits the sample it has undergone a phase shift only (hence the name phase objects sometimes used), and therefore its wavefront has been modified. Placing a wavefront sensor on the sample output should thus allow the optical thickness of the sample to be mapped, and thus a contrast of interest to be generated.

1.4.1. *Necessary approximations*

We consider a simple model for interpreting the measured difference values of the optical path, overlooking the imaging and filtering effects by the microscope objective. The first approach that we can follow for interpreting the measurements consists of considering that at first order, the measured phase shift is due only to photons slowing down when passing through the sample and that no change in direction of propagation occurs during the traversing. Any refraction phenomenon at the interfaces or diffraction by the object is not taken into account: refraction is negligible with small index differences or if the interfaces are orthogonal to the propagation of light; diffraction is visible when the objects become small relative to the resolution limit of the microscope. Under these assumptions, the wavefront sensor directly measures the optical path difference within the sample, according to the diagram in Figure 1.3.

This assumption considers that all photons propagate in the same direction, which is that of the optical axis of the system; the illumination is said to be plane wave illumination. In fact, all of the measurements will be performed following a quasi-planar wave illumination regime via a diameter restriction of the aperture diaphragm of the Köhler illumination of the microscope.

It seems that the simple measurement of the wavefront shape on the sample output provides us with a map of the optical thickness of the sample. In real life, and in particular inside a microscope, it is unrealistic to generate a perfectly plane wavefront incident on the sample. Consequently, we must also record the shape of this incident wavefront – a step that will be called "reference analysis" – which is performed at the beginning of the experiment. It is a priori not necessary to repeat this step as long as the experimental conditions are not modified (temperature, microscope settings, non-uniform conditions at the sample level). The modifications of the wavefront due to the sample, relative to this reference wavefront, will then give the local optical thickness map being sought.

1.4.2. *Experimental configuration*

Figure 1.7 shows the conventional experimental configuration for quantitative phase imaging by wavefront measurement using a wavefront sensor from QLSI technology. This sensor, consisting of the MHM and a CCD camera, is placed on the video output port of a microscope. In fact, all of the images obtained in the following sections will have been obtained from different commercial sensors, whose type will be specified for each case. The CCD sensor of the wavefront sensor is placed in the focal plane of the microscope tube lens so that the sample is imaged on the detector. In fact, the sensor essentially consists of a camera inside which the MHM is inserted. Consequently, its use is identical to that of a conventional camera in terms of handling and fixing on the microscope (C mount). The measurement of the incident light wavefront on the sensor (illumination beam, in green + components due to diffraction by the object, in red) is then carried out according to the methodology explained previously. It is also represented in Figure 1.8, which specifically illustrates the process of quantitative imaging of biological samples.

This figure, taken from Aknoun (2014), effectively resumes the main steps of the reconstruction process of an optical thickness map for a biological sample (here, a living COS-7-type biological cell, the lineage resulting from a kidney of a green monkey from Africa). A recording of the interferogram, which can be seen in the figure, shows the disturbing effect of the presence of inhomogeneities in the sample on the regular alignment of the interference fringes. Then, a spectral demodulation of this interferogram in Fourier space makes it possible to recover the intensity image and to obtain the phase gradients due to the sample in two perpendicular directions. Integration from these two gradients finally results in reconstructing a quantitative phase map of the object. Since the local modulation of the interferogram interfringe is only caused by the local phase shift of the wavefront, and not by its intensity, the phase and intensity measurements are completely uncorrelated. During the whole process, the commercial algorithms used (SID4Bio software, Phasics, France) take into account in an optimal way the preliminary recording of a reference interferogram, acquired from an empty part of the sample under the same conditions used for the latter. As such, only the OPD map due to the sample can be displayed, independently of the characteristics of the light beam that may vary according to the conditions under which the optical system is used. It should be noted that the native light source of the microscope (white halogen lamp, or white LED depending on the microscope used) is employed to make the images due to the achromatic character of the technique. However, it is sometimes useful to use spectral bandpass filters or LEDs of different colors to perform certain measurements in better defined spectral domains, when the application requires it (sensitivity to sample chromaticity, typically).

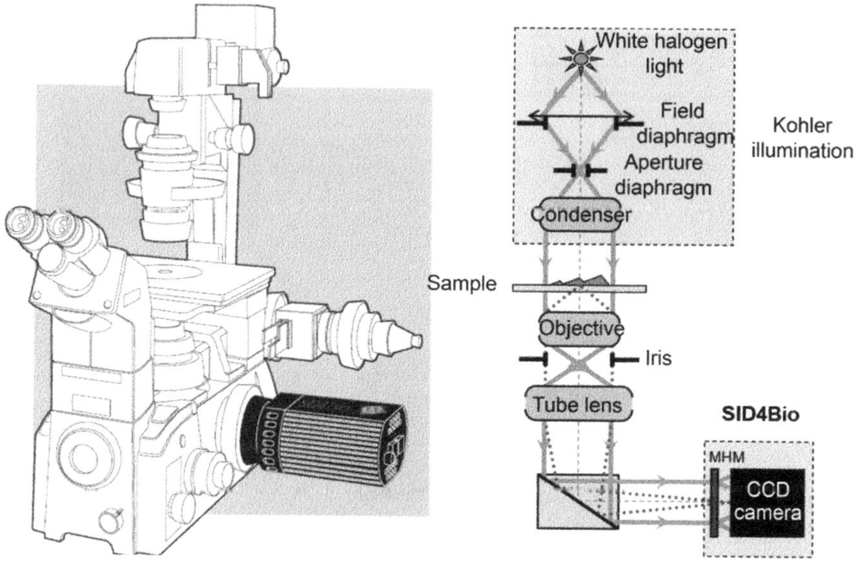

Figure 1.7. *Conventional optical configuration for quantitative phase imaging by QLSI*

1.5. Applications to biological imaging

1.5.1. *High-contrast imaging without labeling*

The first contribution of this imaging technique is to offer remarkable phase contrast, without halo (characteristic of Zernike phase contrast when used without apodized mask) or unidirectional gradient (characteristic of the Normarski/DIC process). Biological samples show sufficient local refractive index inhomogeneities to reveal their internal structure, even when the traversed thicknesses are small. The sensitivity in OPD, of the order of 0.1 nm, is sufficient to clearly characterize the plasma membrane, mitochondria, different types of vesicles (lysosomes, peroxisomes, endosomes, at least a good part of each of them) and of course the nucleus and chromosomes during cell division. It is also possible to distinguish components of the cytoskeleton, such as microtubules and some actin stress fibers, at least in fairly thin areas of the cell further away from the nucleus (Bon et al. 2014). This contrast quality, without even enhancing the quantification inherent to the technique, is already very useful in cell biology to appreciate the state of the cells under the microscope and the results of different treatments (drugs, temperature, illumination at different powers and wavelengths) (Figure 1.9). Similarly, by following the cellular and intracellular dynamics over time, at frequencies that can reach several Hz, the cellular metabolism can be evaluated.

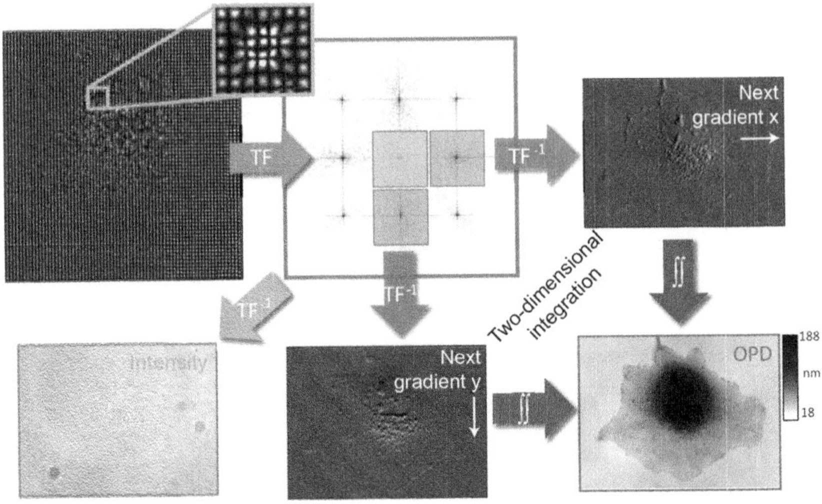

Figure 1.8. *Main steps for reconstructing an OPD distribution from an interferogram recorded by a wavefront sensor (source: Aknoun 2014)*

1.5.2. *Dry mass measurement in living biological cells*

In some specific cases, an optical path difference measurement can provide information about the amount of material present in the sample. For amorphous or crystalline solids, a linear increase in the density of the material is reflected by a linear increase in the real part of the refractive index. Similarly, in the case of a solution, increasing the mass concentration of a solute in a solvent produces a proportional increase in the solution refractive index, according to a coefficient that depends on the solute. Nevertheless, even for biological cells containing a large number of constituents (proteins, lipids, sugars, nucleic acids, etc.), it has been demonstrated that for most eukaryotic cells, considering a single and generic coefficient relating the solution refractive index to the solute mass was valid (Barer 1952).

Consequently, the cell dry mass m, defined as the sum of the masses of any non-aqueous constituent, can be directly calculated from the integral of the distribution of the cell OPD over its projected surface:

$$m = \frac{1}{0.18} \int_S OPD(x,y)\, dxdy \qquad [1.8]$$

where mass is given in picograms, and the integral corresponding to a volume is calculated in μm^3. The coefficient of 0.18 $\mu m^3.pg^{-1}$ is the most commonly used in general by the scientific community dealing with quantitative phase measurement and it can only vary for some particular cell lines. For example, it is equal to 0.19 $\mu m^3.pg^{-1}$ for red blood cells considering that this cell type contains a high hemoglobin content.

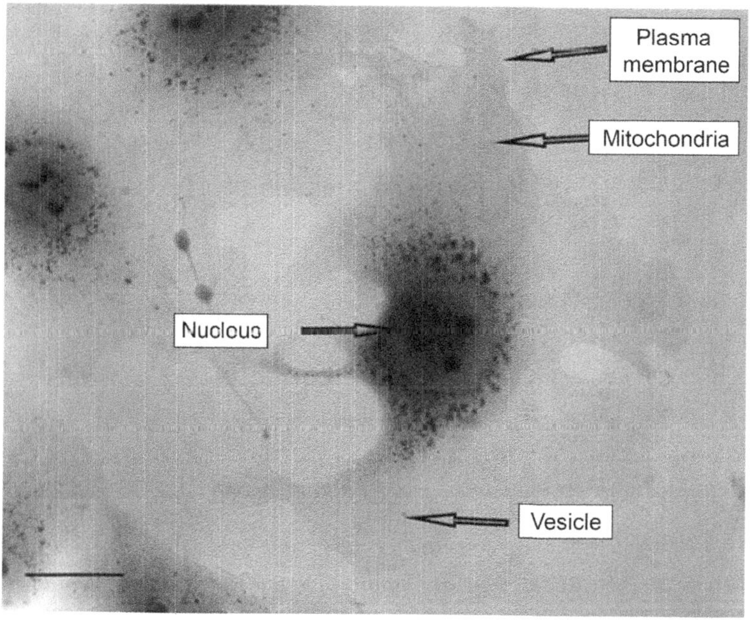

Figure 1.9. *COS-7 cells in culture at 37° C. Quantitative phase image taken with the SID4 HD prototype (2560 x 2160 phase pixels), 100X, NA = 1.3. Scale bar: 10 μm*

The integration of the OPD on the cell surface requires automatic segmentation of the cell edge to define this surface. This operation is facilitated by the fact that the images are of good quality and especially free of halo around the cells. Even in the thinnest areas of the cell edge, where the OPD corresponds only to the plasma membrane composed of a phospolipid bilayer folded over itself, the contrast generated is sufficient for the segmentation algorithm to correctly identify the cell edges. This algorithm, developed jointly with Frédéric Galland (Institut Fresnel, Phyti team), not only allows for this edge detection but also a calibration of the OPD levels. As a matter of fact, it includes a so-called background flattening phase, that is, the possibly local measurement of the residual OPD level between the cells (defined as the image "background"), which will then be used to calibrate the dry mass. The reference analysis step is in fact not efficient enough to ensure zero residual given the sensitivity of the technique. The developed algorithm thus allows the computation of dry mass values that are very accurate and close to biological reality (Aknoun et al. 2015).

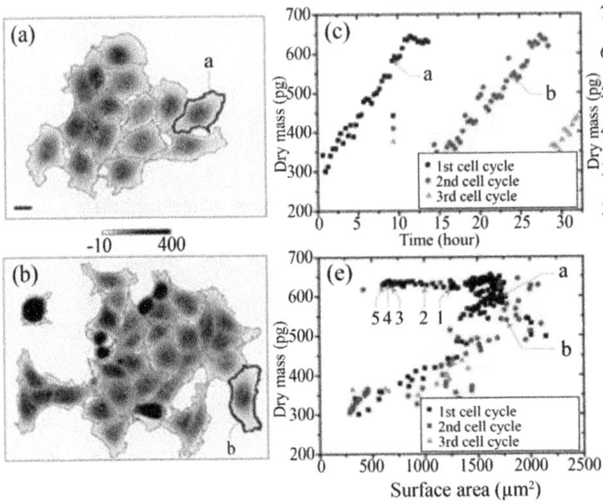

Figure 1.10. *Thirty-four-hour cell cycle monitoring of COS-7 cells*

COMMENTS ON FIGURE 1.10.– *(a) Quantitative phase image taken with SID4Bio, 40X NA 0.75, 37°C and 5% CO_2, scale bar: 20 m. Automatically segmented cells and cell designated by a monitored. (b) Same field of view 15 h later, daughter cell b monitored. (c) Dry mass time monitoring, 1 point every 30 s. Cell a in black, daughter cell b in red. (d) Magnification of the plateau of cell a represented in (c). (e) Representation of the same points in a "projected area versus dry mass" space. (f) Images (raw on the left-hand side and filtered with a high-pass frequency filter on the right side) of cell a at five time points, denoted from 1 to 5 in insets (d) and (e).*

The ability to measure dry mass in an individual living cell by a simple image capture is fundamental, given that it allows the long-term monitoring of dry mass evolution in a cell and/or cell population (Figure 1.10). For example, we have monitored the cell cycle, during which the dry mass of a cell progressively increases until it doubles at the time of mitosis, where it divides into two almost equal daughter cells. Recording a quasi-linear increase in dry mass, before reaching a plateau, is relevant data (Figure 1.10(c)). Each point in this figure is associated with an OPD image of the scene, making it possible to identify which phase of the cell cycle the monitored cell is actually in. This identification is particularly easy at the time of mitosis, where the behavior of chromosomes is visible even at a relatively low magnification of 40X (Figure 1.10(f)).

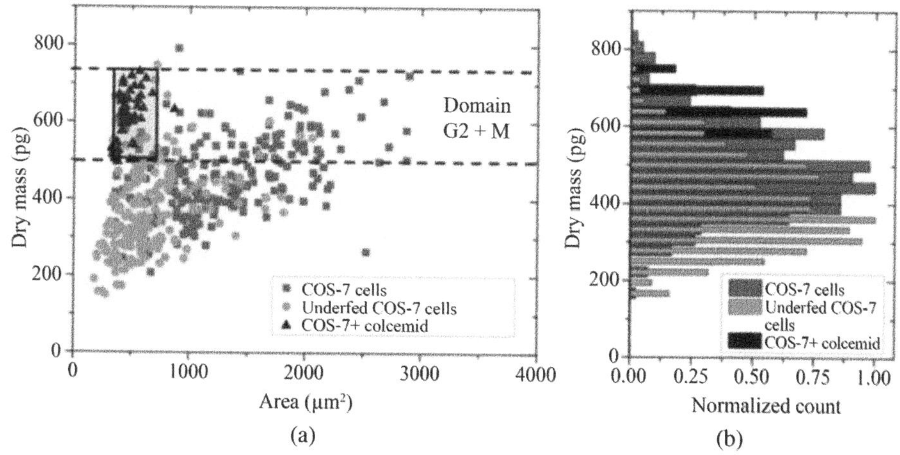

Figure 1.11. *Dry mass and projected area of COS-7 populations. Control cells in red, serum-starved cells in orange and prometaphase-blocked cells in black*

The accuracy of the dry mass measurement, with a standard deviation of the order of 0.2% (Aknoun et al. 2015), enables the impact of treatments on the cells to be highlighted. For example, it is possible to deprive them of feed to a certain extent (percentage reduction of fetal calf serum or FBS in the culture medium, from 10 to 0.5% over 48 h). The metabolic impact of such an action on a cell population is then observed in comparison to control cells (Figure 1.11). The treated cells become smaller, with lower dry mass. Another experiment consists of blocking microtubule polymerization, essential at the time of the separation of the chromosomes between the two future daughter cells (by addition of colcemid, 24 h at 1 mg/L). It is observed that all the cells enter a state of minimal projected surface (they are then spherical) but exhibit maximum dry mass. They are logically blocked in prometaphase. Therefore, from the knowledge of the area/mass characteristics of a given cell population (Figure 1.11(a)), we can statistically classify a cell population according to the cell cycle phases, without the use of labeling. This opens up the possibility of keeping a potential for labeling, for example of the fluorescence type, for the study of other simultaneous cellular functions.

1.5.3. *Rapid imaging for biological phenomena*

We use different QLSI imaging modalities depending on what we want to observe and measure. The primary difference is the sensor. We have the ability to use a high-speed camera, the Phantom Miro M120, which is capable of taking full-field images at 730 Hz. With a 3 x 3 pixel analysis, quantitative phase images are obtained at 640 x 400 pixels at very high frequency.

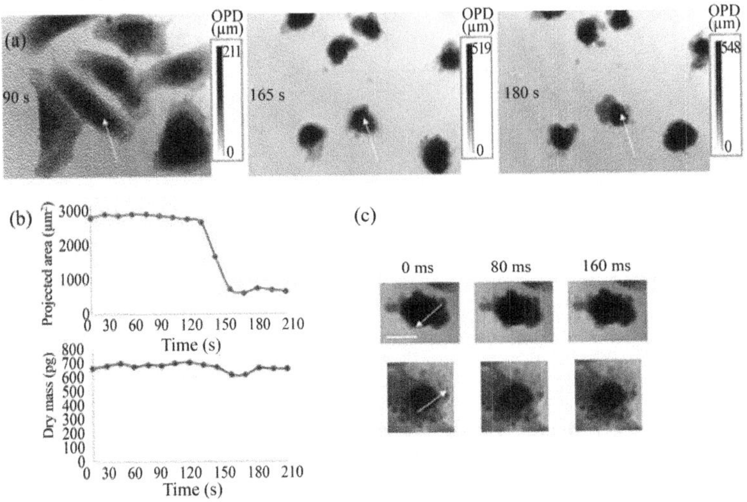

Figure 1.12. *Blebbing in U2-0S cells (human osteosarcoma). Image taken with the fast SID4 element, 40X NA 0.75: (a) one image every 15 s; (b) monitoring of cell projected area and dry mass indicated by white arrow in (a); (c) two cells with blebbing, taken at 100 Hz. Scale bar: 10 μm*

Such a speed allows the observation of very fast phenomena, such as blebbing. This phenomenon corresponds to the prominence of the cell plasma membrane caused by the delocalized uncoupling of the cytoskeleton from the membrane. This sudden onset of blebs, or bulges, is fast and important during division, locomotion or cell apoptosis (programmed cell death). It is not accompanied by loss or gain of material, but by reorganization and flow. It is associated with certain cell types but can be induced by adding calyculin A (20 nM here). If we observe images of cells every 15 s, cells can be seen changing drastically in shape and size, without us understanding what is going on (Figure 1.12(a)). The projected area undergoes an abrupt decrease when the blebbing starts at 120 s of acquisition (Figure 1.12(b)). On the other hand, dry mass remains fairly constant. The cell then changes shape so rapidly that we have no idea where the phenomenon starts each time. If images are taken at higher frequencies, all of the steps can be seen much better and it might be easier to understand the phenomenon more deeply (Figure 1.12(c)). Without reaching up to 730 Hz, a frequency of 100 Hz can also help to average the recordings of interferograms in order to increase the signal/noise ratio, while keeping a high acquisition frequency (100 Hz with seven images, for example).

1.5.4. *Quantitative phase and fluorescence correlative imaging*

Here, we make use of the fact that this technique is achromatic and perfectly usable in the near infrared (NIR) to combine it simultaneously with fluorescence imaging, here in full-field, the latter using the visible spectrum. Figure 1.13 represents the optical scheme of this bimodal imaging. The fact that phase imaging is carried out using transmission while fluorescence uses epi-detection, simplifies the actual simultaneous implementation of the two channels and consequently makes it possible to perfectly superimpose the images acquired by the two cameras (CCD, EMCCD or sCMOS). It is theoretically possible to use a color camera associated with a multiband fluorescence set to simultaneously perform phase imaging and several colors in fluorescence.

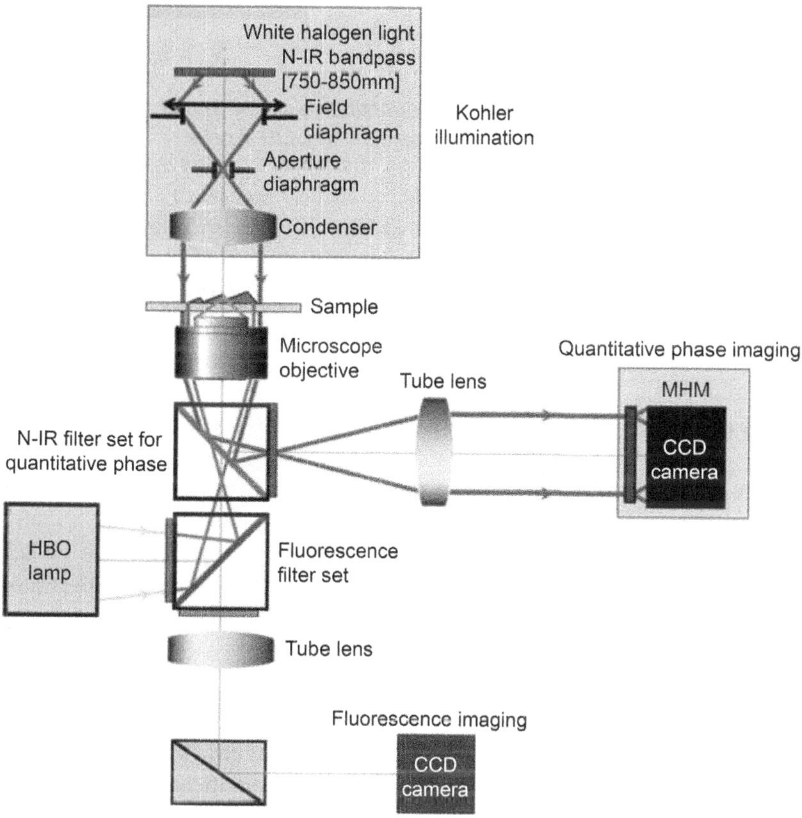

Figure 1.13. *Quantitative phase imaging coupled with fluorescence imaging on a two-stage microscope. The rear video port at the upper stage is used for phase imaging while fluorescence excitation is performed by the lower arm*

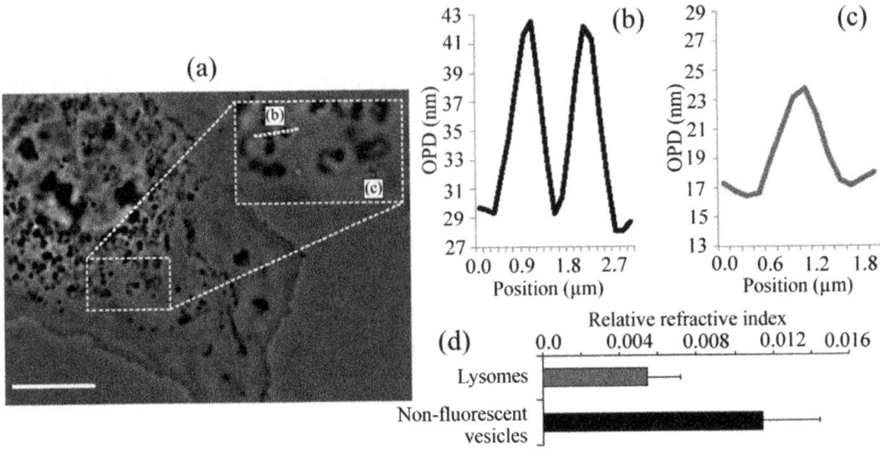

Figure 1.14. *Lysosome quantitative phase imaging compared to other vesicles, in COS-7 cells*

COMMENTS ON FIGURE 1.14.– *(a) An example of phase/fluorescence composite images (in red: RFP, lysosomes), with a magnified view. (b and c) Optical path difference (OPD) profile of vesicles along the white and red dotted lines drawn in (a), respectively. (d) Relative refractive index distribution (Δn/diameter) of fluorescent lysosomes and other non-fluorescent vesicles (mean values and standard deviation), obtained from 70 measurements on independent vesicles of about 1 µm in diameter, showing a significant difference between the two populations. Scale bar: 5 µm.*

We have applied this association to the monitoring and identification of cellular organelles. Fluorescent labeling allowing for optimal specificity and quantitative phase imaging with which a huge number of cellular components can be seen at once; these modalities are perfectly complementary. Figure 1.14(a) illustrates the overlay of a red fluorescent labeling specific to lysosomes as well as quantitative grayscale phase imaging of the overall cell. However, the lysosome labeling does not label all vesicles. A "relative refractive index" of each vesicle considered spherical can then be defined as its OPD divided by its diameter (Figures 1.14(b) and (c)). By computing this relative index from 70 objects of equivalent size (about 1–2 µm, to ensure that we stay above the diffraction limit), a significant difference can be observed between the lysosome population and that of the other vesicles (Figure 1.14(d)).

We also labeled the nucleus and the Golgi apparatus, as shown in Figure 1.15. Again, only one color can be simultaneously taken with the phase, the mitochondria in this case. To better distinguish the overlay, the phase imaging has been inverted to grayscale (the densest optically is the brighter, unlike in Figure 1.14). Mitochondria are still easily detectable in phase imaging.

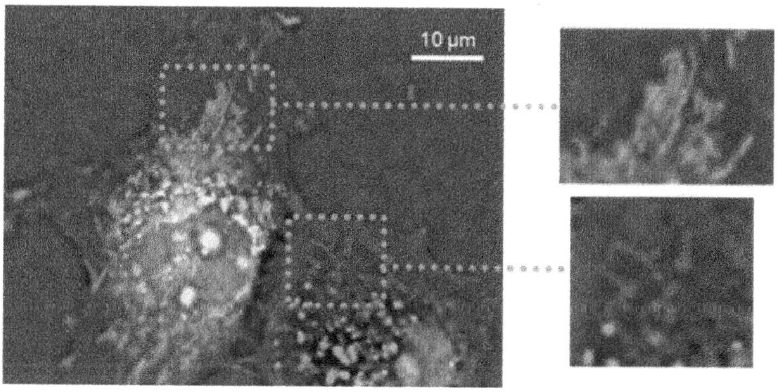

Figure 1.15. *COS-7 labeled at the mitochondria (green), Golgi apparatus (orange) and DNA level, and hence the nucleus (blue), on a grayscale phase imaging background. The cell on the bottom right was not labeled at the mitochondria or Golgi apparatus level due to a transfection rate inducing fluorescent labeling that is not 100%*

1.6. Optical retardance imaging

Until now, to obtain a map of the OPD for a given sample, we have usually measured two successive wavefronts in unpolarized light, namely a first one outside the sample (reference shot) and a second one with sample. The difference between these two measurements gave a map of the OPD of the imaged object (Figure 1.16(a)). A possible variation of the technique consists of using a linearly polarized incident light beam (Figure 1.16(b)). In this case, the first interferogram recording is carried out with polarization along a defined axis, then the second with crossed polarization, perpendicular to the first one. Consequently, if the observed sample is optically isotropic, it will produce the same wavefronts on the sensor. On the other hand, if some area in the sample (blue area on the figure) is optically birefringent, then the refractive index, and thus the retardance, seen by the light field, will be different for the two polarization states under consideration. A comparison between these two wavefronts then allows us to specifically identify any birefringent structure (within the observation plane) of the sample.

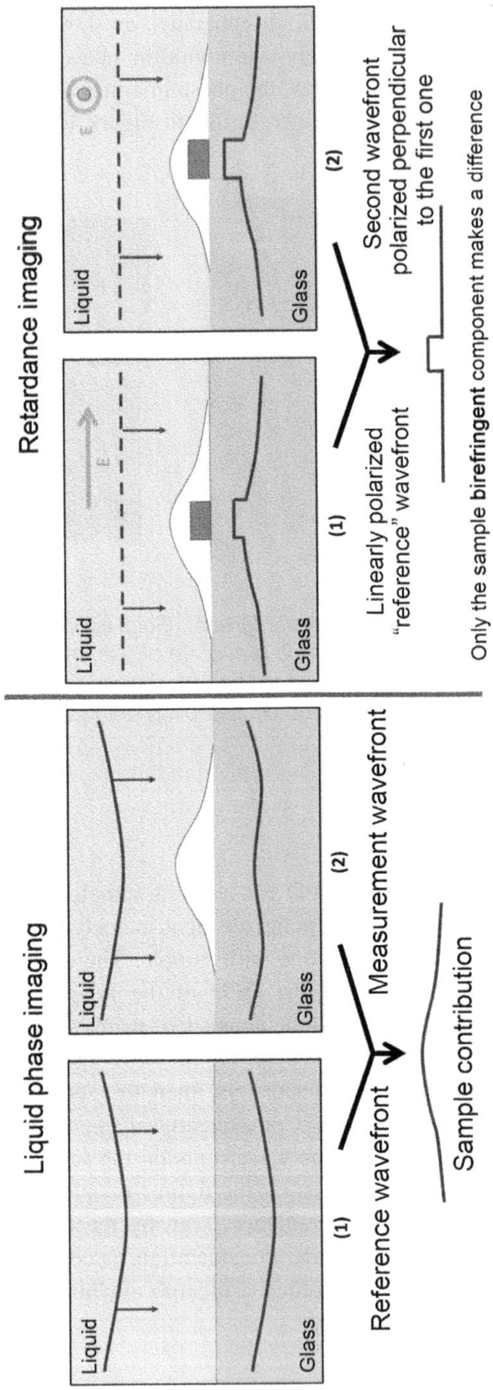

Figure 1.16. *The main reconstruction steps of an OPD distribution from an interferogram recorded by a wavefront sensor (source: Aknoun 2014)*

The evolution of the difference between these two wavefronts depends on the orientations chosen for the crossed polarization axes. Moreover, the orientation of the optical axes of the sample birefringent zones is generally not known. Consequently, it is necessary to perform a set of OPD measurements by varying the linear polarization angle of the beam. As a matter of fact, the OPD of a birefringent medium varies as a function of the angle θ of the polarization direction according to the following equation:

$$OPD(x, y, \theta) = \int_0^h [n(x, y, z, \theta) - n_{med}]\, dz \qquad [1.9]$$

This equation can be rewritten, omitting the spatial coordinates for better readability:

$$OPD(\theta) = \int_0^h (\frac{n_o + n_e}{2} - n_{med})\, dz + \left[\int_0^h (\frac{n_o - n_e}{2})\, dz\right] cos[2(\theta - \theta_0)] \qquad [1.10]$$

where n_o and n_e are the ordinary and extraordinary indexes of the birefringent medium, and θ_0 represents the direction of the principal optical axis of this medium. The first term of the sum giving the OPD corresponds to what would be obtained under unpolarized light, and the second corresponds to a variable part depending on the illumination angle θ.

Figure 1.17(c) shows a typical schematic representation of a curve from six measurements achieved according to six different polarization directions. While the acquisitions can be quickly carried out using automated polarization control systems, the analyses for extracting the retardance maps are much more complex; this is mainly due to the fact that the six OPD images computed for six different polarization angles must be searched for the sine curve crossing the measurement points for each pixel (Figure 1.17(c)). The delay value, for each pixel, is thus obtained as well as the angle θ_0.

Knowledge of these retardance and orientation values can then be used to derive information about the organization of the sample. For example, knowledge of the distribution of θ_0 within amyloid fibers can be used to visualize the organization of these fibers, just as a distribution of retardance in a biological tissue makes it possible to appreciate the orientation of collagen fibers (Figure 1.18), as the signature of the presence of tumor in the tissue (Aknoun et al. 2018).

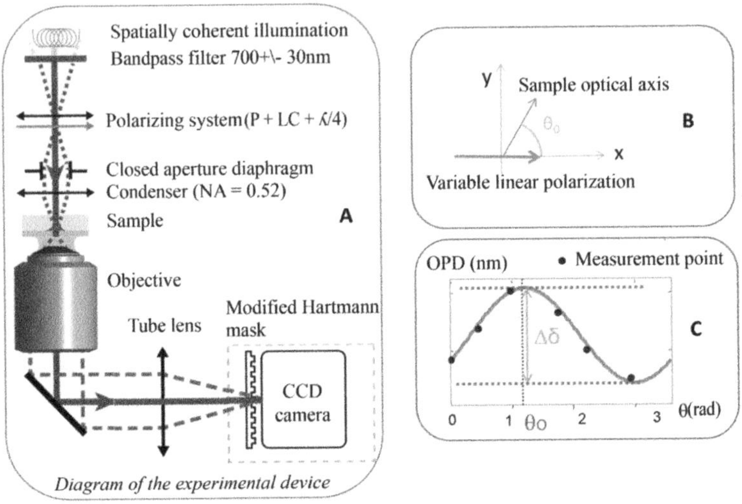

Figure 1.17. *(a) Dedicated retardance imaging configuration. The polarization system is based on liquid crystals enabling control of the polarization direction without mechanical motorization. Representations of the rotating polarization (b) and a typical curve from the measurement points (c)*

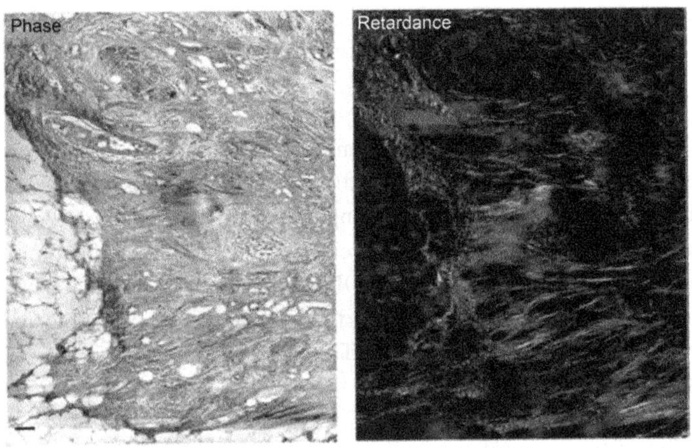

(a) (b)

Figure 1.18. *Example of images obtained from fixed biological tissue. (a) OPD distribution. (b) Optical retardation image showing the presence of collagen fibers whose orientation can be assessed*

1.7. Other applications and new developments

In this chapter, we have focused on the biological applications of the QLSI phase imaging technique. It is nevertheless obvious that this technique can be used with a variety of samples. We can thus clearly identify waveguides buried in a transparent substrate, measure the optical thickness of the core of single-mode optical fiber, that of dielectric thin film up to a graphene monolayer (Khadir et al. 2017). The contactless optical profilometer function is also available, and it has been shown that the technique proves to be particularly effective in detecting very early laser damage (Douti et al. 2015).

Moreover, most liquids, including water, have the property that their refractive index varies with temperature. As such, a hot spot on a sample immersed in water will generate a local perturbation of the water refractive index in the vicinity of the heat source, which can be considered a phase object measurable using the phase imaging technique presented in this chapter. Knowing this phase object, the local temperature can be deduced (Baffou et al. 2012). Therefore, we have been able to demonstrate the possibility of performing local temperature measurements in a sample under a microscope, including control of cell stimulation by temperature (Robert et al. 2018).

Finally, the achromatic character of the QLSI technique is of great interest for measurements under femtosecond illumination, as light pulses of this duration become spectrally broad. We have used this property to visualize the propagation of the Kerr effect within a silica sample in a time-resolved manner (Gallais et al. 2016).

1.8. References

Aknoun, S. (2014). Analyse quantitative d'images de phase obtenues par interférométrie à décalage quadri-latéral. Applications en biologie. PhD thesis, Aix-Marseille Université, Marseille.

Aknoun, S., Bon, P., Savatier, J., Wattellier, B., Monneret, S. (2015a). Quantitative retardance imaging of biological samples using quadri-wave lateral shearing interferometry. *Optics Express*, 23(12), 16383–16406.

Aknoun, S., Savatier, J., Bon, P., Galland, F., Abdeladim, L., Wattellier, B., Monneret, S. (2015b). Living cells dry mass measurements using quantitative phase imaging with quadri-wave lateral shearing interferometry. An accuracy and sensitivity discussion. *Journal of Biomedical Optics*, 20(12), 126009.

Aknoun, S., Aurrand-Lions, M., Wattellier, B., Monneret, S. (2018). Quantitative retardance imaging by means of quadri-wave lateral shearing interferometry for label-free fiber imaging in tissues. *Optics Communications*, 422, 17–27.

Baffou, G., Bon, P., Savatier, J., Polleux, J., Zhu, M., Merlin, M., Rigneault, R., Monneret, S. (2012). Thermal imaging of nanostructures by quantitative optical phase analysis. *ACS Nano*, 6(3), 2452–2458.

Barer, R. (1952). Interference microscopy and mass determination. *Nature*, 169, 366–367.

Berto, P., Gachet, D., Bon, P., Monneret, S., Rigneault, H. (2012). Wide-field vibrational phase imaging. *Physical Review Letters*, 109, 093902.

Bon, P. (2011). Imagerie microscopique de champs électromagnétiques par interférométrie à décalage quadri-latéral. Applications à la biologie. PhD thesis, Aix-Marseille Université, Marseille.

Bon, P., Maucort, G., Wattellier, B., Monneret, S. (2009). Quadriwave lateral shearing interferometry for quantitative phase microscopy of living cells. *Optics Express*, 17(15), 13080–13094.

Bon, P., Monneret, S., Wattellier, B. (2012a). Non-iterative boundary-artifact free wavefront reconstruction from its derivatives. *Applied Optics*, 51(23), 5698–5704.

Bon, P., Savatier, J., Merlin, M., Wattellier, B., Monneret, S. (2012b). Optical detection and measurement of living cell morphometric features with single-shot quantitative phase microscopy. *Journal of Biomedical Optics*, 17(7), 076004.

Bon, S., Lécart, E., Fort, S., Lévêque-Fort, S. (2014). Fast label-free cytoskeletal network imaging in living mammalian cells. *Biophysical Journal*, 106(8), 1588–1595.

Cuche, E., Bevilacqua, F., Depeursinge, C. (1999). Digital holography for quantitative phase-contrast imaging. *Opt. Lett.*, 24, 291–293.

Doualle, T., Gallais, L., Monneret, S., Bouillet, S., Bourgeade, A., Ameil, C., Lamaignere, L., Cormont, P. (2017). CO2 laser microprocessing for laser damage growth mitigation of fused silica optics. *Optical Engineering*, 56(01), 011022.

Douti, L., Chrayteh, M., Aknoun, S., Doualle, T., Hecquet, C., Monneret, S., Gallais, L. (2015). Quantitative phase imaging applied to laser damage detection and analysis. *Applied Optics*, 28(54), 8375–8382.

Gallais, L. and Monneret, S. (2016). Time-resolved quantitative phase microscopy of laser-material interactions using a wavefront sensor. *Optics Letters*, 41(14), 3245–3248.

Khadir, S., Bon, P., Vignaud, D., Galopin, E., McEvoy, N., McCloskey, D., Monneret, S., Baffou, G. (2017). Optical imaging and characterization of graphene and other 2D materials using quantitative phase microscopy. *ACS Photonics*, 4(12), 3130–3139.

Nomarski, G. and Weil, A.R. (1955). Application à la métallographie des méthodes interférentielles à deux ondes polarisées. *Rev. Met. Paris*, 52(2), 121–134.

Primot, J. and Guérineau, N. (2000). Extended Hartmann test based on the pseudoguiding property of a Hartmann mask completed by a phase chessboard. *Appl. Opt.*, 39, 5715–5720.

Primot, J. and Sogno, L. (1995). Achromatic three-wave (or more) lateral shearing interferometer. *J. Opt. Soc. Am. A*, 12(12), 2679.

Radhakrishnan, R., Gallais, L., Monneret, S. (2019). Wavefront sensing applied to determine temperature dependence of liquids. *Applied Optics*, 58(13), 3646–3651.

Robert, H.M.L., Savatier, J., Vial, S., Verghese, J., Wattellier, B., Rigneault, H., Monneret, S., Polleux, J., Baffou G. (2018). Photothermal control of heat-shock protein expression at the single cell level. *Small*, 14(32), 1801910.

Velghe, S., Primot, J., Guérineau, N., Cohen, M., Wattellier, B. (2005). Wave-front reconstruction from multidirectional phase derivatives generated by multilateral shearing interferometers. *Opt. Lett.*, 30, 245–247.

Volkov, V., Zhu, Y., De Graef, M. (2002). A new symmetrized solution for phase retrieval using the transport of intensity equation. *Micron*, 33, 411–416.

Zernike, F. (1935). Das phasenkontrastverfahren bei der mikroskopischen beobachtung. *Z. Tech. Phys.*, 16, 454–457.

2

Holography

Michel GROSS[1] and Nicolas VERRIER[2]

[1] *L2C, CNRS, Université de Montpellier, France*

[2] *IRIMAS, Université de Haute-Alsace, Mulhouse, France*

2.1. Introduction

Contrary to conventional imaging methods, which give a two-dimensional image of an object, holography records the intensity of the optical field scattered/diffracted by the analyzed object. From this record, called a hologram, it is possible to access the optical field amplitude and phase originating from the imaged object. We owe the invention of holography to Denis Gabor who, at the time, was working on improving the resolution of electron microscopes (Gabor 1948; Gabor and Bragg 1949). The principle of the method, illustrated in Figure 2.1, is based on three steps:

1) The holographic recording during which the interferences between a reference wave (solid line in Figure 2.1(a)) and the wave diffracted by the object (dotted line) are recorded on a high-resolution photographic plate. The intensity of this interference pattern, called a hologram, encodes the information on the optical field of the object.

2) The photographic development of the hologram.

3) The reconstruction of the hologram, which consists of an a posteriori refocusing on the object. To this end, the developed hologram is again illuminated by the reference wave and the focus is provided by a relay optic. An example of hologram reconstruction, from (Gabor 1948), is proposed in Figure 2.1(b).

Unconventional Optical Imaging for Biology,
coordinated by Corinne FOURNIER and Olivier HAEBERLÉ.

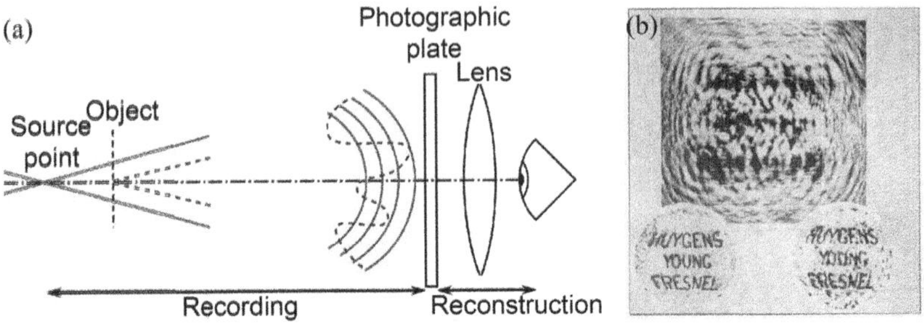

Figure 2.1. *Gabor's experiment. (a) Schematic diagram of Gabor's experiment. (b) Example of hologram from Gabor (1948). For a color version of this figure, see www.iste.co.uk/fournier/unconventional.zip*

In this configuration, the reconstructed hologram is marred by the noise of the twin image corresponding to the blurred image of the analyzed object. To overcome this limitation, other configurations using a reference wave propagating off-axis, have been proposed (Leith and Upatnieks 1962, 1963; Leith et al. 1965). At that time, processing holograms was still completely analog. The development of computational means has quickly made it possible to replace the analog reconstitution of holograms by digitally processing information (Goodman and Lawrence 1967; Kronrod et al. 1972). The transition to digital hologram reconstruction thus opens new possibilities in terms of quality and quantity (optical phase extraction) of the extracted information (Fienup 1982; Liu and Scott 1987; Onural and Scott 1987). Nevertheless, the development phase of the holographic plate and its digitalization are still needed to complete the reconstruction. With the development of coupled charge device (CCD) sensors, holography has seen one of its greatest advances by enabling both digital recording and reconstruction of information (Schnars and Jüptner 1994). Since then, many methods have emerged for the recording and reconstruction of holograms according to the nature of the objects under study and the conditions for acquiring data (Schnars and Jüptner 2002; Verrier and Atlan 2011).

The ability to extract the complex optical field (amplitude and phase) in the sensor plane, and the digital reconstruction of the complex field in the object plane, make holography the method of choice in many areas such as fluid dynamics (Lozano et al. 1999; Pu and Meng 2005), biomedical imaging (Charrière et al. 2006; Kemper and von Bally 2008) or non-destructive structure control (Picart et al. 2005; Iemma et al. 2006).

In the following, we will recall the general principles of holography. We will see how it is possible to reconstruct the complex field of the object wave from the intensity recorded in the holograms. We will also address the constraints related to the acquisition of holograms on a digital sensor. Finally, we will consider the different configurations and their fields of application.

REMARK.– The principles that will be detailed in the majority of the chapters of this book are based on the use of coherent light (laser sources, for example). Electromagnetic waves are spatiotemporal phenomena; two types of coherence can thus be defined: *temporal coherence* and *spatial coherence.*

Temporal coherence is related to the monochromaticity of the source. The finer the source emission spectrum, the greater the source temporal coherence. If the source wavelength is defined as:

$$\lambda = \lambda_{\mathrm{th}} \pm \Delta\lambda \quad [2.1]$$

with λ_{th} the theoretical wavelength of the source and $\Delta\lambda$ its spectral width, the source coherence length is written as

$$L_c = \frac{\lambda_{\mathrm{th}}^2}{\Delta\lambda} \quad [2.2]$$

A perfectly monochromatic source ($\lambda = \lambda_{\mathrm{th}}$) will exhibit an infinite coherence length. In the following discussions presented in this book, we will assume that the temporal coherence of the sources used is infinite. If this is not the case, the results obtained will have to be integrated on an interval $\lambda_{\mathrm{th}} \pm \Delta\lambda$.

Spatial coherence characterizes the ability of one point on the wavefront to interfere with the others. In practice, it is a measure of the cross-correlation of the information originating from two wavefront points. Therefore, a plane wave (most of this research will address this case) and a point source have infinite spatial coherence. In the presence of an extended source (such as a set of point sources), the degree of spatial coherence is degraded by the interference between the different source points. The more extensive a source is, the less spatially coherent it is.

In the rest of this book, we will work with spatially (plane wave or point source) and temporally coherent sources ($\lambda = \lambda_{th}$).

2.2. Principle of holography

In conventional imaging, we record on a photosensitive medium the intensity of light that travels through or that is reflected by an object. The information about the phase of the optical field is lost. This is mainly because the acquisition rates of the state-of-the-art sensors (from a few tens of images per second to a few hundred thousand images per second) are incompatible with the frequencies of the optical waves that we want to measure (of the order of 10^{15} Hz for the visible range of the spectrum).

In order to circumvent this difficulty, holography is based on an interferometric detection method of the information. The light coming from the object is made to interfere with a reference wave presenting the same characteristics as the beam used for illuminating the object. This principle is illustrated in Figure 2.2. Here, the light from a laser (L) is split into two identical waves. One of them illuminates the object (O) and the other is used as a reference wave. The light from the object and the reference wave are then recombined and the interference intensity between these two waves is recorded on a photosensitive sensor (high-resolution photographic plate or digital sensor).

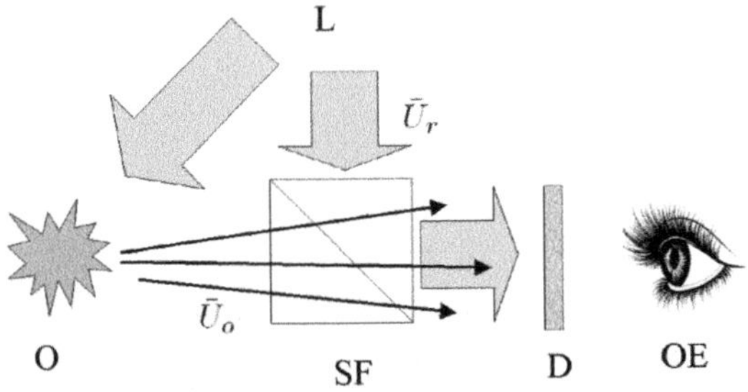

Figure 2.2. *Holography schematic diagram. L: laser, SF: beam splitter cube for superimposing the fields $\bar{U}_o$ and $\bar{U}_r$; O: object; D: detector (photographic plate or digital camera), OE (observer's eye). For a color version of this figure, see www.iste.co.uk/fournier/unconventional.zip*

REMARK.– In fact, the object wave (to be analyzed) is modulated by a reference wave. The aim of this operation, as in electronics, is to detect the whole frequency content of the object signal in a sensor whose spatial and time bandwidths are limited. Hereafter, we will address hologram demodulation, which will lead into extracting the amplitude and the phase.

Consider the optical field $\mathcal{U}_o$ diffracted by the object. At the surface of the sensor, it is expressed by:

$$\begin{aligned} \mathcal{U}_o(x,y,t) &= U_o(x,y)\, e^{j\omega t} \\ \mathcal{U}_o(x,y,t) &= A_o(x,y)\, e^{j\varphi_o(x,y)} e^{j\omega t} \end{aligned} \qquad [2.3]$$

Here, U_o is the slowly varying envelope of the optical field $\mathcal{U}_o$, which oscillates at the angular frequency $\omega \approx 10^{15}$ rad.s^{-1}. The envelope U_o has a strictly positive amplitude A_o and a phase $\varphi_o(x, y)$. Similarly, we can define the reference wave $\mathcal{U}_r$:

$$\begin{aligned} \mathcal{U}_r(x, y, t) &= U_r(x, y)\, e^{j\omega t} \\ \mathcal{U}_r(x, y, t) &= A_r(x, y)\, e^{j\varphi_r(x,y)} e^{j\omega t} \end{aligned} \quad [2.4]$$

As for conventional imaging, the sensors used are not capable of detecting the angular frequency ω (or 2ω for the intensity). On the other hand, slowly variable envelopes can be detected. Therefore, the intensity of the interferences recorded on the sensor can be written as

$$\begin{aligned} I(x, y) &= |U_o(x, y) + U_r(x, y)|^2 \\ &= |U_o(x, y)|^2 + |U_r(x, y)|^2 + U_o^*(x, y)\, U_r(x, y) + U_o(x, y)\, U_r^*(x, y) \end{aligned} \quad [2.5]$$

where * is the complex conjugate. The first two terms of equation [2.5], respectively represent the object wave intensity and the reference wave. They correspond to the zeroth-order of diffraction. The third and fourth terms are, respectively, the –1 and +1 orders of diffraction. They contain the information about the complex field U_o. In fact, if we reconsider equations [2.3] and [2.4], the recorded intensity can be rewritten as

$$I(x, y) = |A_o(x, y)|^2 + |A_r(x, y)|^2 + A_o(x, y)\, A_r(x, y)\, e^{j[\varphi_o(x,y) - \varphi_r(x,y)]} + \text{c.c.} \quad [2.6]$$

with c.c. being the complex conjugate of the +1 order term. Clearly, it appears here that the +1 order term contains the information about the amplitude of the object field and the phase shift between the object wave and the reference wave. Therefore, if the +1 order can be isolated and the reference wave is known, the extracted signal is proportional to the wave originating from the object.

Digital holography will consist of extracting the +1 order signal of [2.5], and from this signal to compute the field everywhere and more particularly in the vicinity of the object. It should be noted here that the measurement is performed on a limited surface (the camera sensor) by sampling and averaging over the pixels of the camera. The amount of information acquired, which is equal to the total number of pixels multiplied by the number of coding bits, and the geometry of the experiment (object and camera size and position) require a large number of constraints both for the selection of the +1 order signal and the reconstruction. We will examine these constraints further in the text.

For now, we focus on the methods for extracting the +1 order of the interference pattern.

2.3. Selection of the +1 order

To select the +1 order signal, two families of methods can be used, off-axis holography and phase-shifting holography.

REMARK.– Here, we will not address iterative phase reconstruction methods. These will be covered in detail in the next chapter.

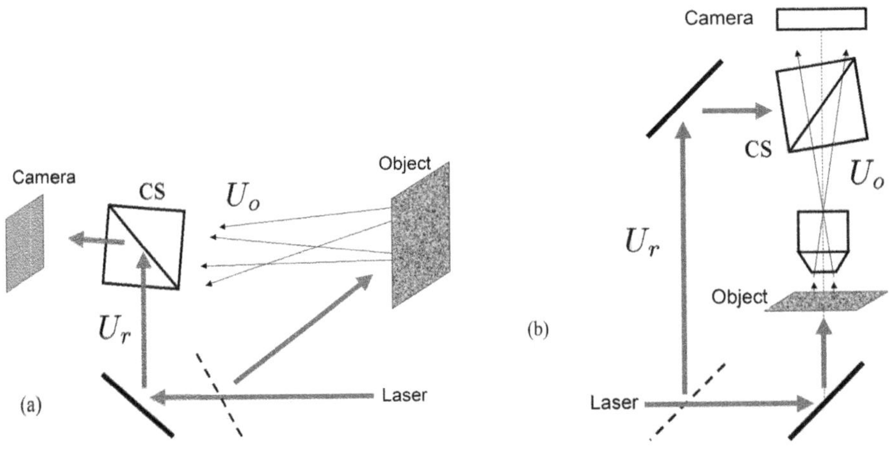

Figure 2.3. *Examples of off-axis holography devices: (a) in free space with reflection illumination and (b) in microscopy based on transmission illumination, with MO the microscope objective and CS the separating cube*

2.3.1. *Off-axis holography*

To enable the reconstruction of the wavefront amplitude and phase, with no twin image artifacts due to the –1 order, Leith and Upatnieks proposed, in the early 1960s, an off-axis holographic recording configuration (Leith and Upatnieks 1962).

Off-axis holography can be used with reflection or transmission illumination, with a holography in the free space as in holographic microscopy. In each case, the objective is to achieve an angular shift of the direction of the reference beam with respect to the average direction of the signal beam. Figure 2.3 shows two configuration examples of off-axis holography. In both cases, the angular shift is obtained by rotating the separation cube CS, which combines the fields U_o and U_r on the camera that records the interference signal $I = |U_r + U_o|^2$.

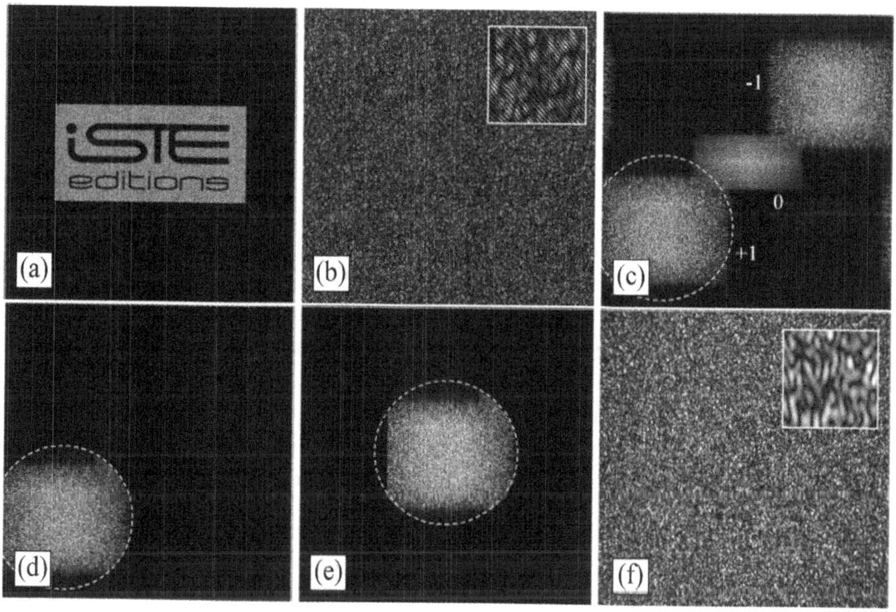

Figure 2.4. *Selection of the +1 order by off-axis holography. (a) Object. (b) Hologram I recorded by the camera. (c) Fourier hologram $\tilde{I}$. (d) Selection of the +1 order. (e) +1 order Fourier hologram +1 $\tilde{I}_{+1}$. (f) +1 order hologram. Inserts (b,f): $\times 4$ magnification*

To understand the principles of off-axis holography, we have simulated an experiment by considering as object a small sheet of paper with the inscription "ISTE editions" (Figure 2.4(a)). The sheet scatters the light in all directions and outside the inscription, the field U_o has a Gaussian amplitude and phase statistics. We have considered that the field U_r is known, and, to simplify, equal to 1. Before rotating the cube, we thus had $U_r(x,y) = 1$ in the camera plane $z = 0$. After rotating the cube, the reference wave becomes $U_r(x,y) = e^{j(k_x x + k_y y)}$ where k_x and k_y are the coordinates of the wave vector along which the reference wave propagates. Equation [2.5] becomes:

$$I(x,y) = 1 + |U_o(x,y)|^2 + \left[U_o(x,y)e^{-j(k_x x + k_y y)} + \text{c.c.}\right] \qquad [2.7]$$

where c.c. is the complex conjugate. Figure 2.4(b) shows the obtained hologram $I(x,y)$. We have considered that the hologram was recorded by a camera with $N \times N$ square pixels (with $N = 1024$) of size $\Delta_x = 5,5$ μm. The coordinates x, y are therefore discrete of step 5.5 μm, and the hologram I is a $1,024 \times 1,024$ matrix. The hologram presents spatial modulations clearly visible in the insert on the top right. These modulations correspond to the interferences between U_r and U_o. To select the +1 order, we have computed the hologram in the Fourier space $\tilde{I}$ by performing a discrete 2D Fourier transform (here denoted by $\mathcal{F}$):

$$\tilde{I}(k_x, k_y) = \mathcal{F}_{k_x,k_y}\left\{I(x,y)\right\} \qquad [2.8]$$

Figure 2.4(c) shows the Fourier hologram $\tilde{I}$ obtained. $\tilde{I}$ is a complex matrix and a logarithmic scale is used for $|\tilde{I}|$. The 0 (center) and ± 1 orders (bottom left, and at the top right) are clearly distinct. It is then possible to select the +1 order by zeroing the other pixels (Figure 2.4(d)), then compensate for the off-axis by moving the +1 order to the center of the Fourier space (Figure 2.4(e)). The +1 order Fourier hologram $\tilde{I}_{+1}(k_x, k_y)$ is thus obtained. The following computations (reconstruction) can be achieved starting from $\tilde{I}_{+1}$ (Figure 2.4(e)), or by performing an inverse Fourier transformation $\mathcal{F}^{-1}$ in order to obtain the +1 order hologram in the direct space $I_{+1}(x, y)$ (Figure 2.4(e)):

$$I_{+1}(x,y) = \mathcal{F}^{-1}_{x,y}\left\{\tilde{I}_{+1}(k_x,k_y)\right\} \qquad [2.9]$$

Spatial filtering and off-axis compensation have transformed the real hologram I, presenting fringes due to the amplitude modulation (Figure 2.4(b)), in a hologram I_{+1} no longer showing fringes and which is complex (Figure 2.4(f)). It is thus possible to access the object wave amplitude and phase in the sensor plane (considering that the reference wave is constant and uniform within this same plane).

In order to be able to separate the 0 and ± 1 orders properly, we have chosen the off-angle so that the +1 order is located at the center of the lower left quarter of the Fourier matrix (Figure 2.4(e)). The shift of order +1 in the Fourier space thus corresponds to $N/4$ pixels along k_x and k_y. The step Δk of the Fourier matrix $\tilde{I}$ verifies:

$$N\Delta_x\Delta_k = 2\pi \qquad [2.10]$$

This step corresponds to the angle $\Delta_\theta = \Delta_k/k$ where $k = 2\pi/\lambda$. We thus have:

$$\begin{aligned} \Delta_k &= 2\pi/(N\Delta_x) \\ \Delta_\theta &= \lambda/(N\Delta_x) \end{aligned} \qquad [2.11]$$

The simulation was therefore achieved for an off-axis angle of about $N\Delta_\theta/4 = \lambda/(4\Delta_x) = 0.028$ rad following each direction.

In order to separate the orders, the area covered by the different orders in the Fourier space must also not be too large so that the different orders do not overlap. These areas depend on the viewing angle of the object from the camera θ_o and the viewing angle of the camera from the object θ_c (Figure 2.5). The area of the ± 1 orders corresponds to the convolution of these two viewing angles ($\approx \theta_o + \theta_c$). The area of the 0th-order signal component (mostly related to the contribution of the object wave intensity) corresponds to the convolution of θ_o with itself ($\approx 2\theta_o$). On the other hand, the area of the zeroth-order reference component is very small. Indeed, if we consider a constant reference wave, it corresponds to a few very bright pixels located at the center of the Fourier space (Dirac peak). In our simulation, given that $U_R = 1$, everywhere, the term $|U_R|^2$ corresponds to the central pixel of Figure 2.4(c), which is indistinguishable from other pixels because of the use of the logarithmic scale for the hologram spectrum. For holographic microscopy (Figure 2.3), the microscope objective (MO) acts as the spatial filter and limits the viewing angle of the object. Since the field U_o necessarily travels through MO, θ_o and θ_c can be calculated, considering that the rear iris of the microscope objective is the object.

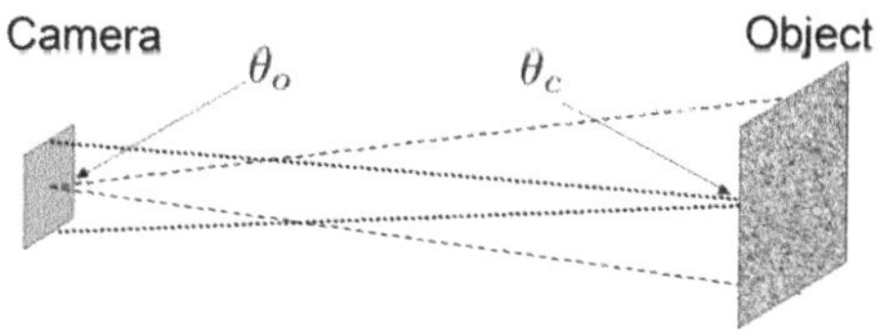

Figure 2.5. *View angles θ_o and θ_c*

The weight of the 0, ± 1 order contributions depends on the average intensities I_o and I_R of the fields U_o and U_R seen by the camera ($I_o = \langle |U_o|^2 \rangle$ and $I_R = \langle |U_R|^2 \rangle$). The total energy (summed over all pixels) associated with the $+1$ (or -1) order term is proportional to $\sqrt{I_o I_R}$, while the total energy of the zeroth-order signal term is I_o, and that of the zeroth-order reference term I_R. If the signal is weak ($|U_o| \ll |U_R|$), the zero-order signal component can be overlooked, and the zeroth order covers only a very small part of the Fourier space. On the other hand, if the object-wave prevails ($|U_o| \gg |U_R|$ et $\theta_o \gg \theta_c$), the zeroth-order signal component covers an area twice the size of the ± 1 orders.

The simulation of Figure 2.4 has been carried out under conditions that made it possible to separate and visualize the 3 orders. The size of the object (Figure 2.4(a)) is 3.7×1.8 mm, it is located at 17.1 cm from the camera, the reference signal ratio is $Io/I_R = 0.3$ and the wavelength $\lambda = 633$ nm.

2.3.2. *Phase-shifting holography*

Phase-shifting holography is the second family of methods used to select the +1 order of [2.5]. Instead of performing the +1 order filtering in the Fourier space just as off-axis holography does, phase-shifting holography performs the filtering in the space of temporal frequencies by calculating the hologram from a sequence of camera images: I_0, I_1, I_2, etc.

Phase-shifting holography uses a device that modifies the reference beam phase φ_n. This can be a piezoelectric transducer (PZT) that moves a mirror (Figure 2.6(a)) located on the reference channel or an electro-optical modulator that modulates the length of the reference arm. This method is simple in its implementation but the desired phase is difficult to obtain with accuracy. An analysis of the interferences existing in the images of the sequence nevertheless leads to measuring the relativistic phase φ_n of each image and selecting the +1 order by an appropriate computation.

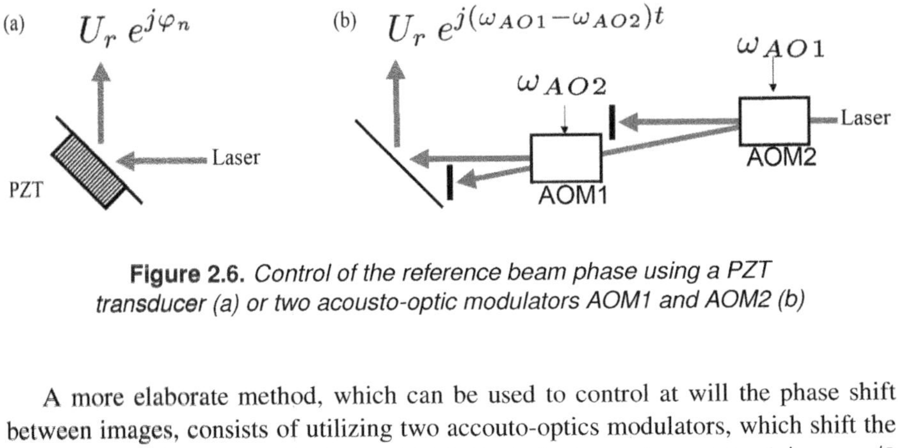

Figure 2.6. *Control of the reference beam phase using a PZT transducer (a) or two acousto-optic modulators AOM1 and AOM2 (b)*

A more elaborate method, which can be used to control at will the phase shift between images, consists of utilizing two accouto-optics modulators, which shift the frequency of U_R as shown in Figure 2.6(b). For inducing a phase shift of $\Delta_\varphi = \pi/2$ between each image to achieve four-phase modulation ($\varphi_n = n\pi/2$), we simply have to shift the frequency of U_R by $+\omega_{AOM1}$ with the first modulator, then $-\omega_{AOM2}$ with the second modulator (where $\omega_{AOM1,2} \simeq$ 80 MHz for typical acousto-optic modulators) by choosing $\omega_{AOM1} - \omega_{AOM2} = \omega_C/4$, where ω_C is the image acquisition frequency of the camera. Therefore, by playing with the frequencies $\omega_{AOM1,2}$, the phase shift Δ_φ can be chosen.

The choice of the value for $\Delta\varphi$ will set the number N of images necessary to travel the 2π angle on which the reference wave phase will evolve during the acquisitions.

By combining the various acquired holograms, we will obtain the demodulated field $I_{\Delta\varphi}$. Here, the demodulation equation is given by

$$I_{\Delta\varphi} = \sum_{k=0}^{N-1} I_k e^{-j2\pi k/N} \qquad [2.12]$$

where I_k represents the kth hologram of the sequence of N holograms. It should be observed that [2.12] corresponds to the temporal Fourier transform of the hologram sequence.

To illustrate how the 0 and −1 orders vanished, we have calculated and visualized in Figure 2.7 the hologram in Fourier space $\tilde{I}_{\Delta\varphi}$ by considering the off-axis configuration of the previous section: the size of the object (Figure 2.4(a)) is 3.7×1.8 mm, and it is located at 17.1 cm from the camera. To restrict the zeroth order spectral spread, we will take into consideration a setup such that the intensity of the reference wave is three times greater than that of the object wave.

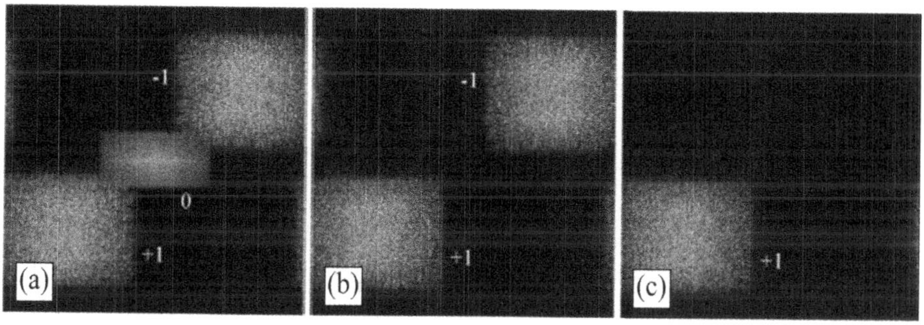

Figure 2.7. *Phase-shift holography. Fourier hologram obtained for one-phase demodulation: $\tilde{I}_{\Delta_\varphi=0}$ (a), two phases (b) and four-phase demodulation (c)*

2.3.2.1. *Using a single hologram*

This situation corresponds to $\Delta_\varphi = 0$ and $I_{\Delta_\varphi=0} = I$, which is given by [2.5]. The three interference orders are present. The simulation (Figure 2.7(a)) gives for $\tilde{I}_{\Delta_\varphi=0}$ the same image as in Figure 2.4(c).

2.3.2.2. *Two-phase demodulation with two images*

In this case, we have the phase shift $\Delta_\varphi = \pi$. Here, [2.12] becomes:

$$I_\pi = I_0 - I_1 \qquad [2.13]$$

For the images I_0 and I_1, [2.5] becomes:

$$\begin{aligned} I_0 &= |U_o|^2 + |U_r|^2 + U_o^* U_r + U_o U_r^* \\ I_1 &= |U_o|^2 + |U_r|^2 - U_o^* U_r - U_o U_r^* \end{aligned} \quad [2.14]$$

which gives, after demodulation

$$I_\pi = 2\left(U_o^* U_r + U_o U_r^*\right) \quad [2.15]$$

The zeroth-order term vanishes, which is confirmed by the calculation of the Fourier hologram $\tilde{I}_\pi$ (Figure 2.7(b)).

2.3.2.3. *Four-phase demodulation with four images*

In this case, the phase shift is $\Delta_\varphi = \pi/2$ and [2.12] is then written as

$$I_{\pi/2} = (I_0 - I_2) - j(I_1 - I3) \quad [2.16]$$

For the images I_0 to I_3, [2.5] becomes

$$\begin{aligned} I_0 &= |U_o|^2 + |U_r|^2 + U_o^* U_r + U_o U_r^* \\ I_1 &= |U_o|^2 + |U_r|^2 + U_o^* U_r + jU_o U_r^* \\ I_2 &= |U_o|^2 + |U_r|^2 + U_o^* U_r - U_o U_r^* \\ I_3 &= |U_o|^2 + |U_r|^2 + U_o^* U_r - jU_o U_r^* \end{aligned} \quad [2.17]$$

which gives, after demodulation

$$I_{\pi/2} = 4\left(U_o U_r^*\right) \quad [2.18]$$

The 0 and -1 orders vanish. Only the first-order remains (Figure 2.7(c)).

Four-phase holography makes it possible to have a much larger field of view since it is no longer necessary to angularly shift the reference beam, nor to satisfy the geometrical conditions of separation of orders 0, ± 1. Nevertheless, it is necessary that the +1 order, which corresponds to the convolution of the view angles $\approx \theta_o$ and θ_c (Figure 2.5), does not exceed the computational grid of the Fourier space. The condition similar to $N\Delta_\theta/2 > \theta_o + \theta_c$ must therefore be respected.

Phase-shifting holography assumes that the object does not move, since U_o must not change during acquisition. Filtering in Fourier space and the reduction of the field of view associated therewith is avoided. By combining phase-shifting holography with off-axis holography, a double filtering is achieved (in the space of temporal and spatial frequencies) and the reference beam completely eliminated, as it is the main source of noise when the holographic signal is low. When the signal is very weak, the signal-to-noise ratio can be significantly improved by performing the demodulation on a large number of images. For example, the four-phase demodulation can be performed with 16 images with

$$H = \sum_{m=0}^{15} j^m I_m \qquad [2.19]$$

This result is valid if all the holograms are, respectively, phase-shifted by $\pi/2$ with respect to each other. Otherwise, equation [2.12] will have to be used and a 16-phase demodulation is carried out.

REMARK.– We perform here an averaging over the field that makes the technique very robust. In this case, and if the phase shift and the off-axis are coupled, it can be shown that the signal-to-noise ratio evolves proportionally to the number of acquisitions (Lesaffre et al. 2013). For more conventional situations where the averaging would be performed on the reconstructed intensity, the signal-to-noise ratio would evolve as the square root of the number of acquisitions.

2.4. Holographic reconstruction

The reconstruction consists of computing the field everywhere and in particular in the vicinity of the object from the hologram recorded with the camera. Since the order +1 term corresponds to the product $U_o U_R^*$ and the reference field U_R is assumed to be known (and most often constant), the order +1 term obtained by off-axis holography (I_{+1}) or by phase-shift holography of ($I_{\pi/2}$) is directly proportional to the field $U_o(x, y)$ on the camera. In order to perform the reconstruction, we thus identify I_{+1} or $I_{\pi/2}$ with the field U_o.

The holographic reconstruction is done by applying the Huygens–Fresnel principle (Figure 2.8) by considering that the hologram behaves like an amplitude and phase-mask illuminated by the reference wave. Each hologram pixel becomes a secondary source, whose amplitude is $U_o(x, y)$ and emits a spherical wave. The backpropagated wave is then the sum of these spherical emitters.

The choice of reconstruction method depends on the geometry of the experiment. In any case, the main limitation of the reconstruction comes from the hologram itself.

Since the hologram has a finite lateral size, the resolution that can be obtained during reconstruction is limited by the numerical aperture associated with the object position and the area of the sensor (angle θ_C in Figure 2.5). Moreover, the spatial filtering used to select the +1 order increases the size of the speckles (Figure 2.4(f)). This reduces the angle of diffraction of the reference wave by the hologram (Figure 2.8(b)) and thus the field of view of the reconstruction. By combining the two effects, it is found that the number of resolved pixels of the reconstructed image cannot be greater than the number of non-zero pixels in Fourier space (Figures 2.4(d) and 2.4(e)).

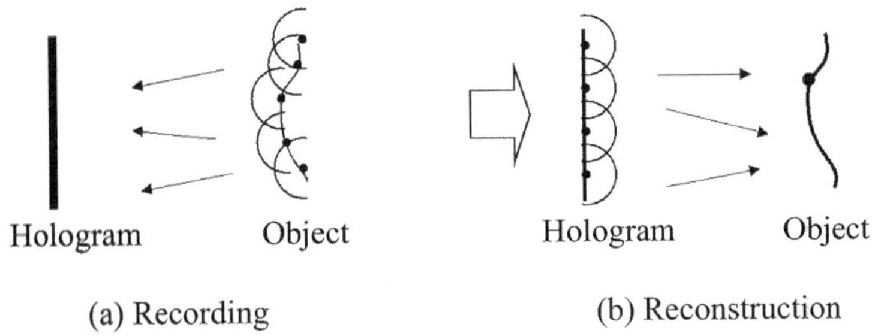

Figure 2.8. *Huygens principle applied to the field computation in the camera plane (a) and to the reconstruction of the field in the object plane (b)*

2.4.1. *Fourier transform reconstruction*

We will present here the single Fourier transform reconstruction, which is the first one that has been proposed. This reconstruction is generally employed for off-axis holography in free space because it is well suited for objects located far from the camera, which may also be larger than the area of the CCD or CMOS (Complementary Metal Oxide Semi-Conductor) sensor. To perform the reconstruction, we will adopt the coordinate system and the method described in Schnars and Jüptner (2002). The reconstructed field at point P with coordinates η, ξ, z is obtained by summing the $U_o(x, y)$ fields of the pixels M of the hologram:

$$U_o(\eta, \xi, z) = \sum_{x,y} \frac{1}{|\mathrm{MP}|} U_o(x, y) \exp(-jk|\mathrm{MP}|) \qquad [2.20]$$

where $k = 2\pi/\lambda$ is the wave vector modulus, and where x, y are the physical coordinates of the camera pixels. It should be noted that all computations will be made considering discrete coordinates except for the z coordinate. Here, we have:

$$\begin{aligned} x &= n\Delta_x \\ y &= m\Delta_x \end{aligned} \qquad [2.21]$$

where n, m are the pixel indices and Δ_x is the size of the pixels assumed to be square. By expanding |MP|, it follows that, for an object located far from the camera[1]:

$$|\mathrm{MP}| \approx z + \frac{(\xi - x)^2}{2z} + \frac{(\eta - y)^2}{2z} \qquad [2.22]$$

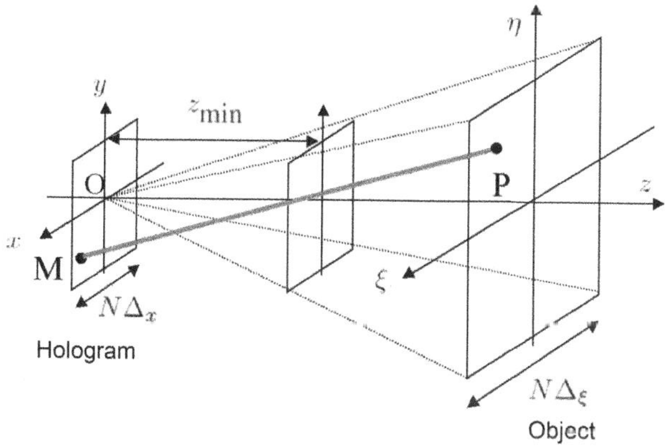

Figure 2.9. *Coordinates used for the reconstruction of a distant object by the method based on a single Fourier transform*

Equation [2.20] becomes:

$$U_o(\eta, \xi, z) = \tfrac{1}{z}\, e^{-jkz}\, e^{-jk(\xi^2+\eta^2)/2z} \sum_{x,y} U_o(x, y)\, e^{-jk(x^2+y^2)/2z}\, e^{-jk(x\xi+y\eta)/z} \qquad [2.23]$$

Let us introduce the coordinates $k_x = k\xi/z$ and $k_y = k\eta/z$. They represent the components along x and y of a vector wave **k** describing the propagation of a field along the direction OP where O is the origin of the coordinates. The factor $e^{jk(x\xi+y\eta)/z}$ becomes $e^{j(k_x x+k_y y)}$. The summation $\sum_{x,y} ...$ corresponds here to the discrete Fourier transform ($\mathcal{F}$) of $U_o(x, y)\, e^{-jk(x^2+y^2)/2z}$. Equation [2.23] becomes:

$$U_o(\xi, \eta, z) = \tfrac{1}{z}\, e^{-jkz}\, e^{-j(k_x^2+k_y^2)z/2k}\, \mathcal{F}_{k_x,k_y}\left\{U_o(x, y)\, e^{-jk(x^2+y^2)/2z}\right\} \qquad [2.24]$$

1 According to the Fresnel theory, it is considered that the object is far from the sensor if the condition $\left[(\xi - x)^2 + (\eta - y)^2\right]^2 / \left(8z^4\right) \ll 1$ is satisfied.

where k_x, k_y are the coordinates of the Fourier space. The hologram field $U_o(x,y)$ is multiplied by the quadratic phase factor $e^{-jk(x^2+y^2)/2z}$, which describes a lens of focal length $-z$ placed within the hologram plane (Goodman 2005). This lens transports the image of the object from the z plane to infinity. The Fourier transform then allows us to obtain the image of the object.

The factors to the left of the FT of [2.24] are global amplitude and phase corrections. The factor $1/z$ describes the decrease in energy with the reconstruction distance. The factor e^{-jkz} describes the phase variation along z for a propagation along z. The factor $e^{-j(k_x^2+k_y^2)z/2k}$ is a phase correction, quadratic in k_x and k_y. It describes the phase delay of a field that is propagating in the k_x, k_y direction between the planes $z = 0$ and z, with respect to the field propagating along z. We will find this phase factor during the reconstruction by the angular spectrum. Very often, these global corrections are not calculated because they do not change the intensity of the reconstructed image.

2.4.1.1. *Computational grid*

The coordinates ξ and η of [2.24] are discrete with steps $z\Delta_\theta$ where Δ_k is given by [2.11]. The computational grid used for the reconstruction (Figure 2.9) therefore has the shape of a pyramid whose top is located at O and whose aperture angle $\theta = N\Delta_\theta$ is equal to the diffraction angle of a camera pixel λ/Δ_x: it also follows that the optical etendue $S\Omega$ associated with a pixel and the aperture angle of the reconstruction grid (solid angle $\Omega = \theta^2$) is $S\Omega = \Delta_x^2\theta^2 = \lambda^2$. Similarly, the optical etendue $S\Omega$ associated with the focusing of the field during reconstruction can be considered. The area is then that of the reconstructed pixel $S = \Delta_\xi^2$, and the solid angle then corresponds to the hologram seen from the object: $\Omega = (N\Delta_x/z)^2$. Once more, an optical etendue $S\Omega = \lambda^2$ is found. This result means that the reconstruction step Δ_ξ is equal to the diffraction limit associated with the area of the hologram.

2.4.1.2. *Reconstruction with or without spatial filtering*

To illustrate the reconstruction with a single Fourier transform, we have performed the reconstruction of the object and of Figure 2.4(b) (3.7×1.8 mm object located at 17.1 cm from the camera) starting from the hologram I_{+1} in Figure 2.4(f), which is obtained after spatial filtering and off-axis compensation.

The single Fourier transform reconstruction is often used in off-axis geometry without performing spatial filtering. To test this reconstruction, we started with the hologram I shown in Figure 2.4(b). Since the reference wave is off axis, the object image, which is reconstructed from the +1 term of [2.7] ($U_o(x,y)\ e^{-j(k_x x+k_y y)}$), is not at the center of the grid but at the bottom left (Figure 2.10(b)). The order -1 term ($U_o^*(x,y)\ e^{+j(k_x x+k_y y)}$) gives the out-of-focus image visible in the upper-right corner. The use of fast Fourier transform algorithms for the reconstruction of holograms places periodicity conditions on the computational domain (Cooley and Tukey 1965). Thus, the portion of the image of order –1 which goes beyond the computational grid on the right-hand side reappears at the top left. The white square at the center of the image corresponds to the zero-order term associated with the reference beam ($|U_r|^2$) whose intensity is greater.

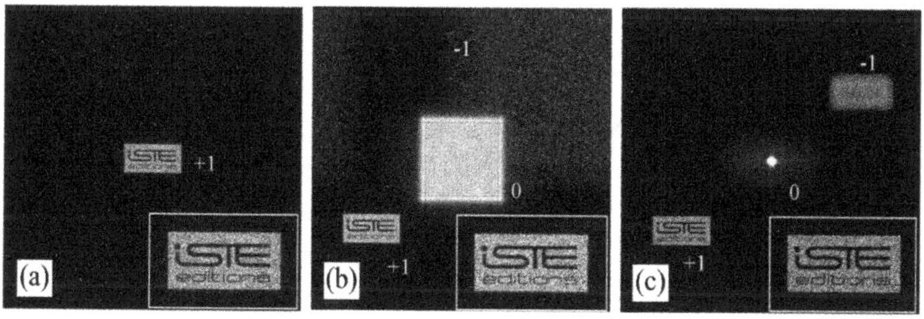

Figure 2.10. *Holographic image reconstructed by the single Fourier transform method with +1 order selection and off-axis compensation (a) or without +1 order selection (b, c), and with plane wave (a, b) or spherical wave (c) reference. Inserts:* $\times 2$ *magnification during reconstruction*

By using an off-axis reference, the images associated with the 0, ± 1 terms of [2.5] (and [2.24]) can be separated without performing spatial filtering.

To simplify the discussion, we have so far considered that the reference U_r was a plane wave. In practice, it often proves useful to use an experimental device where the reference beam is spherical (Figure 2.11). The reconstruction can be done by [2.24] provided that z be replaced by z' with

$$z' = \left(z^{-1} - r^{-1}\right)^{-1} \tag{2.25}$$

where r is the curvature of the reference wave. As shown in Figure 2.10(c) which was obtained with $z = 17.1$ cm, $r = 16.1$ cm, and $z' = -2.82$ m, the reconstructed image is strictly identical to the image obtained, in the plane of the hologram, in plane wave. By choosing $r \simeq z$, we have obtained here 0 and –1 order images, which occupy less space on the computational grid. The bright area in the center of the image corresponds to the order 0 term associated with the reference ($|U_R|^2$), while the lower intensity fuzzy area that surrounds it corresponds to the zeroth order term associated with the object ($|U_o|^2$). As indicated above, the weight of the different components of the image in Figure 2.10(c) can be modified by adjusting the relative weights of the signal U_o and the reference U_r. It is often useful to use a spherical wave reference because this allows for a better separation of the orders 0, ± 1 and leads to a larger field of view.

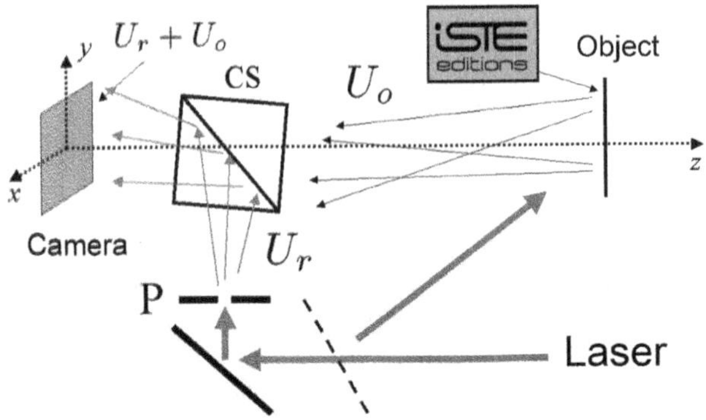

Figure 2.11. *Example of off-axis holography device with spherical wave reference generated by the filter hole P*

It should be noted that the reconstruction achieved by [2.24] is valid only for large z. Indeed, the phase lens of focal length z (i.e. $e^{-jk(x^2+y^2)/2z}$) diverges when z tends to zero. In practice, it can be considered that z is large enough when the transverse size of the reconstruction grid is larger than the hologram: $N\Delta_\xi > N\Delta_x$ (Figure 2.9), that is, when the reconstructed pixels are larger than the camera pixels $\Delta_\xi > \Delta_x$. This condition corresponds to

$$z > z_{\text{min}} = N\Delta_x^2/\lambda \qquad [2.26]$$

In our simulation, this condition is satisfied since we have $z = 17.1$ cm and $z_{min} = 4.9$ cm.

2.4.2. *Two Fourier transform reconstruction (angular spectrum)*

When the reconstruction distance z is small, the 1FT-reconstruction does not work because the phase factor $e^{-jk(x^2+y^2)/2z}$ of [2.24] diverges. In this case, it can be useful to use angular spectrum reconstruction. We refer to it here as angular spectrum because this is the term used in the literature, but in reality it would be better call it reconstruction by plane wave field decomposition or a two Fourier transform reconstruction.

The field $U_o(x, y, z)$ that propagates through the whole space can be decomposed into plane waves:

$$U_o(x, y, z) = \sum_{k_x, k_y} a(k_x, k_y)\, e^{j(k_x x + k_y y)}\, e^{-jk_z z} \qquad [2.27]$$

where k_x, k_y and k_z are the components of the wave vector $\mathbf{k}$ with $k = |\mathbf{k}| = 2\pi n/\lambda$, where n is the optical index of the medium between the hologram and the object. Consider the hologram plane $z = 0$. Equation [2.27] becomes: $U_o(x, y, 0) = \mathcal{F}_{x,y}^{-1}\{\, a(k_x, k_y)\, \})$. We thus have $a = \mathcal{F}_{k_x,k_y}\{\, U_o\}$ where:

$$U_o(x, y, z) = \mathcal{F}_{x,y}^{-1}\left[\, e^{-jk_z z}\, \mathcal{F}_{k_x,k_y}\, (U_o(x, y))\, \right] \qquad [2.28]$$

where k_z is dependent on k_x and k_y, since $k_x^2 + k_y^2 + k_z^2 = k^2$:

$$k_z = \sqrt{k^2 - k_x^2 - k_y^2} \qquad [2.29]$$

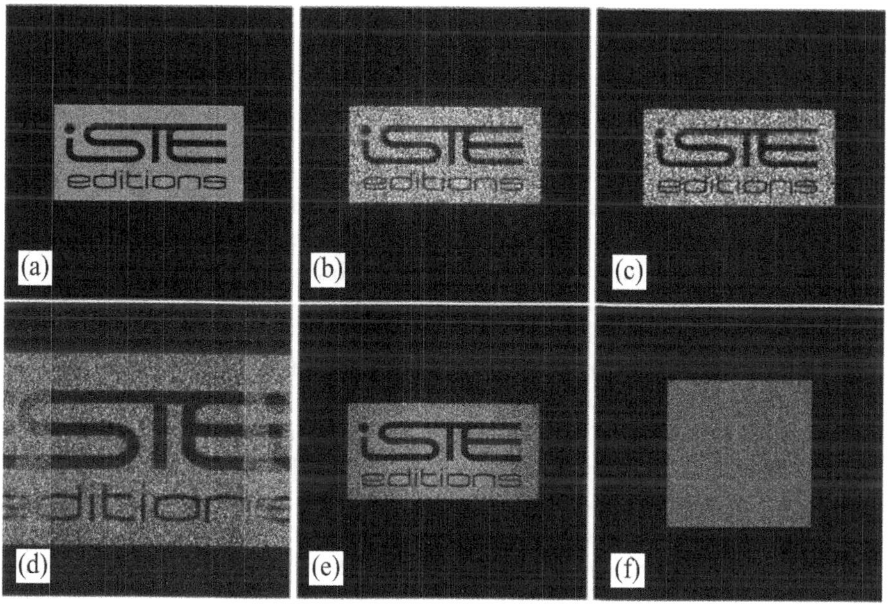

Figure 2.12. *2FT reconstruction. (a) Object. (b) Reconstructed field $U_o(x, y, z)$ by [2.30]. (c) ×3.5 magnification of the same object reconstructed with 1FT. (d, e) Reconstruction of an object twice as large on a 1,024 × 1,024 pixel grid (d) and on a 2,048 × 2,048 grid extended by zero padding (e). 2,048 × 2,048 hologram used for the zero-padding reconstruction (f)*

When the field propagation from the object to the camera is achieved under the conditions of [2.22] (i.e. with small angles), which is generally the case when holography is made in free space (outside microscopy), equation [2.28] can be written as:

$$U_o(x,y,z) \propto \mathcal{F}^{-1}_{x,y} \left\{ e^{+j(k_x^2+k_y^2)z/2k} \, \mathcal{F}_{k_x,k_y} \left[U_o(x,y) \right] \right\} \qquad [2.30]$$

Equation [2.28] (or the simplified equation [2.30]) describes the backpropagation of the camera field (plane $z = 0$) to the plane z of the object.

The reconstruction equations [2.28] and [2.30] have $U_o(x, y)$ as a starting point. When off-axis holography is used to select the order +1, the component of order +1 in the Fourier space $\tilde{I}_{+1}(k_x, k_y)$ is obtained as an intermediate result. This component can be treated as the Fourier field, and used as a starting point for the computation:

$$\tilde{I}_{+1}(k_x, k_y) \equiv \tilde{U}_o(k_x, k_y) = \mathcal{F}_{k_x,k_y} \left\{ U_o(x,y) \right\} \qquad [2.31]$$

Similarly to single Fourier transform reconstruction, the computations are done with discrete x, y coordinates of step Δx. It should be noted that the step is the same in the camera plane ($z = 0$) and in the z plane where the reconstruction is performed. The number of $N \times N$ pixels in the computational grid is generally chosen as being equal to the number of pixels of the camera. This means that the reconstruction is done over a parallelepiped, which corresponds to the shadow of the camera sensor.

To illustrate the two Fourier transform (FT) reconstruction, we have completed the reconstruction of the object in Figure 2.4(a) (3.7×1.8 mm object located at 17.1 cm from the camera) on which we had selected the +1 order by spatial filtering to obtain $\tilde{I}_{+1} \equiv \tilde{U}_o$ (Figure 2.4(e)). The reconstructed image (Figure 2.12(b)) is similar to the image that we have reproduced here in Figure 2.12(a). The specks are larger because spatial filtering acts as a low-pass filter that eliminates high spatial frequencies. It should be noted that the simulation has been carried out under conditions where it is possible to make a 1FT reconstruction. The image obtained with 1FT in Figure 2.12(g) is 3.5 times smaller but contains the same information. To better understand this, we have enlarged the 1FT image by a factor of $\times 3.5$ and obtained the image of Figure 2.12(c), which is very similar to the image in Figure 2.12(b).

2.4.3. *Two Fourier transform reconstruction with* zero padding

If the object is larger than the camera, the 2FT (2 Fourier transforms) reconstruction cannot be used because the object is larger than the computational grid. The result is an incomplete picture in which the areas of the image are located outside the computational grid yield images as shown in Figure 2.12(d), which was obtained by performing the reconstruction of an object similar to the one shown in Figure 2.12(a) but twice as large.

One way to solve this incompatibility is based on using the *zero padding* method, which consists of considering a larger hologram. The pixels located at the center of the hologram are measured by the camera, while the edge pixels are set to zero (Figure 2.12(f)). With the frequency support extended, the effects of the circularity condition of fast Fourier transform algorithms are limited. The 2FT reconstruction can then be carried out without problems, as shown in Figure 2.12(e).

2.4.4. *Two Fourier transform reconstruction with the addition of a digital lens*

In order for the 2FT reconstruction to be done with pixels whose size does not depend on z, the reference beam has to be a plane wave. Otherwise, the reconstruction grid is distorted and the pixel size depends on z. This defective planarity of the reference wave can be offset by multiplying the hologram by the digital lens $e^{jk(x^2+y^2)/(2r)}$, which compensates for the curvature r of the reference beam.

It also proves useful to voluntarily introduce a digital lens to adjust the pixel size in the reconstruction plane z. This is called variable magnification reconstruction. The latter consists of multiplying the hologram by a numerical lens $e^{jk(x^2+y^2)/(2r)}$ and then performing a 2FT reconstruction. The reconstructed field becomes

$$U_o(x', y', z') \simeq \mathcal{F}^{-1}_{x,y}\left\{e^{+j(k_x^2+k_y^2)z'/2k}\mathcal{F}_{k_x,k_y}\left[e^{-jk(x^2+y^2)/2r}U_o(x,y,z)\right]\right\} \quad [2.32]$$

where $z' = (1/z - 1/r)^{-1}$. The step of the transverse coordinates x', y' becomes $\Delta'_x = z/z'$. It depends on r and can therefore be adjusted at will. Variable magnification reconstruction is useful for color holography, for combining holographic images recorded at different wavelengths.

There is one final situation where the addition of a digital lens is necessary: namely for holographic microscopy. Indeed, the microscope lens that images the object on the camera adds to the object field the curvature $e^{jk(x^2+y^2)/(2r)}$ where r is the distance between the camera and the MO. Furthermore, when there is no object, the illumination beam is transformed into a spherical wave of curvature r (Figure 2.3(b)). The field therefore has to be multiplied by $e^{-jk(x^2+y^2)/(2r)}$. It is then possible to use 2FT reconstruction to image the object. However, it should be noted that the 2FT reconstruction is achieved from the camera image to the object. This means that the reconstruction step is equal to the size of the camera pixels divided by the imaging magnification of the MO lens. The pixels are therefore small. Since the field propagation is no longer done relying on the small-angle approximation, the equation for the 2FT reconstruction [2.28] should be used.

2.5. Associated holographic configurations and applications

So far, we have discussed the main properties of holography, describing the extraction of the complex optical field by spatial or temporal filtering, and the digital reconstruction/refocusing of holograms.

We will now present the main configurations and their fields of application.

2.5.1. *In-line holography*

2.5.1.1. *Principle*

In-line holography is directly inspired by Gabor's experiment (Gabor 1948). A schematic diagram of the experimental configuration is illustrated in Figure 2.13.

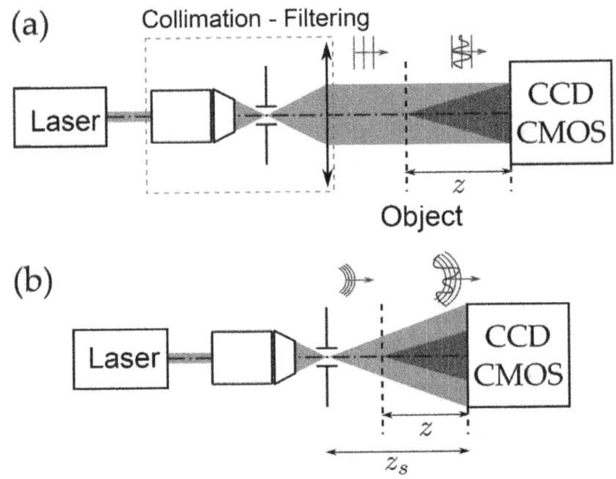

Figure 2.13. *In-line holography schematic diagram. (a) Wave plane object illumination. (b) Spherical wave object illumination. For a color version of this figure, see www.iste.co.uk/fournier/unconventional.zip*

The wave traveling from a laser is focused by means of a microscope objective, or a short focal length lens, through a pinhole. The purpose of this step is to spatially filter the beam. Two cases can then be considered: the filtered beam is collimated to illuminate the object (Figure 2.13(a)) or the object is illuminated with the spherical wave exiting from the pinhole (Figure 2.13(b)). This is referred to as lensless imaging in this case. In these two configurations, the object illumination wave (in red in Figure 2.13) is also used as the reference wave. The interferences between the wave diffracted/scattered by the objects under study (in blue) and the reference wave (the portion of the illumination beam that has not been perturbed by the object) are recorded on a CCD or CMOS sensor devoid of collection optics.

2.5.1.2. *Limitations and constraints related to the experimental setup*

As can be seen in Figure 2.13, the in-line holography assembly is simple. Some precautions should nevertheless be taken concerning acquisitions and hologram reconstruction.

Let us revisit equation [2.5], which gives the intensity recorded in the sensor plane. In an in-line holography setup, the 0, +1 and –1 order terms propagate along the same axis. It is therefore impossible to filter them, whether it is by spatial or temporal filtering. We thus no longer consider order filtering. The reconstructions are then marred by "twin image" noise. This problem is illustrated by Figure 2.14. Indeed, it is as if, during reconstruction, the image of the object located at distance $+z$ that we want to reconstruct (order +1) was superimposed to the twin image of a symmetrical object located at distance $-z$ (–1 order).

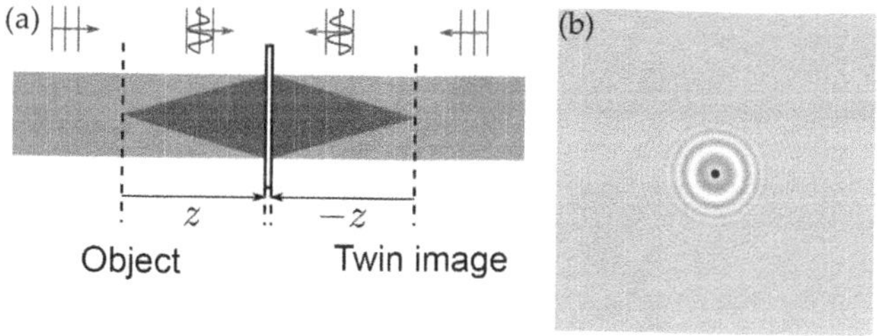

Figure 2.14. *Illustration of the "twin image" problem in in-line holography. For a color version of this figure, see www.iste.co.uk/fournier/unconventional.zip*

This is highlighted in Figure 2.14(b), which illustrates the reconstruction of the image of a spherical bead acquired in in-line holography. It can be observed that the image of the bead is well reconstructed but that it is superimposed on the fringes corresponding to the object located at a distance $-z$ from the hologram. This effect is all the more detrimental when the goal is to image objects whose lateral sizes are much larger than those of the sensor pixels. The twin image effect will be weaker when observing small objects located far away from the sensor. The use of iterative reconstruction algorithms can result in removing the twin image and reconstructing the amplitude and phase of the wave object (Gerchberg and Saxton 1972; Fienup 1982; Latychevskaia 2019).

Another limitation of in-line holography is that the object illumination wave is also the reference wave. For the reference wave not to be hidden, it is necessary that the imaged objects occupy only a small area of the field (Meng et al. 1993; Malek et al. 2004). The illumination must be done in transmission and the objects are small (beads, drops, bacteria). In addition, the relative weights of the signal field and the reference field cannot be modified. Finally, the reconstructed field in the object plane corresponds to the superposition of the field scattered/diffracted by the object and the illumination field. This is why the reconstructed field is non-zero and uniformly flat away from the bead in Figure 2.14(b).

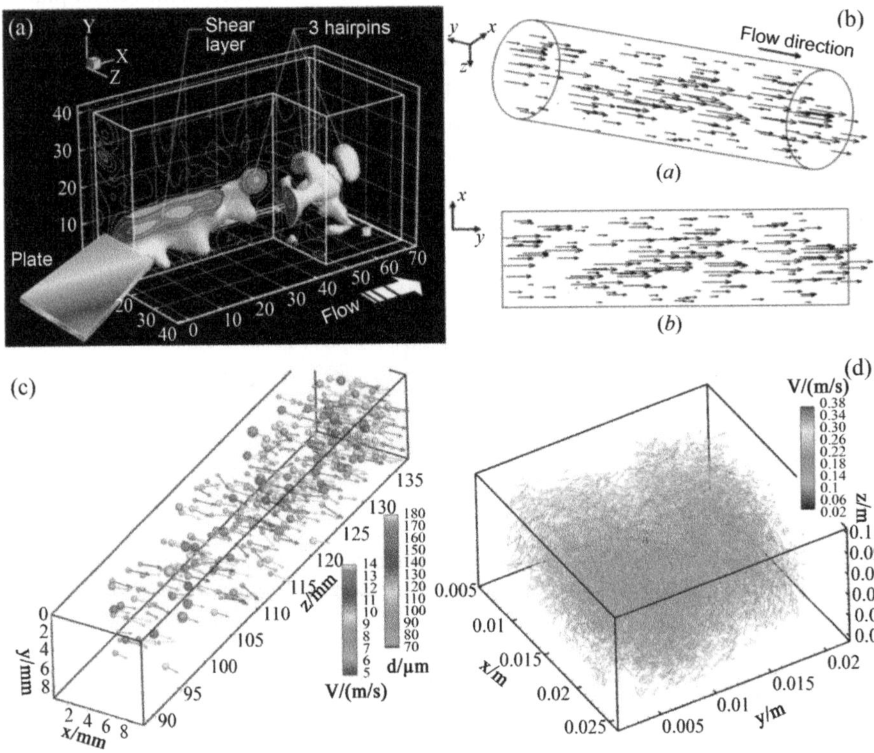

Figure 2.15. *Some results obtained in in-line holography for characterizing fluids. For a color version of this figure, see www.iste.co.uk/fournier/unconventional.zip*

2.5.1.3. *Some applications*

In its in-line setup (Figure 2.13), holography allows for the extraction of 3D information in severe experimental environments. In fact, a single optical access is necessary. Moreover, as the reference wave and the object wave share the same optical axis, this assembly is very robust to variations in experimental conditions (temperature, vibrations, etc.). These characteristics make in-line holography a method of choice for 3D flow characterization. The latter are seeded with microtrackers which, if properly selected, make it possible to extract 3D flow characteristics (3D positions, associated velocities, etc.).

Some results obtained with an in-line holographic configuration are proposed in Figure 2.15. Hologram acquisition and reconstruction result here in characterizing in 3D: (a) vorticity in flows (Pu and Meng 2005); (b) the trajectories of tracers in microchanneling (Ichi Satake et al. 2006); (c) bubbles in laminar flows (Wu et al. 2015); and (d) bubbles in swirling flows (Wu et al. 2020).

2.5.2. *Off-axis holography*

2.5.2.1. *Principle*

To overcome the limitations of the in-line setup previously presented, Leith and Upatnieks have proposed a modification of the holographic assembly based on the use of an external reference wave which interferes with the object wave (Leith and Upatnieks 1962). The two waves are recombined by introducing a small angle, which causes a spatial modulation in the hologram. This is the configuration discussed in section 2.3.1 and is represented schematically in Figure 2.3 for a sample imaged in free-space reflection (a) or in microscopy transmission (b). The holography setup is most often based on a Mach–Zehnder interferometer. The wave from a laser is split into two waves by means of a beam-splitter cube or a semi-transparent mirror (dotted line in Figure 2.3). One of these two waves will be used as a reference wave while the other will illuminate, in transmission or reflection, the object to be analyzed. The diffracted wavefront U_o and the reference wave U_r are finally recombined by means of the recombining cube CS and interfere in the camera plane. The cube CS is angularly tilted to introduce a spatial modulation on the hologram. This modulation is visible in the insert in Figure 2.4(b), which shows a magnification of the intensity $|U_r + U_o|^2$ calculated in the camera plane.

As we have shown in section 2.3.1, this setup makes it possible to extract the amplitude and phase of the field scattered/diffracted/reflected by the object using spatial filtering in Fourier space (Cuche et al. 1999).

2.5.2.2. *Constraints related to the experimental setup and precautions during reconstruction*

Off-axis holography is often used to image objects whose lateral sizes are larger than those of the sensor. In this case, hologram reconstruction with the 1FT method described in section 2.4.1 is preferred. To use this method, particular attention should be paid to ensure that the object to be characterized is at a distance greater than $z_{min} = \frac{N\Delta x^2}{\lambda}$ from the sensor as shown in Figure 2.9 and the discussion, which has led to establishing [2.25].

Off-axis holography can be used to image objects with sizes similar to those of the sensor. In this case, we should use the 2FT reconstruction described in section 2.4.2, or reconstruction methods based on the representation of the Fresnel integral as a convolution product (Verrier and Atlan 2011). For intermediate sized objects (larger than the sensor but not very large), we can use zero-padding 2FT reconstruction described in section 2.4.3 or the variable magnification reconstruction method, which can adapt the reconstructed field to the experimental situation under consideration (Zhang et al. 2004; Chang Li et al. 2009; Restrepo and Garcia-Sucerquia 2010). This method consists of multiplying the hologram by a numerical lens and then performing a 2FT reconstruction, as indicated in section 2.4.4.

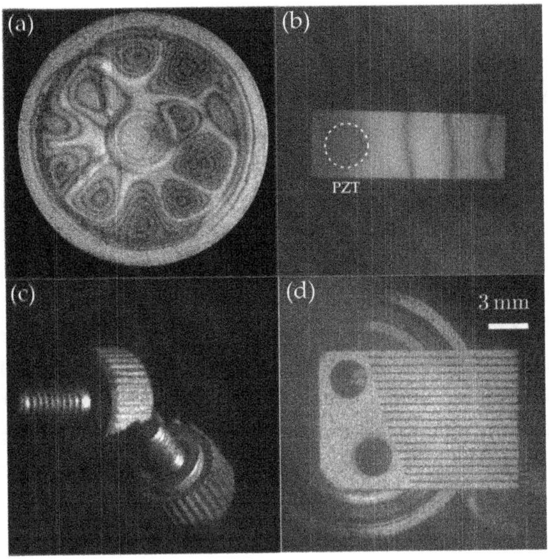

Figure 2.16. *Some results obtained with off-axis holography with 1FT reconstruction*

COMMENT ON FIGURE 2.16.– *(a) Time-averaged imaging of the membrane of a vibrating speaker (Picart et al. 2005). (b) Imaging of the vibration modes of a tab by heterodyne holography (from Verrier et al. (2013)). (c) Screw picture (McElhinney et al. 2008). (d) Reconstruction of a lamellophone (from Bruno et al. (2014)).*

2.5.2.3. *Some applications*

As we have seen so far, holography is well suited for imaging small objects. However, it is also possible to image large-sized objects compared to the lateral sizes of the sensor. In fact, if we choose a 1FT reconstruction (suitable for large objects located far away from the sensor), the computational grid depends on the axial position of the object (Figure 2.9). This property allows us to consider the use of holography in fields such as non-destructive testing, particularly for parts submitted to vibration, and inspection. Figure 2.16 presents some applications of off-axis holography with 1FT reconstruction. It is thus possible to analyze vibrating structures: by time-averaged holography (Picart et al. 2005) (Figure 2.9(a)) or heterodyne holography (Verrier et al. 2013) (Figure 2.9(b)). In this case, the analysis of the vibration modes in the structure can provide information on possible structural defects. It is also possible to visually inspect large objects as shown (Figures 2.9(c) and (d)).

2.5.3. *Holographic microscopy and quantitative phase imaging*

2.5.3.1. *Principle*

We have seen that off-axis holography setups enabled by means of spatial or temporal information filtering, extracting the amplitude and phase of the optical field from an object. We have seen applications for imaging with large objects and non-destructive testing.

The ability to extract the complex field and thus the amplitude and phase of the object wave open up new perspectives for unlabeled imaging of phase-shifting structures, such as those seen in biomedical imaging. These studies are most often achieved by combining holography and microscopy. The schematic diagram of a holographic microscopy setup is proposed in Figure 2.3(b) for a transmission setup. Clearly, it is visible that the setup is very close to an off-axis holography setup in free space such as Figure 2.3(a). The main difference lies in adding a microscope objective for collecting the optical field propagating from the object. It should be noted that using a condenser is not essential as long as we make sure that the illumination of the object is plane. In a reflection configuration, the device is similar but the objective is used both as a condenser for the illumination and a lens to collect the field and image the object.

Most often, the objective forms the object image on the camera and holography is used to extract the amplitude and the phase of the optical field produced by the object. Holography thus makes it possible to quantitatively measure the phase. It may happen that the object is out of focus outside the imaging plane. In order to obtain the object image, a reconstruction will be carried out after extraction of the complex optical field. This reconstruction can also be used to obtain images of the object field in planes located in the vicinity of the object so that a 3D image of the field diffracted/scattered by the object is obtained.

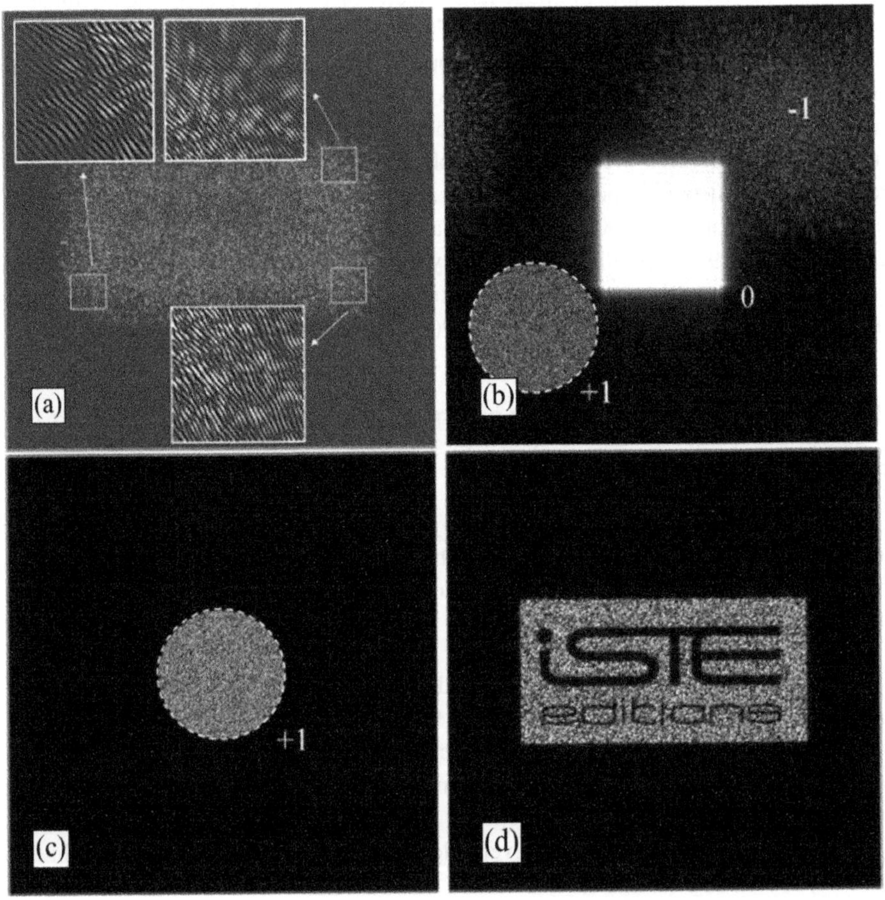

Figure 2.17. *Holographic microscopy reconstruction. (a) Hologram $H(x, y)$. Inserts: $\times 4$ magnifications of $H(x, y)$ of the indicated regions. (b) 1FT reconstruction of the MO iris. (c) Selection and translation of the +1 order component; we obtain: $FT(\, U_o(x', y')\,)$. (d) Reconstructed field*

There are a number of points that have to be considered here. The microscope objective, which collects the field and images the object, introduces a phase curvature (i.e. a digital lens) that should be compensated before any reconstruction is carried out. This point has been described in the 2FT reconstruction part of section 2.4.4. Moreover, the rear pupil of the lens constitutes a circular diaphragm, which limits the extent of the signal field in the Fourier space. To analyze this effect, we have performed a simulation and imaged with a $\times 10$ magnification lens the sheet with "ISTE imaging" written on whose size has been reduced by a factor of $\times 10$. The sheet has been placed out of focus and the image of the sheet appears blurred on the hologram (Figure 2.17(a)). Because of the off-axis reference, the hologram $H(x, y)$ presents visible fringes in the inserts in Figure 2.17(a). After compensating for the phase introduced by the lens, we have calculated the hologram $\tilde{H}(k_x, k_y)$ in Fourier space. The +1 order component of the object field is a circular disk with a sharp edge. This disk corresponds to the image of the rear iris of the lens. In fact, the holographic microscopy device in Figure 2.3(b) can be seen as a holography device in free-space that images the rear iris of the MO objective and the operations we have carried out (multiplication by a quadratic phase and Fourier transform) constitute a 1FT reconstruction of the iris. The digital lens that compensates for the phase introduced by the lens corresponds here exactly to the lens that enables the 1FT reconstruction of the iris image. To visualize this, we should simply consider a thought experiment achieved with a vertical plane wave incident on the MO lens in Figure 2.3(b). This wave is focused by the lens in the plane of the rear iris at the center of the iris. The digital lens that reconstructs the iris has the same focal length as the lens that compensates the phase induced by the objective. The diameter of the +1 order disk (250 pixels) in Figure 2.17(c) corresponds to a view angle of $250\Delta_\theta = 0.0336$ rad (see [2.11]), that is, an objective located 17 cm from the camera and whose iris is 5.72 mm in diameter. In holographic microscopy, the diameter of the +1 order disk is generally much smaller than the computational grid (here $1,024 \times 1,024$). This means that the camera performs an oversampling of the hologram and there is no loss of information.

The reconstruction is made by propagating the image field from the camera to the object (Figure 2.17) using a 2FT computation. The reconstruction pixels are small because they are obtained by dividing the camera pixels by the imaging magnification (here $\times 10$). The result is that the angles are large (here $\times 10$ larger) and the exact reconstruction kernel $e^{-jk_z z}$ must be used (see [2.27] and [2.29]). The reconstruction distances are also small since z_{min} given by [2.26] is here $\times 100$ times smaller.

The holographic microscopy simulation was carried out here with a reconstruction distance $z = 0.5\ z_{min} = 245\ \mu$m, while the free space simulations have been performed for $z = 3.5\ z_{min} = 17.1$ cm. With the highly diffusing object located at $z = 0.5\ z_{min}$ from the camera, it would not have been possible to properly separate the 0, ± 1 orders in the free space. In holographic microscopy, it is possible to correctly distinguish the orders because the lens iris limits the range of the ± 1 orders to a disk with a 300-pixel diameter in Fourier space.

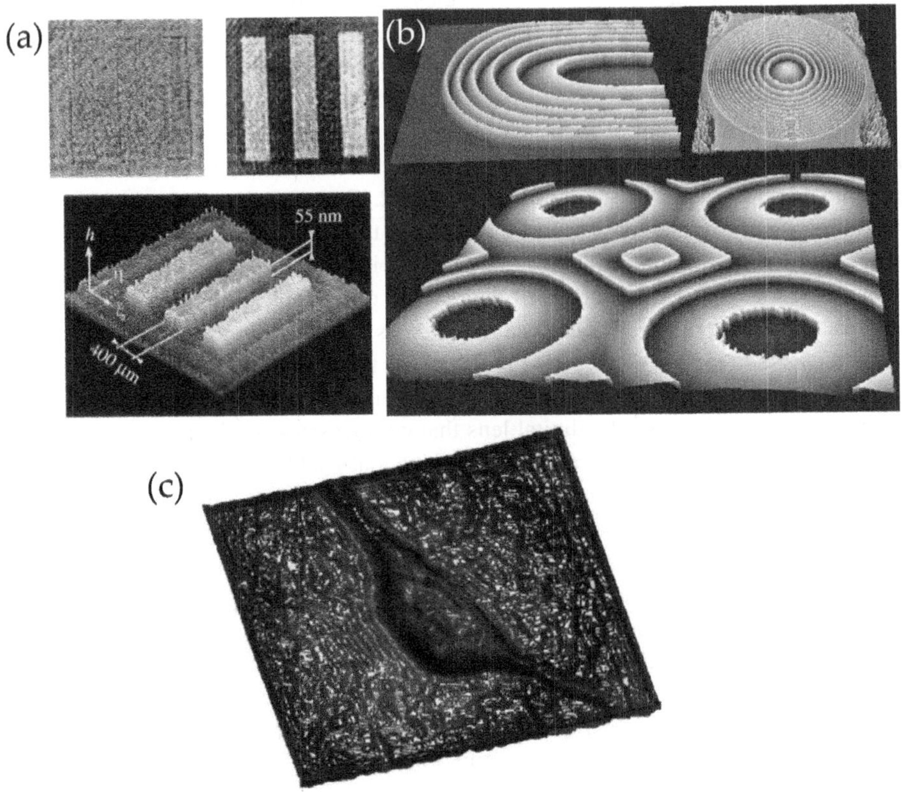

Figure 2.18. *A few results obtained with quantitative phase holography imaging. (a) Phase resolution test pattern characterization (taken from Cuche et al. (1999)). (b) Microoptical components characterization (according to Charriere et al. (2006)). (c) Reconstruction of the topology of an ovarian cancer cell (from Kim et al. (2006)). For a color version of this figure, see www.iste.co.uk/fournier/unconventional.zip*

2.5.3.2. *Some applications*

Holography makes it possible to extract the amplitude and the phase of the optical field scattered/diffracted by an object. It is therefore used to perform quantitative imaging of the optical phase (Park et al. 2018). This information is of great interest for label-free imaging of transparent structures.

In this case, the phase information makes it possible to identify the optical step difference. This latter will lead to obtaining the thickness and the refractive index of the medium under study.

Some applications of holography for phase quantitative imaging, such as for characterizing a phase test pattern (a), the analysis of optical components (b) or cellular imaging (c) are proposed in Figure 2.18.

2.6. Conclusion

In this chapter, we have laid the foundation for digital holography. This technique is used to measure the amplitude and phase of a laser field scattered/diffracted by an object on a matrix detector, and then to reconstruct through computations the field produced by the object at any point in space. Since the detectors are only sensitive to the average optical field strength (average because the field evolves at typically 10^{15} Hz), holography makes use of the interference with a known reference field, originating from the same laser, to code the field amplitude and phase in the form of interference fringes.

The first reconstruction stage, which is described in section 2.3, consists of extracting from the hologram the field amplitude and phase at the surface of the detector. This extraction is done by filtering in the space of spatial frequencies: off-axis holography, section 2.3.1, or temporal holography or phase-shift holography, section 2.3.2.

Once this field is known, it is possible to reconstruct the object field at any point in space from Maxwell's equations. In practice, a scalar field is considered for simplicity (overlooking polarization) and the equations of optics are used: the Huygens–Fresnel principle or plane wave decomposition. The different reconstruction methods are described in detail in section 2.4. Since the hologram is measured on a matrix detector (the camera), the calculations are done with matrices. Two types of transformations are carried out with them, a multiplication by a phase mask (most often quadratic) and Fourier transform (FT). The 1FT reconstruction (section 2.4.1) is done with: 1 phase mask + 1FT; 2FT reconstruction (section 2.4.2) with: 1FT + mask + 1FT; variable magnification and microscopy reconstructions (section 2.4.4) with: 1 mask + 1FT + 1 mask + 1FT.

The choice of reconstruction method to be used depends on the geometry of the experiment. In many situations, several methods can be used and lead to equivalent results. 2FT reconstruction with zero padding (see section 2.4.3) for example can be used in all cases, provided the size of the computational grid is enlarged, which can lead to very cumbersome computations. The main limitation to the quality of reconstruction derives from the measurement itself. The measurement is discrete (there is sampling from the pixels), it is made over a limited area (the camera), with averaging of the intensity over the pixels. All of this results in limitations with the resolution, the size of the reconstructed area and possibly by aliasing effects.

Holography is often described as a three-dimensional measurement. This is not quite the case, since holography records holograms on a 2D detector with a number of limited pixels. Holography is capable of calculating plane fields in front of, behind or on the object, but the information contained in each plane is the same since it is possible to shift from one plane to the other by performing reversible transformations (FT, multiplication by a phase mask), unitary in the mathematical sense. It should be noted that in this chapter, we have neglected discussions that concern measurement sensitivity, photon noise and the coherent character of holographic detection.

After having laid the most important theoretical foundations of digital holography, we presented a brief review of some applications in section 2.5.

2.7. References

Bruno, F., Laudereau, J.-B., Lesaffre, M., Verrier, N., Atlan, M. (2014). Phase-sensitive narrowband heterodyne holography. *Appl. Opt.*, 53(7), 1252–1257.

Chang Li, J., Tankam, P., Jie Peng, Z., Picart, P. (2009). Digital holographic reconstruction of large objects using a convolution approach and adjustable magnification. *Opt. Lett.*, 34(5), 572–574.

Charrière, F., Pavillon, N., Colomb, T., Depeursinge, C., Heger, T.J., Mitchell, E.A., Marquet, P., Rappaz, B. (2006). Living specimen tomography by digital holographic microscopy: Morphometry of testate amoeba. *Opt. Express*, 14(16), 7005–7013.

Cooley, J.-W. and Tukey, J.-W. (1965). An algorithm for the machine calculation of complex Fourier series. *Math. Comput.*, 19, 297–301.

Cuche, E., Bevilacqua, F., Depeursinge, C. (1999). Digital holography for quantitative phase-contrast imaging. *Opt. Lett.*, 24(5), 291–293.

Fienup, J.R. (1982). Phase retrieval algorithms: A comparison. *Appl. Opt.*, 21(15), 2758–2769.

Gabor, D. (1948). A new microscopic principle. *Nature*, 161(4098), 777–778.

Gabor, D. and Bragg, W.L. (1949). Microscopy by reconstructed wave-fronts. *Proceedings of the Royal Society of London. Series A. Mathematical and Physical Sciences*, 197(1051), 454–487.

Gerchberg, R. and Saxton, W. (1972). A practical algorithm for the determination of the phase from image and diffraction plane pictures. *Optik*, 35(237), 237–246.

Goodman, J.W. (2005). *Introduction to Fourier Optics*, 3rd edition. Roberts & Company Publishers, Greenwood Village.

Goodman, J.W. and Lawrence, R.W. (1967). Digital image formation from electronically detected holograms. *Applied Physics Letters*, 11(3), 77–79.

Ichi Satake, S., Kunugi, T., Sato, K., Ito, T., Kanamori, H., Taniguchi, J. (2006). Measurements of 3D flow in a micro-pipe via micro digital holographic particle tracking velocimetry. *Measurement Science and Technology*, 17(7), 1647–1651.

Iemma, U., Morino, L., Diez, M. (2006). Digital holography and Karhunen–Loeve decomposition for the modal analysis of two-dimensional vibrating structures. *Journal of Sound and Vibration*, 291(1–2), 107–131.

Kemper, B. and von Bally, G. (2008). Digital holographic microscopy for live cell applications and technical inspection. *Appl. Opt.*, 47(4), A52–A61.

Kim, M.K., Yu, L., Mann, C.J. (2006). Interference techniques in digital holography. *Journal of Optics A: Pure and Applied Optics*, 8(7), S518–S523.

Kronrod, M.A., Merzlyakov, N.S., Yaroslavskii, L.P. (1972). Reconstruction of a hologram with a computer. *Soviet Physics Technical Physics*, 17, 333.

Latychevskaia, T. (2019). Iterative phase retrieval for digital holography: Tutorial. *J. Opt. Soc. Am. A*, 36(12), D31–D40.

Leith, E.N. and Upatnieks, J. (1962). Reconstructed wavefronts and communication theory. *J. Opt. Soc. Am.*, 52(10), 1123–1130.

Leith, E.N. and Upatnieks, J. (1963). Wavefront reconstruction with continuous-tone objects. *J. Opt. Soc. Am.*, 53(12), 1377–1381.

Leith, E.N., Upatnieks, J., Haines, K.A. (1965). Microscopy by wavefront reconstruction. *J. Opt. Soc. Am.*, 55(8), 981–986.

Lesaffre, M., Verrier, N., Gross, M. (2013). Noise and signal scaling factors in digital holography in weak illumination: Relationship with shot noise. *Appl. Opt.*, 52, A81–A91.

Liu, G. and Scott, P.D. (1987). Phase retrieval and twin-image elimination for in-line fresnel holograms. *J. Opt. Soc. Am. A*, 4(1), 159–165.

Lozano, A., Kostas, J., Soria, J. (1999). Use of holography in particle image velocimetry measurements of a swirling flow. *Experiments in Fluids*, 27(3), 251–261.

Malek, M., Allano, D., Coëtmellec, S., Lebrun, D. (2004). Digital in-line holography: Influence of the shadow density on particle field extraction. *Opt. Express*, 12(10), 2270–2279.

McElhinney, C.P., Hennelly, B.M., Naughton, T.J. (2008). Extended focused imaging for digital holograms of macroscopic three-dimensional objects. *Appl. Opt.*, 47(19), D71–D79.

Meng, H., Anderson, W.L., Hussain, F., Liu, D.D. (1993). Intrinsic speckle noise in in-line particle holography. *J. Opt. Soc. Am. A*, 10(9), 2046–2058.

Onural, L. and Scott, P.D. (1987). Digital decoding of in-line holograms. *Optical Engineering*, 26(11), 1124–1132.

Park, Y., Depeursinge, C., Popescu, G. (2018). Quantitative phase imaging in biomedicine. *Nature Photonics*, 12(10), 578–589.

Picart, P., Leval, J., Mounier, D., Gougeon, S. (2005). Some opportunities for vibration analysis with time averaging in digital fresnel holography. *Appl. Opt.*, 44(3), 337–343.

Pu, Y. and Meng, H. (2005). Four-dimensional dynamic flow measurement by holographic particle image velocimetry. *Appl. Opt.*, 44(36), 7697–7708.

Restrepo, J.F. and Garcia-Sucerquia, J. (2010). Magnified reconstruction of digitally recorded holograms by Fresnel–Bluestein transform. *Appl. Opt.*, 49(33), 6430–6435.

Schnars, U. and Jüptner, W. (1994). Direct recording of holograms by a ccd target and numerical reconstruction. *Appl. Opt.*, 33(2), 179–181.

Schnars, U. and Jüptner, W. (2002). Digital recording and numerical reconstruction of holograms. *Measurement Science and Technology*, 13(9), R85.

Verrier, N. and Atlan, M. (2011). Off-axis digital hologram reconstruction: Some practical considerations. *Appl. Opt.*, 50(34), H136–H146.

Verrier, N., Gross, M., Atlan, M. (2013). Phase-resolved heterodyne holographic vibrometry with a strobe local oscillator. *Opt. Lett.*, 38(3), 377–379.

Wu, Y., Wu, X., Yao, L., Gréhan, G., Cen, K. (2015). Direct measurement of particle size and 3D velocity of a gas solid pipe flow with digital holographic particle tracking velocimetry. *Appl. Opt.*, 54(9), 2514–2523.

Wu, Y., Zhang, H., Wu, X., Cen, K. (2020). Quantifying bubble size and 3D velocity in a vortex with digital holographic particle tracking velocimetry (DHPTV). *Flow Measurement and Instrumentation*, 76, 101826.

Zhang, F., Yamaguchi, I., Yaroslavsky, L.P. (2004). Algorithm for reconstruction of digital holograms with adjustable magnification. *Opt. Lett.*, 29(14), 1668–1670.

3

Inverse Problems for Image Reconstruction in Holography

Ferréol SOULEZ and Éric THIÉBAUT
Université de Lyon, Université Lyon 1, ENS de Lyon, CNRS,
Centre de recherche astrophysique de Lyon, Saint-Genis-Laval, France

3.1. Introduction

In the field of experimental physics, we seek to estimate parameters of interest based on observations of the object under study. In most cases, it is possible to build a numerical model of the observations according to the parameters of interest (see section 3.2). Equipped with this *direct model* and taking into account the data, the estimation of the parameters of interest is tantamount to solving an *inverse problem*. Even if the direct model is invertible, it may be preferable to take into account the non-uniform quality of data (see section 3.4) and impose constraints that can either be hard (see section 3.5) or soft (see section 3.7) to determine a good estimator for the object of interest. This estimator must have good properties, being both optimal with respect to error (and noise) propagation and well defined in the presence of incomplete data (e.g. amplitude measurements only or truncated field of view). The framework of *inverse problems* described in this chapter is very general and is particularly suited to the reconstruction of images from holographic data. For a more general presentation of inverse problems, the reader should refer to the forthcoming book on the subject coordinated by Paul Escande and Emmanuel Soubies, due to be published in the SCIENCES collection by ISTE Ltd.

Unconventional Optical Imaging for Biology,
coordinated by Corinne FOURNIER and Olivier HAEBERLÉ. © ISTE Ltd 2024.

3.1.1. *Notations*

We use lowercase letters for functions and scalars (e.g. o and λ), bold lowercase for vectors (e.g. $\boldsymbol{o}$), calligraphic capital letters for operators acting on functions (e.g. $\mathcal{M}$) and capital letters for matrices (e.g. $\mathbf{H}$). Regardless of the context, *vectors* are collections of values (e.g. a dataset, a sampled object, etc.), while *matrices* are linear mappings that produce vectors when applied to vectors. We denote by $\boldsymbol{x}^\top$ the adjoint (i.e. the conjugate transpose) of $\boldsymbol{x}$, $\|\boldsymbol{x}\|_2 = \sqrt{\boldsymbol{x}^\top \boldsymbol{x}}$ the Euclidean norm of $\boldsymbol{x}$ and $\|\boldsymbol{x}\|_\mathbf{W} = \sqrt{\boldsymbol{x}^\top \mathbf{W} \boldsymbol{x}}$ a weighted version of this norm (with the positive semi-definite Hermitian matrix $\mathbf{W}$). $\langle \boldsymbol{x}, \boldsymbol{y} \rangle = \boldsymbol{x}^\top \boldsymbol{y}$ is the scalar product between vectors $\boldsymbol{x}$ and $\boldsymbol{y}$ and $\boldsymbol{x} \times \boldsymbol{y}$ their element-wise product (Hadamard). With these notations, a wave $w \in \mathbb{W}$ is a complex-valued function of 2D side coordinates $\boldsymbol{x} = [x_1, x_2]^\top$. Due to the finite amount of energy carried by the wave, w is square integrable, so $\mathbb{W}$ is the Hilbert space of the integrable square functions of $\mathbb{R}^2$ in $\mathbb{C}$. The discretized version of this wave is the vector $\boldsymbol{w} = [w_1, \dots, w_N]^\top \in \mathbb{C}^N$ of the N pixels being considered (e.g. in the memory storage order).

3.2. Direct model

Any digital imaging device produces discrete measurements $\boldsymbol{d} \in \mathbb{K}^N$ with $\mathbb{K} = \mathbb{C}$ or $\mathbb{R}$ depending on the device and N the number of detector pixels. A correct interpretation of the measurements $\boldsymbol{d}$ requires taking into account the physical process of image formation and noise statistics. This is expressed by the following equation which connects the object of interest $o \in \mathbb{W}$ and the measurements $\boldsymbol{d} \in \mathbb{R}^N$:

$$\boldsymbol{d} = \mathcal{M}(o) + \boldsymbol{e} \qquad [3.1]$$

In this equation, $\mathcal{M}$: $\mathbb{W} \to \mathbb{K}^N$ represents the *direct model* as a mapping from $\mathbb{W}$, the Hilbert space of square-integrable functions of $\mathbb{R}^2$ in $\mathbb{C}$, to $\mathbb{K}^N$. The *vector* $\boldsymbol{e} \in \mathbb{K}^N$ is an error term that accounts for random noise and modeling approximations. When the complex wavefront can be measured (e.g. in off-axis holography), the direct model $\mathcal{M}$ is simply a discrete version of $\mathcal{H}$: $\mathbb{W} \to \mathbb{W}$ the linear operator of wave propagation toward the image plane (e.g. the Fraunhofer or Fresnel operators or that of the angular spectrum). When only the complex wavefront intensity is recorded (in line holography, for example), $\mathcal{M}$ can be described as the composition of two operations: the wave propagation implemented by $\mathcal{H}$ and the conversion of the complex amplitude into intensity. The resulting direct model is then nonlinear and $\mathbb{K} = \mathbb{R}$; if we neglect the detector sampling, it is given by:

$$\mathcal{M}(o) = |\mathcal{H}(o)|^2 \qquad [3.2]$$

In practice, the object of interest o is discretized and the operator $\mathcal{H}$ is approximated by a discrete linear operator (i.e. a *matrix* in our formalism) denoted by $\mathbf{H}$. In the linear and nonlinear cases, the data model is then written as:

$$\boldsymbol{d} = \mathbf{H}\,\boldsymbol{o} + \boldsymbol{e}, \qquad \text{(linear model, with } \mathbb{K} = \mathbb{C}\text{)} \qquad [3.3]$$

$$\boldsymbol{d} = |\mathbf{H}\,\boldsymbol{o}|^2 + \boldsymbol{e}, \qquad \text{(nonlinear model, with } \mathbb{K} = \mathbb{R}\text{)} \qquad [3.4]$$

In this last expression, the squared modulus $|\ldots|^2$ is applied element-wise. The discretization of $\mathcal{H}$ must be carefully carried out to account for the higher spatial frequencies allowed by the configuration, while avoiding moiré effects (Soulez 2021). Independently of the propagation regime being considered (Fraunhofer, Fresnel or Rayleigh–Sommerfeld), the propagation operator $\mathcal{H}$ is unitary which means that its adjoint is simply the *backpropagation operator*: $\mathbf{H}^\top = \mathbf{H}^{-1}$.

Considering an object $\boldsymbol{o}$ discretized over N pixels, the size of matrix $\mathbf{H}$ is $N \times N$. Under typical experimental conditions, N can have a value of several millions and $\mathbf{H}$ contains so many values that this matrix can neither be stored nor inverted in practice. It is however possible to quickly compute the result of the propagation by $\mathbf{H}$ and the backpropagation by $\mathbf{H}^\top$ of any vector $\boldsymbol{x} \in \mathbb{C}^N$. This is of paramount importance because iterative methods for solving inverse problems, described in this chapter, only require applying $\mathbf{H}$ and its adjoint $\mathbf{H}^\top$.

EXAMPLE.– In the case of the simplest imaging system, the operator $\mathcal{H}$ operates the convolution of the object of interest by the impulse response (*point spread function* (PSF)) of the device. The Fourier transform for converting the convolution into a simple termwise multiplication, a discretized approximation of $\mathcal{H}$ and its adjoint are provided by

$$\mathbf{H} = \mathbf{F}^{-1}\,\mathrm{diag}(\widehat{\boldsymbol{h}})\,\mathbf{F} \qquad [3.5]$$

$$\mathbf{H}^\top = \mathbf{F}^{-1}\,\mathrm{diag}(\widehat{\boldsymbol{h}}^\star)\,\mathbf{F} \qquad [3.6]$$

where $\mathbf{F}$ is the discrete Fourier transform, $\widehat{\boldsymbol{h}} = \mathbf{F}\,\boldsymbol{h}$ is the Fourier transform of $\boldsymbol{h}$ the impulse response of the system and $\widehat{\boldsymbol{h}}^\star$ its (termwise) conjugate. Virtually, $\mathbf{F}$ and $\mathbf{F}^{-1}$ are $N \times N$ matrices but, in practice, can be applied by an algorithm (*fast Fourier transform* (FFT)), which is fast ($\sim N\,\log_2(N)$ operations instead of N^2) and barely requires any storage.

A version in NumPy (*numerical Python*) of functions operating the effects of $\mathbf{H}$ and $\mathbf{H}^\top$ would be, for example,

```
mtf = fft(psf)
def H(x): return ifft(mtf{*}fft(x))
def Ht(x): return ifft(conj(mtf){*}fft(x)),
```

where `psf` is the variable storing $\boldsymbol{h}$ the PSF (an image by the system of a point source), `mtf` (for *modulation transfer function*) the variable storing $\widehat{\boldsymbol{h}}$ the discrete Fourier transform of $\boldsymbol{h}$, `H(x)` and `Ht(x)` the functions acting as $\mathbf{H}$ and $\mathbf{H}^\top$ on an image `x`, `fft` and `ifft` the functions implementing the (fast) discrete Fourier transform and its inverse, and `conj` the function returning the (element-wise) conjugate of its argument. It should be noted that applying the operators $\text{diag}(\widehat{\boldsymbol{h}})$ and $\text{diag}(\widehat{\boldsymbol{h}}^\star)$ is tantamount to multiplying their argument elementwise by $\widehat{\boldsymbol{h}}$ and $\widehat{\boldsymbol{h}}^\star$, which is automatically done by the operator `*` of NumPy. Also observe the strong analogy between the expressions and the numerical code. A quick analysis of the code proposed above shows that the only storage needed is that of `mtf`, that is N complex values (instead of N^2 for explicitly storing the coefficients of the operators).

3.3. Experimental application

All sections of this chapter will be illustrated by numerical reconstructions of simulated data. The instrumental configuration, shown in Figure 3.2, is identical for all reconstructions. It simulates an in-line configuration with a laser of wavelength $\lambda = 532$ nm illuminating a target placed at a distance $z = 265$ mm from a camera with $1{,}024\times1{,}024$ pixels of size $6.7\times6.7\,\mu\text{m}^2$ with a filling factor of 1. According to Soulez (2021), the resolution of this imaging system can be estimated to be 20 µm at the center and 10 µm at the edge of the detector. This ensures that the Fresnel approximation is valid for the direct model. Throughout this chapter, the wave propagation operator $\mathbf{H}$ is thus a Fresnel transform.

To avoid the so-called *inverse crime* (i.e. the reconstruction of the object from simulated data with exactly the same numerical model as the one assumed for the direct model), data are generated with the band-limited angular spectrum propagation model (Matsushima and Shimobaba 2009) on a wide field of view of 8192×8192 3.35 µm pixels to avoid moiré effects. The data are contaminated by additive Gaussian noise of 30 dB. The target, shown in Figure 3.1(a), is a transparent object from an SVG version of the USAF-1951 chart (Soulez 1951), discretized to the resolution of 3.35 µm/pixel and extended to $8{,}192 \times 8{,}192$ pixels by mirror-type boundary conditions.

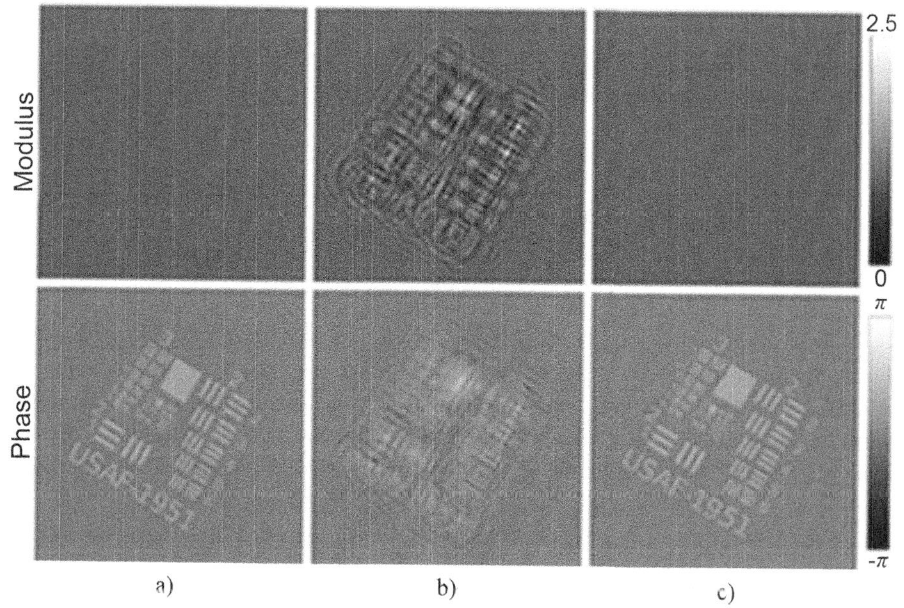

Figure 3.1. *(a) Object used in the simulation. (b) Wave in the diffracted plane with a noise of 30 dB. (c) Backpropagation of (b) in the object plane*

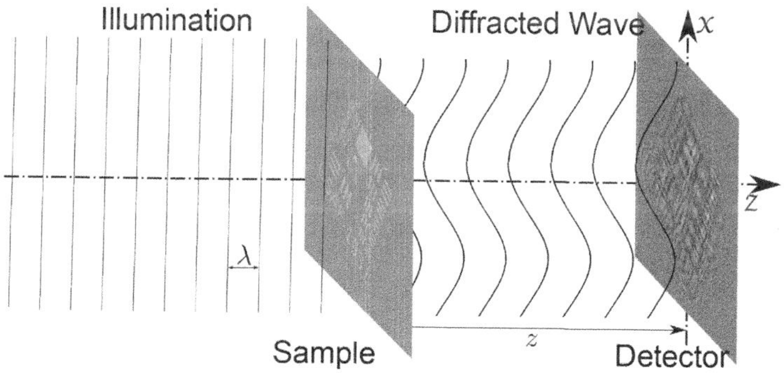

Figure 3.2. *Simulated experimental setup*

The quality of the reconstructed objects compared to the original object o_{gt} (where *gt* means *ground truth*) is evaluated by the reconstruction signal to noise ratio (SNR):

$$\mathrm{SNR}(\boldsymbol{o}) = 10 \log_{10}\left(\frac{\|\boldsymbol{o}_{\mathrm{gt}}\|_2^2}{\|\boldsymbol{o}_{\mathrm{gt}} - \boldsymbol{o}\|_2^2}\right) \qquad [3.7]$$

All of the simulations and reconstructions presented in this chapter have been achieved with MATLAB™ using the GlobalBioIm library (Soubies et al. 2019) and the code used for generating all of the figures is available at the COMCI repository (Soulez n.d.).

3.4. Maximum likelihood approach

3.4.1. *Formal expression*

In order to obtain a good reconstruction of the object $\boldsymbol{o}$ taking the measurements $\boldsymbol{d}$ and the direct model $\mathcal{M}$ into account, a given number of practical difficulties must be addressed. First, independently of the model, the noise term $\boldsymbol{e}$ is unknown, therefore equations [3.3] or [3.4] have infinite solutions in $\boldsymbol{o}$. Furthermore, not all noise realizations have the same probability. All of this can be taken into account when searching for the solution based on *maximum likelihood* (denoted ML), that is the solution that maximizes the probability of having observed the data and that is defined by:

$$\begin{aligned} \boldsymbol{o}^{(\mathrm{ML})} &= \arg\max_{\boldsymbol{o}} \Pr(\boldsymbol{d} \,|\, \boldsymbol{o}) \\ &= \arg\min_{\boldsymbol{o}} \bigl\{ \mathcal{L}(\boldsymbol{o}) = c_1 - c_2 \log \Pr(\boldsymbol{d} \,|\, \boldsymbol{o}) \bigr\} \end{aligned} \qquad [3.8]$$

The co-log-likelihood function $\mathcal{L}(\boldsymbol{o})$ can be interpreted as a way to measure the deviation between the data $\boldsymbol{d}$ and the model $\mathcal{M}(\boldsymbol{o})$, the solution $\boldsymbol{o}^{(\mathrm{ML})}$ being the one that minimizes this distance. The expression of $\mathcal{L}(\boldsymbol{o})$ depends on noise statistics which is described by $\Pr(\boldsymbol{d} \,|\, \boldsymbol{o})$, the probability density of observing the data $\boldsymbol{d}$ knowing the object $\boldsymbol{o}$. In the above definition of $\mathcal{L}(\boldsymbol{o})$, $c_1 \in \mathbb{R}$ and $c_2 > 0$ are arbitrary constants because their choice does not affect the solution. These two constants are usually chosen to simplify the expression of $\mathcal{L}(\boldsymbol{o})$.

3.4.2. *Noise statistics and likelihood*

For a photon counting detector, the counts measured per pixel are mutually independent, each having a Poisson distribution of likelihood given by the direct model. By taking $c_2 = 1$ and wisely choosing c_1, the likelihood penalty can be written as:

$$\mathcal{L}(\boldsymbol{o}) = \sum_{n=1}^{N} \{\mathcal{M}_n(\boldsymbol{o}) - d_n \log\bigl(\mathcal{M}_n(\boldsymbol{o})\bigr)\} \qquad [3.9]$$

where $\mathcal{M}_n(\boldsymbol{o})$ and d_n, respectively represent the nth values of $\mathcal{M}(\boldsymbol{o})$ and $\boldsymbol{d}$. The first one gives the average number of photoelectrons captured by the nth pixel plus, possibly, the average number of electrons due to the detector dark current (Winick 1986).

In practice, a more general and yet fairly good approximation of statistical noise can be derived by assuming that, knowing the object, the perturbation $\boldsymbol{e}$ is additive, centered and Gaussian. Taking $c_2 = 2$ and an appropriate value of c_1, the likelihood penalty is then written as

$$\mathcal{L}(\boldsymbol{o}) = \|\boldsymbol{d} - \mathcal{M}(\boldsymbol{o})\|^2_{\mathbf{W}} \quad [3.10]$$

where $\mathbf{W}$ is the data precision matrix knowing the object (Trouvé et al. 2014). If there are no missing data (see section 3.4.5), $\mathbf{W} = \mathbf{C}^{-1}$ with $\mathbf{C}$ the noise covariance matrix.

3.4.3. *Backpropagation*

When the complex wavefront is recorded, the direct model is linear and given by equation [3.3]. Under the Gaussian approximation of noise, the likelihood function is then written as $\mathcal{L}(\boldsymbol{o}) = \|\boldsymbol{d} - \mathbf{H}\,\boldsymbol{o}\|^2_{\mathbf{W}}$, which is quadratic and convex with respect to the object of interest $\boldsymbol{o}$. The maximum likelihood solution can then be expressed by imposing first-order optimality conditions $\mathbf{0} = \partial\mathcal{L}(\boldsymbol{o})/\partial\boldsymbol{o} = 2\,\mathbf{H}^\top\,\mathbf{W}\,(\mathbf{H}\,\boldsymbol{o} - \boldsymbol{d})$. Reordering the terms leads to the following *normal equations*:

$$\left(\mathbf{H}^\top\,\mathbf{W}\,\mathbf{H}\right)\boldsymbol{o} = \mathbf{H}^\top\,\mathbf{W}\,\boldsymbol{d} \quad [3.11]$$

which are necessarily verified by the maximum likelihood solution $\boldsymbol{o}^{(\mathrm{ML})}$. If the data precision matrix $\mathbf{W}$ and the propagation operator $\mathbf{H}$ are both invertible, the solution to equation [3.11] is unique:

$$\boldsymbol{o}^{(\mathrm{ML})} = \mathbf{H}^{-1}\,\boldsymbol{d} = \mathbf{H}^\top\,\boldsymbol{d} \quad [3.12]$$

where the simplification of the right-hand side term follows from the fact that $\mathbf{H}$ is unitary.

REMARK.– Interestingly, if the noise is i.i.d. (*independent and identically distributed*), then $\mathbf{W} \propto \mathbf{I}$ with $\mathbf{I}$ the identity matrix. Then solving normal equations [3.11] amounts to finding the minimum of $\|\mathbf{H}\,\boldsymbol{o} - \boldsymbol{d}\|^2_2$ in $\boldsymbol{o}$. If $\mathbf{H}$ is invertible, the solution to this simple linear least-squares problem is given by equation [3.12]; if $\mathbf{H}$ is not invertible (and therefore not unitary), then:

$$\boldsymbol{o}^{(\mathrm{ML})} = \mathbf{H}^\dagger\,\boldsymbol{d} \quad [3.13]$$

is the minimal norm solution to the linear least squares problem, $\mathbf{H}^{\dagger}$ being the pseudo-inverse of $\mathbf{H}$. Since, in our context, $\mathbf{H}^{\dagger} = \mathbf{H}^{\top}$, the backpropagation solution in [3.12] can also be considered as the *least-norm maximum likelihood solution* when the model is linear and the noise is assumed to be i.i.d. and Gaussian.

The wavefront phase and modulus measured in the presence of 30 dB of noise are represented in Figure 3.1 with the wavefront backpropagated within the object plane. Maximum likelihood reconstruction (i.e. backpropagation) comes close to the real image. A reconstruction of this quality is made possible because the problem is well-conditioned (because all eigenvalues of $\mathbf{H}$ are equal to one in our context) meaning that no information has been attenuated by propagation.

3.4.4. *Iterative methods for maximum likelihood estimation*

In the general case, computing the maximum likelihood solution is not as simple as the backpropagation given by [3.13]. This can be either because there is no closed form expression of the minimum of $\mathcal{L}(o)$ (e.g. for the Poisson statistic or when the model is nonlinear) or because the solution to the normal equations in [3.11] cannot possibly be computed in practice (e.g. when $\mathbf{H}^{\top}\,\mathbf{W}\,\mathbf{H}$ is too large to be stored and/or inverted by direct numerical methods).

In the linear case, the normal equations [3.11] can be solved by iterative methods such as the linear conjugate gradient algorithm (Hestenes and Stiefel 1952), which only requires coding $\mathbf{H}$, $\mathbf{H}^{\top}$ and $\mathbf{W}$ as numerical functions (see the example in section 3.2).

In the nonlinear case (either because the Poisson statistic is assumed for data or because the model is nonlinear), the solution to the maximum likelihood can only be found by means of a numerical iterative nonlinear optimization method with limited memory, such as the algorithms L-BFGS (Liu and Nocedal 1989) or VMLM-B (Thiébaut 2002) (see section 3.10).

3.4.5. *Extrapolation of the field of view*

As explained in Soulez (2021), the effective field of view of a holographic device can be much larger than the physical size of the detector. In numerical simulations (see Figures 3.3(a) and (b)) where the object is larger than the field of view of the camera, artifacts due to this truncation are clearly visible when simply backpropagating the data (see Figure 3.3(c)).

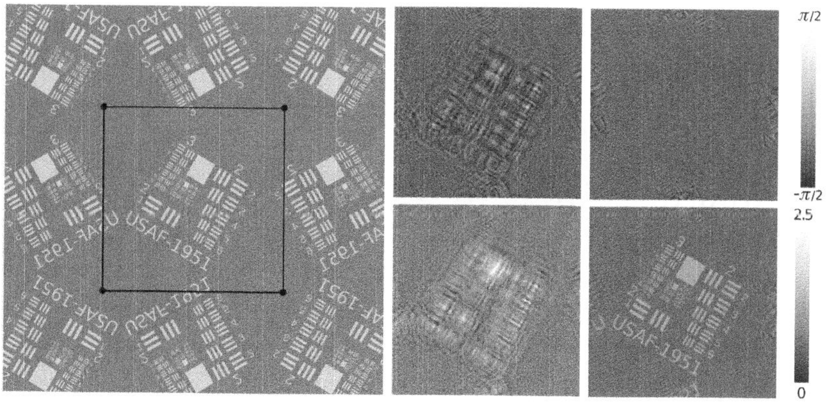

(a) (b) (c)

Figure 3.3. *(a) Phase of the extended object used in simulation, the black square represents the detector field of view. (b) Measured modulus (top) and phase (bottom). (c) Backpropagation modulus (top) and phase (bottom) of (b)*

The field of view extrapolation consists of reconstructing an object larger than the detector field. To keep a propagation operator $\mathbf{H}$ that is invertible, the data must be artificially completed to cover the same field of view. This operation, called *padding*, produces modified data $\tilde{\boldsymbol{d}}$ that have arbitrary values for the unmeasured pixels, that is, outside the detector field of view. These unmeasured pixels should not introduce information that could possibly propagate during the reconstruction. In other words, the likelihood function (in [3.9] or [3.10]) must remain unaffected by these unmeasured pixels. In the case of independent Gaussian noise, this is formally equivalent to expressing the precision matrix $\mathbf{W}$ as:

$$W_{n,n'} = \begin{cases} 1/\sigma_n^2 & \text{if } n' = n \text{ and the } n\text{th pixel is measured} \\ 0 & \text{otherwise} \end{cases} \quad [3.14]$$

where σ_n^2 is the noise variance at pixel n. It should be noted that the above precision matrix is diagonal, which implies independent noise. Because of the extension of the field of measures, $\mathbf{W}$ is not invertible but its pseudo-inverse has a simple expression:

$$W_{n,n'}^{\dagger} = \begin{cases} \sigma_n^2 & \text{if } n' = n \text{ and the } n\text{th pixel is measured} \\ 0 & \text{otherwise} \end{cases} \quad [3.15]$$

Since, in our context, $\mathbf{H}$ is invertible, and such that $\mathbf{H}^{-1} = \mathbf{H}^\top$, the solution to the minimal-norm normal equations [3.11] is simplified into:

$$o^{(\mathrm{ML})} = \mathbf{H}^\top \boldsymbol{r}, \text{ with } \boldsymbol{r} = \mathbf{W}^\dagger \mathbf{W} \widetilde{\boldsymbol{d}} \qquad [3.16]$$

because $(\mathbf{H}^\top \mathbf{W} \mathbf{H})^{-1} = \mathbf{H}^\top \mathbf{W}^\dagger (\mathbf{H}^\top)^{-1}$. It should be observed that the product $\mathbf{W}^\dagger \mathbf{W}$ is a diagonal matrix with diagonal values equal to 1 for the measured pixels and 0 for the unmeasured pixels. Therefore, $\boldsymbol{r} = \mathbf{W}^\dagger \mathbf{W} \widetilde{\boldsymbol{d}}$ corresponds to the data completed with zeros at the position of the unmeasured pixels regardless of the values initially chosen for these unmeasured pixels:

$$\left[\boldsymbol{r} = \mathbf{W}^\dagger \mathbf{W} \widetilde{\boldsymbol{d}}\right]_n = \begin{cases} d_n & \text{if the } n\text{-th is measured} \\ 0 & \text{otherwise} \end{cases} \qquad [3.17]$$

Consequently, the solution in the sense of maximum likelihood and minimal norm given by [3.16] is simply provided by the backpropagation of $\boldsymbol{r}$, the data completed by zeros (*zero padding*). This solution, illustrated by Figure 3.4(a), shows strong artifacts at the edges of the detector. These artifacts can be intuitively understood as being caused by diffraction from the detector edges, since *zero padding* is equivalent to assuming that no wave is transmitted outside the detector, as explained below.

REMARK.– If $\mathbb{Q} = \ker(\mathbf{A})$, the kernel of $\mathbf{A} = \mathbf{H}^\top \mathbf{W} \mathbf{H}$ is introduced, then by definition:

$$(\mathbf{H}^\top \mathbf{W} \mathbf{H})\, \boldsymbol{q} = \mathbf{A}\, \boldsymbol{q} = \mathbf{0}, \quad \forall \boldsymbol{q} \in \mathbb{Q} = \ker(\mathbf{A}) \qquad [3.18]$$

Consequently:

$$(\mathbf{H}^\top \mathbf{W} \mathbf{H})\, (o^{(\mathrm{ML})} + \boldsymbol{q}) = \mathbf{H}^\top \mathbf{W} \widetilde{\boldsymbol{d}}, \quad \forall \boldsymbol{q} \in \mathbb{Q} = \ker(\mathbf{A}) \qquad [3.19]$$

In other words, the kernel $\mathbb{Q}$ contains all the objects whose contribution, after propagation in the detector plane, is zero at the locations of the measured pixels. Since $\mathbf{H}$ is unitary, the subspace $\mathbb{Q}$ is generated by backpropagating the set of extended images that are zero at the measured pixels and have unmeasured pixels with any value. This means that backpropagation of the zero-padded data $\widetilde{\boldsymbol{d}}$ is a maximum likelihood solution (but not necessarily a minimum norm solution) regardless of the values of the unmeasured pixels. Therefore, it is possible to reduce edge artifacts by carefully choosing the values of the unmeasured pixels. Using the knowledge that the target is transparent at a distance z, we show in Figure 3.4(b) the solution in the maximum likelihood sense, with the extended values calculated as $\exp(\imath\, k\, z)$

with $k = 2\pi/\lambda$. Such a reconstruction shows virtually no artifacts. Even if the reconstructions presented in Figures 3.4(a) and 3.4(b) do not have the same visual quality, they are both maximum likelihood solutions (i.e. with $\mathcal{L}(\boldsymbol{o}) \approx \min_{\boldsymbol{o}} \mathcal{L}(\boldsymbol{o})$ for both). We shall see in section 3.7.2 that a well-chosen *regularization* is a better alternative to data extension as this can help to effectively reduce artifacts while ensuring the uniqueness of the solution.

3.5. Phase reconstruction: a nonlinear problem

In most in-line setups, only light intensity is recorded. The direct model is nonlinear and given by [3.4]. Backpropagating the square root of the measured intensity in the object plane gives rise to the well-known twin image problem that can be seen in Figure 3.5(a), where the reconstructed image is superimposed over an out-of-focus version of itself. This is due to the fact that reconstructing the object in this way is tantamount to considering that the unmeasured wavefront phase is zero everywhere. Correctly reconstructing the object requires estimating the wavefront phase in the detector plane and corresponds to a problem that belongs to the phase reconstruction class of problems (*phase retrieval*).

The first numerical method capable of recovering the complex wavefront from intensity measurements was the Gerchberg–Saxton algorithm (Gerchberg and Saxton 1972). This method reconstructs the complex wavefront in the object plane from the measured intensities $\boldsymbol{d}_{\text{img}}$ and $\boldsymbol{d}_{\text{obj}}$ in the image plane and in the object plane, respectively. The Gerchberg–Saxton algorithm consists of propagating the wavefront between each plane while forcing the wavefront modulus to be equal to the square root of the intensity measured in the corresponding plane. The Gerchberg–Saxton algorithm is iterative and, at iteration k, the next iterate is given by

$$\boldsymbol{o}^{(k+1)} = \mathbf{H}^{-1} P_{\mathbb{S}_{\text{img}}}\big(\mathbf{H}\, P_{\mathbb{S}_{\text{obj}}}\big(\boldsymbol{o}^{(k)}\big)\big) \qquad [3.20]$$

or, by:

$$\boldsymbol{o}^{(k+1)} = P_{\mathbb{S}_{\text{obj}}}\big(\mathbf{H}^{-1} P_{\mathbb{S}_{\text{img}}}\big(\mathbf{H}\,\boldsymbol{o}^{(k)}\big)\big) \qquad [3.21]$$

where $P_{\mathbb{S}_{\text{obj}}}$ and $P_{\mathbb{S}_{\text{img}}}$ are the projection operators that impose the constraints in the object and image planes, respectively. These projections can be expressed as follows:

$$P_{\mathbb{S}}(\boldsymbol{x}) = \arg\min_{\boldsymbol{y}\in\mathbb{C}^N} \left(\imath_{\mathbb{S}}(\boldsymbol{y}) + \frac{1}{2}\,\|\boldsymbol{y} - \boldsymbol{x}\|^2 \right) \qquad [3.22]$$

where $\imath_{\mathbb{S}}$ is the characteristic function of the set $\mathbb{S}$ defined by:

$$\imath_{\mathbb{S}}(\boldsymbol{x}) = \begin{cases} 0 & \text{if } \boldsymbol{x} \in \mathbb{S} \\ \infty & \text{otherwise} \end{cases} \qquad [3.23]$$

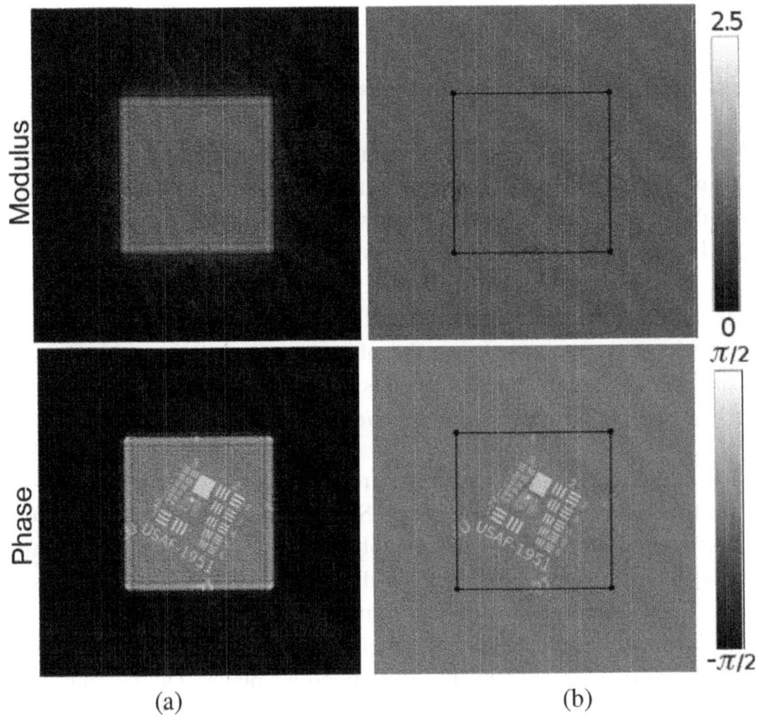

Figure 3.4. *(a) Backpropagation modulus (on top) and phase (bottom) of Figure 3.3(b) padded with zeros to the size of Figure 3.3(a) (SNR reconstruction = 0.42 dB). (b) Backpropagation modulus and phase of Figure 3.3(b) completed with* $\exp(\imath\, k\, z)$ *(SNR reconstruction = 10.30 dB)*

The iterates given by [3.20] and by [3.21] only differ in the order in which the constraints are applied. In near- or far-field regimes, the propagation operator $\mathbf{H}$ is unitary and $\mathbf{H}^{-1} = \mathbf{H}^{\top}$ corresponds to the backpropagation operator. Equation [3.20] shows that the Gerchberg–Saxton algorithm is an instance of a *fixed-point method* for solving the implicit equation $\mathbf{H}\,\boldsymbol{o} = P_{\mathbb{S}_{\mathrm{img}}}\left(\mathbf{H}\,P_{\mathbb{S}_{\mathrm{obj}}}(\boldsymbol{o})\right)$.

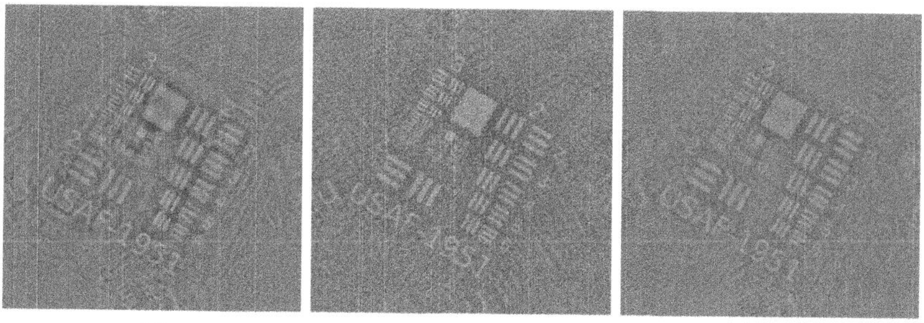

(a) (b) (c)

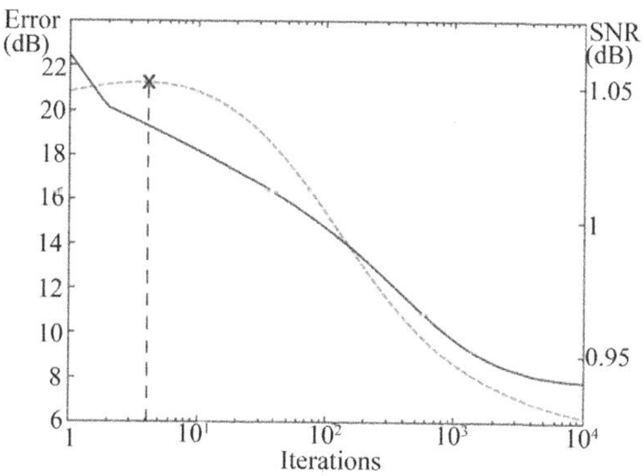

(d)

Figure 3.5. *(a) Backpropagation phase of the square root of the intensity showing the twin image artifact. (b, c) Phases after 10,000 and four iterations (minimum error), respectively. (d) Minimized error by the ER (solid line) and reconstruction SNR algorithm (gray dashed line) according to the number of iterations. The reconstruction SNR is maximal at the fourth iteration (indicated by the cross)*

Considering $\mathbb{S} = \{\boldsymbol{y} \in \mathbb{C}^N : |\boldsymbol{y}|^2 = \boldsymbol{d}\}$, the set of complex amplitudes whose squared modulus is equal to the measured intensities $\boldsymbol{d} \in \mathbb{R}^N$, the projection onto $\mathbb{S}$ is separable according to the pixels and, for the nth pixel, the projection is written as

$$\left[P_{\mathbb{S}}(\boldsymbol{x})\right]_n = \underset{y \in \mathbb{C}: |y|^2 = d_n}{\arg\min} \; \|x_n - y\|^2 = \begin{cases} \frac{x_n}{|x_n|}\sqrt{d_n} & \text{if } |x_n| > 0 \\ \sqrt{d_n} & \text{otherwise} \end{cases} \qquad [3.24]$$

Note that, when $x_n = 0$, the phase of the result of the projection can be arbitrarily chosen (we will assume it to be zero here). We also observe that $\mathbb{S}$ is not a convex set (except if $\boldsymbol{d} = \boldsymbol{0}$). Consequently, the convergence of the Gerchberg–Saxton algorithm to a global optimum can not be ensured (Noll and Rondepierre 2015). This algorithm nevertheless ensures that the squared error defined by

$$E^{(k)} = \left\| o^{(k)} - P_{\mathbb{S}_{\text{obj}}}\left(o^{(k)}\right) \right\|^2 + \left\| \mathbf{H}\, o^{(k)} - P_{\mathbb{S}_{\text{img}}}\left(\mathbf{H}\, o^{(k)}\right) \right\|^2 \qquad [3.25]$$

decreases at each iteration, that is $E^{(k+1)} \leq E^{(k)}$. Hence, the acronym ER (*error reduction*) used for this family of algorithms.

In the simulations presented here, we know that the object is transparent and therefore we can assume that $\boldsymbol{d}_{\text{obj}} = \mathbf{1}$, that is $[\boldsymbol{d}_{\text{obj}}]_n = 1$ $(\forall n)$, without actually doing the measurements. The quadratic error defined by [3.25] as well as the reconstruction SNR are illustrated in Figure 3.5(d). While the error $E^{(k)}$ effectively decreases along with the iterations, the reconstruction error (measured by the SNR) increases after an optimum reached well before convergence (at the fourth iteration in this example). This means that the ER algorithm results in overfitting the measurements (*over-interpretation*): the differences between the ER solution in Figure 3.5(b) and the best iteration in Figure 3.5(c) are essentially fine structures arising from noise. The information introduced by the constraint $\boldsymbol{d}_{\text{obj}} = \mathbf{1}$ is thus insufficient to correctly solve the phase reconstruction problem from noisy data.

3.6. Alternating projection methods

Imposing the value of the intensity in the object plane (for instance, $\boldsymbol{d}_{\text{obj}} = \mathbf{1}$ in the ER method) is equivalent to introducing several priors by means of the projection $P_{\mathbb{S}_{\text{obj}}}$. In the object plane, the set $\mathbb{S}_{\text{obj}}$ and the projection $P_{\mathbb{S}_{\text{obj}}}$ can be redefined according to prior knowledge of the object: phase shift or absorption by the constant object, finite support, etc.. These approaches have given rise to the ER method described above and to the *hybrid input-output* (HIO) algorithm by Fienup (1980, 1982), which both belong to the family of alternating projection algorithms. The introduction of prior knowledge or constraints into alternating projection algorithms can be generalized by *maximum a posteriori* (MAP) methods described in section 3.7.2.

3.6.1. *From alternating projection to criterion minimization*

Gerchberg–Saxton and Fienup algorithms belong to the family of alternating projection methods. The iterations given by [3.21] can be seen as an instance of the *backward-backward* algorithm for solving the following optimization problem (Soulez et al. 2016; Combettes and Pesquet 2011):

$$o^{+} = \underset{o \in \mathbb{C}^N}{\arg\min} \left\{ \imath_{\mathbb{S}_{\text{obj}}}(o) + \inf_{y} \left(\imath_{\mathbb{S}_{\text{img}}}(y) + \tfrac{1}{2} \left\| \mathbf{H}\, o - y \right\|^2 \right) \right\} \qquad [3.26]$$

This formulation brings forward several flaws in the Gerchberg–Saxton and Fienup algorithms:

– the data are introduced via the intensity projection of [3.24], which does not take into account noise statistics and therefore the uneven quality of the measurements;

– prior knowledge is imposed in the form of hard constraints preventing the use of soft constraints such as taking into account an a priori statistic of the object;

– even when all projections are convex (the intensity projection certainly is not), the solution to problem [3.26] is not unique (when the intersection of subspaces is not reduced to a singleton) or may not even exist (when the subspaces are disjoint);

– the objective function of problem [3.26] is not symmetric with respect to the constraints on the object and image domains – consequently, iterating [3.20] instead of [3.21] is tantamount to minimizing a different objective function;

– the *backward-backward* algorithm is known to be not very efficient, compared for example to the Douglas–Rachford algorithm (Soulez et al. 2016), which is also more general (the latter would work with types of functions other than domain indicators).

In order to overcome these limitations, it is necessary to: (i) consider objective functions that correctly take into account noise statistics and (ii) impose additional soft constraints that are more flexible and can help in choosing from all the solutions that are compatible with the measurements (when the intersection of the subspaces is not unique) or choose a good compromise (when the intersection of the subspaces is empty).

3.6.2. *Maximum likelihood approach*

The correct way to take into account the noise statistic is to use the likelihood function $\mathcal{L}(\boldsymbol{o})$ defined in [3.8] instead of the intensity indicator function $\imath_{\mathbb{S}_{\mathrm{img}}}(\mathbf{H}\,\boldsymbol{o})$. Replacing $\imath_{\mathbb{S}_{\mathrm{img}}}(\mathbf{H}\,\boldsymbol{o})$ by $\mathcal{L}(\boldsymbol{o})$ in [3.24] generalizes the notion of projection and introduces the *proximal operator* of the function $\mathcal{L}(\boldsymbol{o})$:

$$\mathrm{prox}_{\mathcal{L}}(\widetilde{\boldsymbol{o}}) \stackrel{\mathrm{def}}{=} \underset{\boldsymbol{o}\in\mathbb{C}^N}{\arg\min}\Big(\mathcal{L}(\boldsymbol{o}) + \tfrac{1}{2}\,\|\boldsymbol{o} - \widetilde{\boldsymbol{o}}\|_2^2\Big) \qquad [3.27]$$

There exist analytical expressions of the proximal operator for Gaussian and Poissonian likelihood functions (Soulez et al. 2016). Equipped with these proximal operators, the error reduction algorithm [3.20] can be rewritten to take into account measurement statistics:

$$\boldsymbol{o}^{(k+1)} = \mathbf{H}^{-1}\ \mathrm{prox}_{\mathcal{L}}\big(\mathbf{H}\,P_{\mathbb{S}_{\mathrm{obj}}}(\boldsymbol{o}^{(k)})\big) \qquad [3.28]$$

Unfortunately, when the functions involved are not characteristic functions, as defined in [3.23], this version of the *backward-backward* algorithm does not converge to the desired solution which is that of the maximum likelihood (Combettes and Pesquet 2011), that is to say the minimum of $\mathcal{L}(o)$ in $o \in \mathbb{S}_{\text{obj}} \subset \mathbb{C}^N$, and which is expressed by:

$$\begin{aligned} o^{(\text{CML})} &= \underset{o \in \mathbb{S}_{\text{obj}}}{\arg\min}\, \mathcal{L}(o) \\ &= \underset{o \in \mathbb{C}^N}{\arg\min} \big\{ \mathcal{L}(o) + \imath_{\mathbb{S}_{\text{obj}}}(o) \big\} \end{aligned} \qquad [3.29]$$

where CML stands for *constrained maximum likelihood.*

There are several algorithms for minimizing the sum of a differentiable function such as $\mathcal{L}(o)$ and a non-differentiable function such as $\imath_{\mathbb{S}_{\text{obj}}}(o)$: the *forward-backward* algorithm or Beck and Teboulle's Fast Iterative Shrinkage-Thresholding Algorithm (FISTA) (Beck and Teboulle 2009) (see Combettes and Pesquet (2011) for more details). When the proximal operators of the two functions of [3.29] have an analytical form, it is also possible to apply the Douglas–Rachford (DR) algorithm (Soulez et al. 2016). ER, FISTA and DR reconstructions are presented in Figure 3.6 alongside the SNR of their reconstruction according to the number of iterations. Under low-noise conditions, the best iterations provided by these algorithms are all similar. Their iterations follow different paths: the best SNR is achieved in 26 iterations for DR, 50 iterations for FISTA and 120 iterations for ER. However, it should be noted that not stopping the iterations may worsen the SNR, which is a clear indication that the minimization of the criterion given in equation [3.29] is not enough to define the *best solution*, which is not satisfactory.

3.7. Improving over the maximum likelihood

In the previous sections, we have seen that taking the measurement statistics into consideration makes it possible to minimize the likelihood penalty $\mathcal{L}(o)$ instead of $\imath_{\mathbb{S}_{\text{img}}}(\mathcal{M}(o))$, that is, instead of strictly imposing that the model $\mathcal{M}(o)$ is equal to the measured data $\boldsymbol{d}$. We will now focus on the *hard* a priori constraints set by the term $\imath_{\mathbb{S}_{\text{obj}}}(o)$ and examine means to impose *soft* constraints instead.

3.7.1. *Penalized maximum likelihood*

The most general way to take into account a priori knowledge about the object o consists of introducing a penalty called the *regularization term*. This term, say $\mathcal{R}(o)$, is added to the likelihood penalty $\mathcal{L}(\boldsymbol{o})$, formally defined by [3.8], to establish an a posteriori objective function $\mathcal{C}(\boldsymbol{o})$ and define the solution of the regularized problem as

$$\boldsymbol{o}^{(\text{rgl})} = \underset{\boldsymbol{o}\in\mathbb{C}^N}{\arg\min}\Big\{\mathcal{C}(\boldsymbol{o}) = \mathcal{L}(\boldsymbol{o}) + \mu\,\mathcal{R}(\boldsymbol{o})\Big\} \qquad [3.30]$$

where $\mu \geq 0$ is a *hyperparameter* that can be used to adjust the trade-off between the constraints brought by the measurements and those of the a priori. The regularization penalty $\mathcal{R}(\boldsymbol{o})$ must be smaller when the object $\boldsymbol{o}$ conforms to the a priori. The introduction of a regularization penalty $\mathcal{R}(\boldsymbol{o})$ can be seen as a generalization of the characteristic function $\imath_{\mathbb{S}_{\text{obj}}}(\boldsymbol{o})$ used in section 3.6 to impose *hard constraints* on the object. This regularization is however more flexible and, as described later, can also be used to apply a wide variety of *soft constraints* such as smoothing, sparsity, etc.

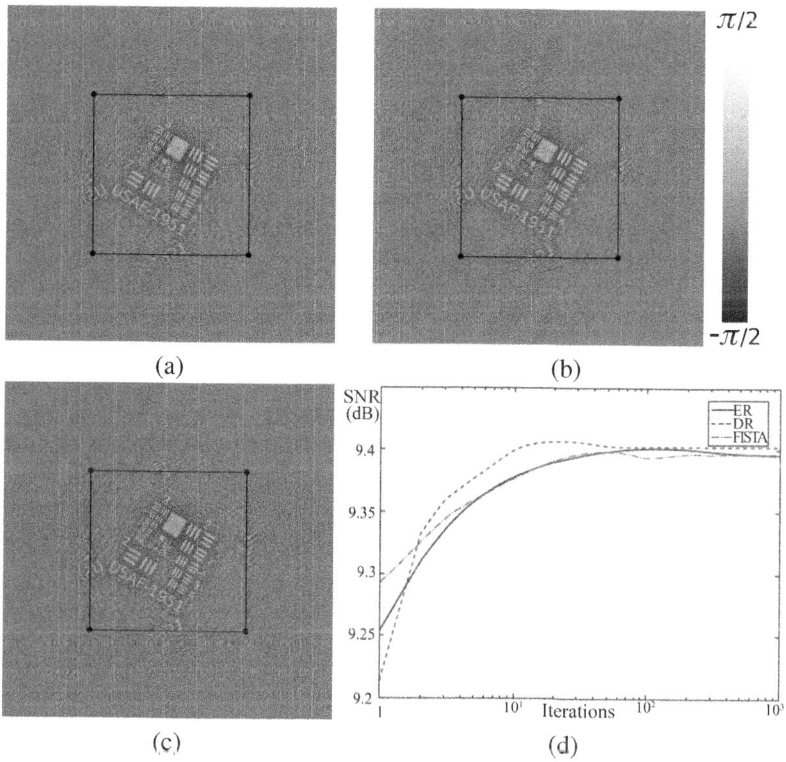

Figure 3.6. *Phases reconstructed with the best SNR achieved by: (a) FISTA, (b) DR, (c) ER. SNR of the reconstructed phases according to the number of iterations by the different methods (d)*

3.7.2. *Bayesian interpretation: maximum a posteriori*

According to Bayes' rule, the a posteriori probability of the object $\boldsymbol{o}$ knowing the data $\boldsymbol{d}$ can be put in the form:

$$\Pr(\boldsymbol{o}\,|\,\boldsymbol{d}) = \frac{\Pr(\boldsymbol{d}\,|\,\boldsymbol{o})\,\Pr(\boldsymbol{o})}{\Pr(\boldsymbol{d})} \qquad [3.31]$$

where $\Pr(\boldsymbol{o})$ is the a priori probability of the object $\boldsymbol{o}$, whereas $\Pr(\boldsymbol{d})$ is known as the *evidence*. Since evidence is positive and does not depend on $\boldsymbol{o}$, the so-called MAP solution, which is the one that maximizes a posteriori the probability, can be expressed as follows:

$$\begin{aligned} \boldsymbol{o}^{(\mathrm{MAP})} &\stackrel{\mathrm{def}}{=} \operatorname*{arg\,max}_{\boldsymbol{o}\in\mathbb{S}_{\mathrm{obj}}} \Pr(\boldsymbol{o}\,|\,\boldsymbol{d}) = \operatorname*{arg\,max}_{\boldsymbol{o}\in\mathbb{S}_{\mathrm{obj}}} \Pr(\boldsymbol{d}\,|\,\boldsymbol{o})\,\Pr(\boldsymbol{o}) \\ &= \operatorname*{arg\,min}_{\boldsymbol{o}\in\mathbb{S}_{\mathrm{obj}}} \{\mathcal{C}_{\mathrm{MAP}}(\boldsymbol{o}) = \mathcal{L}(\boldsymbol{o}) - c_2 \log \Pr(\boldsymbol{o})\} \end{aligned} \qquad [3.32]$$

where, according to [3.8], $c_2 > 0$ and $\Pr(\boldsymbol{d}\,|\,\boldsymbol{o}) \propto \exp\big(-\mathcal{L}(\boldsymbol{o})/c_2\big)$. By comparing equations [3.30] and [3.32], it can be understood that the solution $\boldsymbol{o}^{(\mathrm{rgl})}$ to [3.30] is also the solution $\boldsymbol{o}^{(\mathrm{MAP})}$ if it is assumed that the a priori probability is $\Pr(\boldsymbol{o}) \propto \exp\big(-(\mu/c_2)\,\mathcal{R}(\boldsymbol{o})\big)$. Defining the solution according to [3.30] can thus be seen as a generalization of the MAP solution defined by [3.32].

3.8. Regularization functions and a priori

In this section, we summarize the most relevant regularizations for image reconstruction. Historically, regularization has been introduced to address ill-conditioned inverse problems (Tikhonov 1963). In the context of holographic imaging, introducing an a priori is necessary to deal with degeneration (truncated hologram) but also has a positive effect on the quality of the restored object, as illustrated by the results presented in section 3.10.

3.8.1. *Quadratic regularization*

Regularization was first introduced by Tikhonov (1963) to prevent the amplification of noise in ill-conditioned linear inverse problems. This regularization function is the quadratic penalty:

$$\mathcal{R}_{\ell 2}(\boldsymbol{o}) = \|\mathbf{D}\,\boldsymbol{o}\|_2^2 \qquad [3.33]$$

where $\mathbf{D}$ is a linear operator. By taking $\mathbf{D} = \mathbf{I}$, the identity matrix, priority is given to solutions where all the values of $\boldsymbol{o}$ have the same order of magnitude. By taking $\mathbf{D} \approx \nabla$, a numerical approximation of the spatial gradient operator, smooth solutions are enforced.

Such a quadratic regularization, also called ℓ_2 regularization or *ridge regression*, has the right property to lead to a closed form expression $\boldsymbol{o}^{(\mathrm{rgl})}$ when combined with a linear model and a Gaussian likelihood as defined in [3.10]:

$$\begin{aligned} \boldsymbol{o}^{(\mathrm{rgl})} &= \underset{\boldsymbol{o}\in\mathbb{C}^N}{\arg\min} \left\{ \|\boldsymbol{d} - \mathbf{H}\,\boldsymbol{o}\|_{\mathbf{W}}^2 + \mu\, \|\mathbf{D}\,\boldsymbol{o}\|_2^2 \right\} \\ &= \left(\mathbf{H}^\top \mathbf{W}\,\mathbf{H} + \mu\,\mathbf{D}^\top\mathbf{D}\right)^{-1} \mathbf{H}^\top \mathbf{W}\,\boldsymbol{d} \end{aligned} \qquad [3.34]$$

From a Bayesian point of view (see section 3.7.2), using the quadratic regularization defined in [3.33] amounts to assuming that the object is a realization of a zero-mean Gaussian process and with covariance $\mathrm{Cov}(\boldsymbol{o}) = \left((\mu/c_2)\,\mathbf{D}^\top\mathbf{D}\right)^{-1}$ such that $-c_2 \log \Pr(\boldsymbol{o}) \propto \|\boldsymbol{o}\|_{(\mu\,\mathbf{D}^\top\mathbf{D})}^2$. In this context, by taking $\mathbf{D} \approx \nabla$ we assume a priori that the spatial gradients of the object are i.i.d., Gaussian and centered, or equivalently, that the object has zero mean and that its average power spectral density follows a power law:

$$\langle \widehat{o} \rangle = \mathbf{0} \qquad [3.35]$$

$$\left\langle |\widehat{o}(\boldsymbol{\omega})|^2 \right\rangle \propto \|\boldsymbol{\omega}\|^{-2} \qquad [3.36]$$

where $\langle \ldots \rangle$ denotes the expected value and $\widehat{o}$ the Fourier transform of $\boldsymbol{o}$.

3.8.2. *Edge-preserving smoothing*

Quadratic regularizations are easy in their implementation but yield results that are either too smooth or polluted by bouncing effects around the protruding areas such as edges. To overcome these problems, regularizations known as *edge-preserving* have been proposed (Charbonnier et al. 1997). For example:

$$\mathcal{R}_{\mathrm{EP}}(\boldsymbol{o}) = \sum_{n=1}^{N} \sqrt{\|\mathbf{D}_n\, \boldsymbol{o}\|^2 + \epsilon^2} \qquad [3.37]$$

where $\epsilon > 0$ is a positive threshold and $\mathbf{D}_n$ a linear operator such that $\mathbf{D}_n\,\boldsymbol{o}$ is a numerical approximation (e.g. using finite differences) of the spatial gradients of the object $\boldsymbol{o}$ at the nth pixel along each dimension. This regularization yields smooth solutions while preserving sharp edges at locations where the spatial gradient norm is greater than ϵ.

Endowed with such a regularization, the solution is governed by the values of two hyper-parameters: μ and ϵ. Moreover, this solution does not have any analytical expression whether the direct model is linear or not. Nonetheless, provided that $\epsilon > 0$ and that $\mathcal{L}(\boldsymbol{o})$ is a convex and differentiable function, efficient algorithms exist for finding this solution (see section 3.10.3). At the limit, $\epsilon \to 0^+$, $\mathcal{R}(\boldsymbol{o})$ behaves as the *total variation* (TV) discussed later (see section 3.8.5), which is convex but not differentiable.

3.8.3. *Sparsity*

A way to avoid *overfitting* (measurement overinterpretation) and the resulting noise amplification is to assume that the object of interest can be described by fewer significant variables than the number N of elements of $\boldsymbol{o}$. For instance, it can be assumed that the object $\boldsymbol{o}$ contains only a few non-zero pixels. Since the number of non-zero values in a vector is given by its pseudo-norm ℓ_0, the following regularization function could be chosen:

$$\mathcal{R}_{\ell 0}(\boldsymbol{o}) = \|\boldsymbol{o}\|_0 = \sum_{n}^{N} \begin{cases} 1 & \text{if } o_n \neq 0 \\ 0 & \text{if } o_n = 0 \end{cases} \qquad [3.38]$$

Unfortunately, with such a regularization function, the criterion in [3.30] becomes non-convex and solving the problem is tantamount to minimizing the criterion for all possible configurations (i.e. for all possible subsets of variables set to zero). To get around this combinatorial problem (known as NP-hard), the simplest way is to relax the ℓ_0 norm by replacing it by the nearest convex norm, that is, the ℓ_1 norm. This leads to the following adjustment:

$$\mathcal{R}_{\ell 1}(\boldsymbol{o}) = \|\boldsymbol{o}\|_1 = \sum_{n}^{N} |o_n| \qquad [3.39]$$

When $\boldsymbol{o}$ is real, this regularization, also called LASSO or *basis pursuit*, yields sparse solutions, namely with a limited number of non-zero values. With an example involving a two-parameter object $\boldsymbol{o} = [o_1, o_2]^\top$, Figure 3.7 shows the level curves of the likelihood functions $\mathcal{L}(\boldsymbol{o})$ (in green) and of the regularization $\mathcal{R}(\boldsymbol{o})$ (in red) when the regularization is ℓ_2 (Figure 3.7(a)) or ℓ_1 (Figure 3.7(b)). For these two regularizations, the paths of the solutions to [3.30] defined by varying the hyperparameter μ are plotted as blue dashed curves. With the regularization ℓ_1, the solution path reaches the horizontal axis when μ is large enough, which leads to a sparse solution (here with $o_2 = 0$). On the other hand, the elements o_1 and o_2 of the solutions obtained with the ℓ_2 regularization are always non-zero regardless of the value of μ.

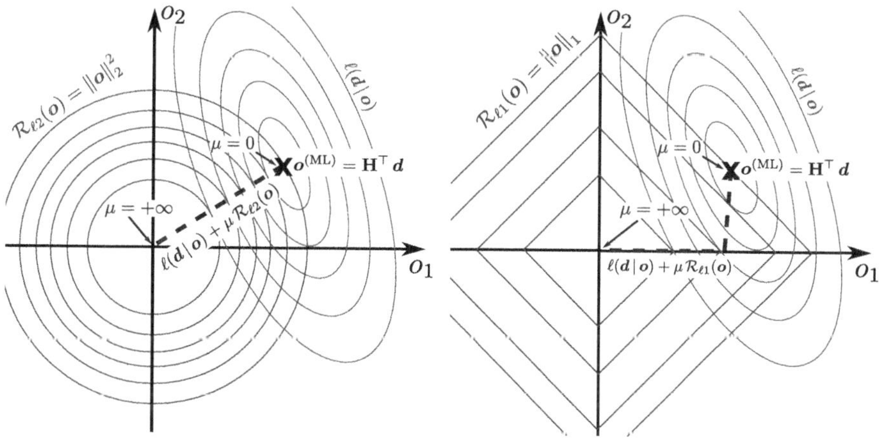

(a) ℓ_2 regularization (quadratic) (b) ℓ_1 regularization

Figure 3.7. *Level curves of likelihood functions $\mathcal{L}(\boldsymbol{o})$ (in green) and of regularization functions $\mathcal{R}(\boldsymbol{o})$ (in red) along the paths followed by the solutions (in blue) to [3.30] by varying the hyperparameter μ for quadratic (a) and ℓ_1 regularization (b). For a color version of this figure, see www.iste.co.uk/fournier/unconventional.zip*

If ℓ_1 regularization is chosen, there is no closed form expression for the solution to [3.30] and nonlinear iterative numerical methods should be used to find the solution. Since the ℓ_1 norm is non-differentiable at 0, so-called *proximal splitting* methods (Combettes and Pesquet 2011) are important methods for finding the solution. Fortunately, the proximal operator of the ℓ_1 norm is extremely easy to calculate (at each pixel n):

$$\begin{aligned}\mathrm{prox}_{\mu \ell_1}(\widetilde{o}_n) &= \underset{o_n \in \mathbb{R}}{\arg\min}\Big(\mu\,|o_n| + \tfrac{1}{2}\,\|o_n - \widetilde{o}_n\|_2^2\Big) \\ &= \mathrm{sign}(\widetilde{o}_n)\,\max\left(|\widetilde{o}_n| - \mu, 0\right)\end{aligned} \qquad [3.40]$$

This operation performs a *soft thresholding* of the values of $\widetilde{\boldsymbol{o}}$.

3.8.4. *Joint parsimony*

When the object has complex values, the absolute value in [3.39] becomes the modulus $|o_n| = \sqrt{\mathrm{Re}(o_n)^2 + \mathrm{Im}(o_n)^2}$ and the proximal operator of the ℓ_1 norm multiplied by μ is then given by:

$$\mathrm{prox}_{\mu\,\ell_1}(\widetilde{o})_n = \begin{cases} \left(1 - \dfrac{\mu}{|\widetilde{o}_n|}\right) \widetilde{o}_n & \text{if } |\widetilde{o}_n| > \mu \\ 0 & \text{otherwise} \end{cases} \qquad [3.41]$$

which is a generalization to complex-valued vectors of the soft thresholding defined by [3.40].

It is clear that the output of the proximal operator in equation [3.41] is zero for a significant number of elements (all pixels n such that $|\widetilde{o}_n| \leq \mu$). This operator therefore has the same property for imposing a certain sparsity of the solution as in the real-valued case. It should be observed that a complex is merely a pair of real numbers; this type of joint sparsity operator can be generalized to any multivalued signal.

Consider a multivariate object $\boldsymbol{o} \in \mathbb{R}^{N \times M}$ such that a multispectral or polarimetric image that has M channels of N pixel each. When such an object is known to be sparse along the spatial dimension but not along the spectral dimension, then a good regularization can be provided by the following *joint sparsity* function (also known as *group sparsity*) (Fornasier and Rauhut 2008):

$$\mathcal{R}_{\mathrm{joint}}(\boldsymbol{o}) = \sum_{n=1}^{N} \sqrt{\sum\nolimits_{m=1}^{M} o_{n,m}^2} \qquad [3.42]$$

The expression of this sparsity regularization function is very similar to the sparsity function for complex-valued images (which can be assimilated to two-channel multi-spectral images) and its proximal operator is therefore very similar:

$$\mathrm{prox}_{\mu\,\mathcal{R}_{\mathrm{joint}}}(\widetilde{o})_{n,m} = \begin{cases} \left(1 - \dfrac{\mu}{\widetilde{\beta}_n}\right) \widetilde{o}_{n,m} & \text{if } \widetilde{\beta}_n > \mu \\ 0 & \text{otherwise} \end{cases} \qquad [3.43]$$

with $\widetilde{\beta}_n = \sqrt{\sum_{m=1}^{M} o_{n,m}^2}$ the Euclidean norm of the vector whose elements are the values of the nth pixel in the M channels under consideration.

3.8.5. *Total variation*

TV (Rudin et al. 1992) is a very popular regularization for image reconstruction. This regularization favors piecewise constant images and is defined by:

$$\mathcal{R}_{\text{TV}}(o) = \sum_{n=1}^{N} \sqrt{\|\mathbf{D}_n\, o\|^2} \qquad [3.44]$$

where $\mathbf{D}_n$ is the linear operator computing the spatial gradient at the nth pixel (as in [3.37]). This regularization function is convex but non-differentiable at zero. Focusing on piecewise constant images is equivalent to considering an image with sparse spatial gradients. TV can then be seen as a joint sparsity regularization applied to spatial gradients. The proximal operator of the TV has however no analytic expression[1]. Many algorithms are based either on the proximal operator of the TV, numerically computed by the Chambolle–Pock algorithm (Chambolle and Pock 2010), or on methods that introduce auxiliary variables such as the *alternating direction method of multipliers* (ADMM) (see section 3.10.2.2) for solving inverse problems regularized by TV.

3.8.6. Plug and play *regularization*

The computation of the proximal operators as defined by [3.27] amounts to solving a *denoising problem*, that is, an inverse problem in which the direct model is the identity. This equivalence has given rise to the notion of *plug and play* (PnP) a priori (Venkatakrishnan et al. 2013; Sun et al. 2019). The key idea of the PnP approach consists of replacing in an iterative algorithm the proximal operator by a state-of-the-art denoising algorithm, such as BM3D (Danielyan et al. 2012), or debuggers based on (deep) learning (Zhang et al. 2021). Nevertheless, these methods do not necessarily have a corresponding regularization function and therefore cannot always be interpreted as the resolution of a well-defined optimization problem.

3.9. Choosing the optimization algorithm for the solution of the inverse problem

In the previous sections, we described the key elements of an *inverse problem* approach for processing holographic data: a likelihood term $\mathcal{L}(o)$ combining a model of the image formation (section 3.2) and noise statistics (section 3.4.2), and a priori

1 Since $\mathbf{D}_n$ is not semi-orthogonal, the proximal operator of [3.43] cannot be extended to the total variation.

knowledge imposed through hard constraints (section 3.5) and regularization functions (section 3.7). To determine the solution to such an inverse problem, a numerical optimization algorithm has to be used to minimize the objective function defined by [3.30].

First of all, the large number of parameters being sought (that is the number N of pixels $\boldsymbol{o}$) prevents the use of algorithms whose memory requirements grow at $\mathcal{O}(N^2)$, such as the *Simplex* method from Nelder and Mead (1965), Newton's method or the Levenberg–Marquardt method (Press et al. 1992). *Limited memory* methods should be used, since their memory requirements are only a few times N. Optimization methods of the latter class of algorithms must be chosen according to the properties of the objective function to be minimized:

– *Convexity*: if the objective function is not convex, then the convergence of iterative methods to a global optimum cannot be ensured and it is necessary to rely on global methods (such as stochastic methods, for instance) whose costs in terms of operations are often prohibitive.

– *Differentiability*: differentiable functions can be minimized with the use of continuous optimization methods such as limited-memory quasi-Newton methods (VMLM, LBFGS, etc.) or nonlinear conjugate gradients. Otherwise, we must resort to primal-dual methods (DR, FISTA or ADMM) involving proximal operators. These methods are often in the first order (not making use of the objective function curvature) and are therefore much less efficient in terms of convergence speed than second-order methods, such as limited-memory quasi-Newton or nonlinear conjugate gradient methods.

– An existing *analytical expression for the proximal operator*: when one of the terms of the objective function is not differentiable and has no known analytical expression for its proximal operator, the solution to this proximal operator must be estimated numerically in an internal loop, at the expense of additional computations.

– *Fast to compute*: in iterative methods each function is evaluated many times. If such evaluations are too costly in computational terms (due to the complexity of the direct model, for instance), stochastic gradient methods can prove helpful depending on the underlying structure of the problem (Tang et al. 2020).

In addition, hard constraints (if any) will also determine the choice of algorithm according to their properties:

– *linear equality constraints* of the form $\mathbf{A}\,\boldsymbol{o} = \boldsymbol{b}$ such as the normalization constraint: $\sum_{n=1}^{N} o_n = 1$;

– *nonlinear equality constraints* such as constraints on the intensity: $|o_n|^2 = 1$, $\forall n$;

– *linear inequality constraints* of the form $\mathbf{A}\,\boldsymbol{o} \geq \boldsymbol{b}$ such that non-negativity constraints: $o_n \geq 0$, $\forall n$ (assuming that $\boldsymbol{o} \in \mathbb{R}^N$);

– *separable constraints* which are performed independently on each element o_n such as support constraints: $o_n = 0, \forall n \notin \mathbb{S}$ where $\mathbb{S}$ refers to the object support.

3.10. Practical examples

In this section, we illustrate the effects of the different regularizations of section 3.8 for the phase reconstruction problem. These examples also cover most of the different strategies available for solving the problem described by [3.30], according to the properties of the objective function (especially if it is differentiable) and constraints. All of these examples involve the same dataset utilized in section 3.5 and simulated for the configuration described in section 3.3. In each experiment, the hyperparameter μ has been set to approximately maximize the reconstruction SNR. It should be noted that in this section, we consider a nonlinear model $\mathcal{M}(\boldsymbol{o}) = |\mathbf{H}\,\boldsymbol{o}|^2$ with Gaussian noise. In other words, the likelihood penalty is given by:

$$\mathcal{L}(\boldsymbol{o}) = \left\| \boldsymbol{d} - |\mathbf{H}\,\boldsymbol{o}|^2 \right\|_{\mathbf{W}}^2 \qquad [3.45]$$

3.10.1. *Unconstrained and differentiable problem*

3.10.1.1. *Quadratic regularization (Tikhonov)*

Knowing a priori that the target is smooth (see Figure 3.3(a)), a quadratic regularization function, as defined in [3.33], is selected with $\mathbf{D} \approx \nabla$ approximating the spatial gradient operator. The objective function is then written as

$$\mathcal{C}_{\ell_2}(\boldsymbol{o}) = \mathcal{L}(\boldsymbol{o}) + \mu\, \|\mathbf{D}\,\boldsymbol{o}\|_2^2 \qquad [3.46]$$

The reconstructed complex image is the minimum of this function. Since $\mathcal{C}_{\ell_2}(\boldsymbol{o})$ is differentiable, the most suitable optimization method is a memory-limited quasi-Newton method such as VMLM or L-BFGS, also known as variable-metric and memory-limited methods (Nocedal and Wright 2006). In short, at each iteration, these methods employ an approximation of the inverse of the Hessian (second derivative) of the objective function to determine a good search direction and then perform a rough minimization along this direction to effectively reduce the objective function. The Hessian approximation is based on the gradient variation of the objective function during the previous M iterations. Therefore, such methods only require computing the objective function and its gradient and have storage requirements of the order of $\mathcal{O}(M\,N)$ instead of $\mathcal{O}(N^2)$ for a Newton-type method. Even with $M \ll N$, say $M = 3$ to 10, memory-limited quasi-Newton methods prove to be very efficient and are well suited for solving large-sized nonlinear optimization problems whose objective function is differentiable. The object reconstructed with $\mu = 1$ after $1,000$ iterations is shown in Figure 3.8(a). Its SNR $= 9.22\,\text{dB}$ is lower than that of the maximum likelihood reconstructions presented in section 3.6.2, indicating that a quadratic regularization is not suitable for the type of object being considered here.

3.10.1.2. *Edge-preserving regularization*

Since the target is composed of areas where the phase is piecewise constant, an edge-preserving regularization as defined in [3.37] should be better suited than quadratic smoothing for this type of object. The solution is then written as

$$\boldsymbol{o}^{(\mathrm{EP})} = \underset{\boldsymbol{o}\in\mathbb{C}^N}{\arg\min}\left\{ \mathcal{C}_{\mathrm{EP}}(\boldsymbol{o}) = \mathcal{L}(\boldsymbol{o}) + \mu \sum_{n=1}^{N} \sqrt{\left\|\mathbf{D}_n\, \boldsymbol{o}\right\|^2 + \epsilon^2} \right\} \qquad [3.47]$$

The objective function $\mathcal{C}_{\mathrm{EP}}(\boldsymbol{o})$ is differentiable and can also be minimized by a variable-metric method such as VMLM. The object reconstructed with $\mu = 10^{-2}$ and $\epsilon = 10^{-3}$ after $1,000$ iterations is shown in Figure 3.8(b). With $\mathrm{SNR}(\boldsymbol{o}^{(\mathrm{EP})}) = 9.94\,\text{dB}$, this reconstruction is much better than with quadratic regularization and the target is reconstructed even far from the boundaries of the detector field of view. However, the estimated modulus is not equal to the unit everywhere as it should be for a transparent object and significant artifacts are visible around the 2-2 group.

3.10.2. *Constrained problems*

3.10.2.1. *Constrained differentiable problems*

A closer look into the reconstruction defects obtained by edge-preserving regularization will allow us to hopefully improve the quality of the result by using additional a priori on the object. The knowledge that the object is transparent cannot be used with an algorithm such as VMLM-B because the hard constraint $|o_n|^2 = 1$, $\forall n$ is nonlinear. We can nevertheless use the a priori knowledge that the object phase is either 0 or 1 radian. Such a bi-level constraint is difficult to implement and would require specific methods such as *graph-cut* algorithms (Boykov et al. 2001). However, this constraint can be relaxed and we can impose only that the phase be between 0 and $\pi/2$, which is equivalent to the separable bound constraints $\mathrm{Re}(o_n) \geq 0$ and $\mathrm{Im}(o_n) \geq 0$, $\forall n$. The solution is then written as

$$\boldsymbol{o}^{(\mathrm{BEP})} = \underset{\boldsymbol{o}\in\mathbb{B}}{\arg\min}\left\{ \mathcal{C}_{\mathrm{BEP}}(\boldsymbol{o}) = \mathcal{L}(\boldsymbol{o}) + \mu \sum_{n=1}^{N} \sqrt{\left\|\mathbf{D}_n\, \boldsymbol{o}\right\|^2 + \epsilon^2} \right\} \qquad [3.48]$$

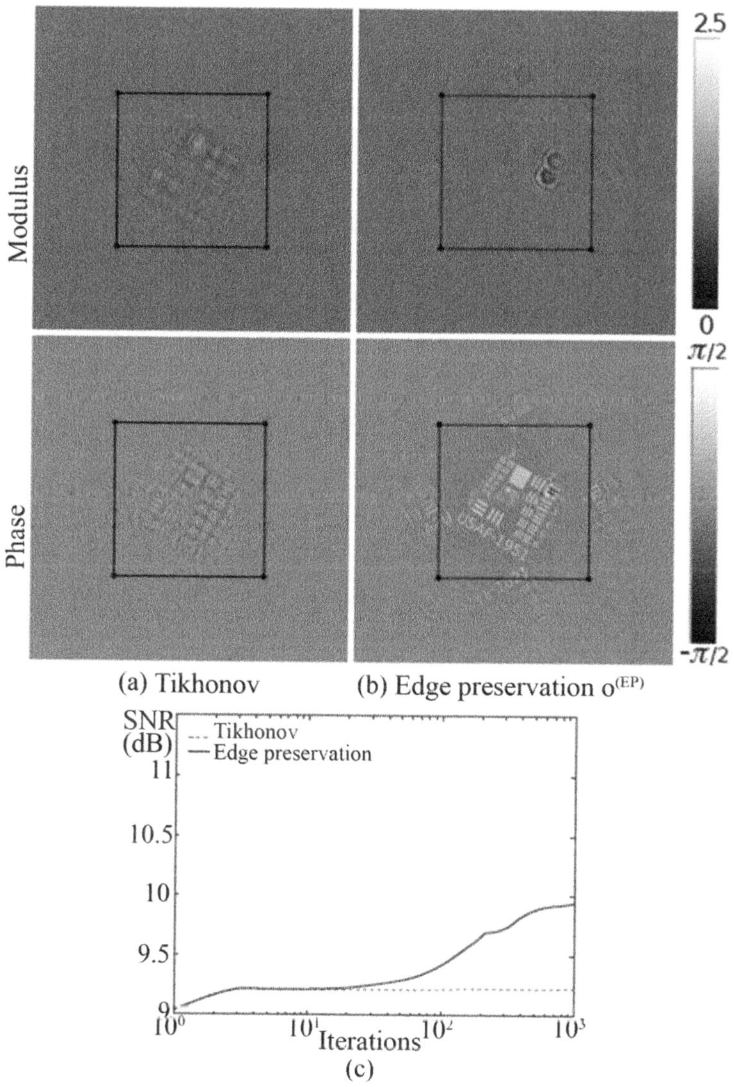

Figure 3.8. *Regularized reconstruction: (a) Tikhonov; (b) edge preservation after 1,000 iterations. (c) Reconstruction SNR according to iterations*

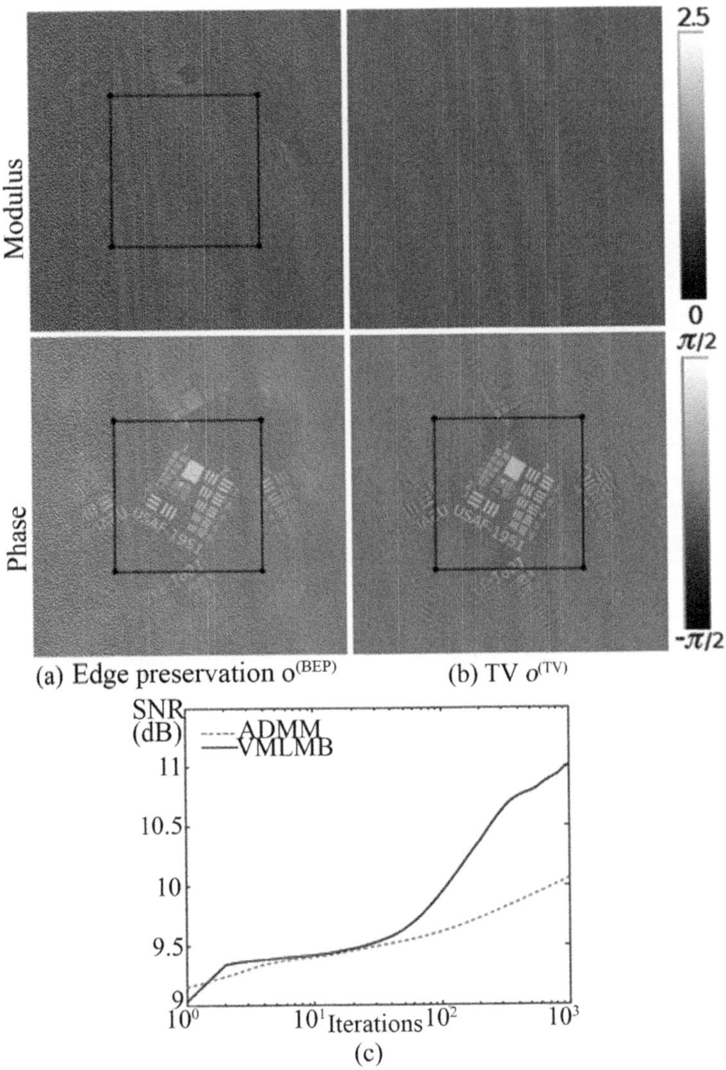

Figure 3.9. *Constrained reconstruction after 1,000 iterations by: (a) VMLM-B for edge-preserving regularization (section 3.10.2) and (b) ADMM for TV regularization (section 3.10.2.2). (c) Reconstruction SNR according to iterations*

with $\mathbb{B} = \{o \in \mathbb{C}^N : \mathrm{Re}(o_n) \geq 0, \mathrm{Im}(o_n) \geq 0 =, \forall n\}$ the subset of $\mathbb{C}^N$ whose elements have complex pixels with positive real and imaginary parts (and thus $0 \leq \arg(o_n) \leq \frac{\pi}{2}, \forall n$). To solve the above problem, we use VMLM-B, a variant of the VMLM algorithm that can take separable bound constraints into account (Thiébaut 2002). With $\mathrm{SNR}(\boldsymbol{o}^{(\mathrm{BEP})}) = 11.01$ dB after $1,000$ iterations, the reconstructed object reaches a better reconstruction quality as can be seen from Figure 3.9(a).

3.10.2.2. *Non-differentiable problems*

The TV described in section 3.8.5 seems the most appropriate regularization to apply the constraint according to which the object under consideration is piecewise constant. As it is also known that the object is transparent, we have combined TV with the hard constraint that the modulus of the complex object must be equal to one everywhere and considered the following problem:

$$\boldsymbol{o}^{(\mathrm{TV})} = \underset{\boldsymbol{o} \in \mathbb{C}^N}{\arg\min} \Big\{ \mathcal{C}_{\mathrm{TV}}(\boldsymbol{o}) = \mathcal{L}(\boldsymbol{o}) + \mu \, \mathcal{R}_{\mathrm{TV}}(\boldsymbol{o}) + \imath_{\mathbb{M}}(\boldsymbol{o}) \Big\} \qquad [3.49]$$

where $\mathbb{M} = \{\boldsymbol{o} \in \mathbb{C}^N : |o_n| = 1, \forall n\}$ is the set of complexes of unit modulus. Given that the function $\mathcal{R}_{\mathrm{TV}}$ is not differentiable and that $\imath_{\mathbb{M}}$ is not continuous, the objective function $\mathcal{C}_{\mathrm{TV}}(\boldsymbol{o})$ cannot be minimized by a variable metric method. A primal-dual scheme that can be implemented through the ADMM method (Boyd et al. 2010) is very well adapted for such a problem where the objective function is the sum of non-differentiable functions, which have analytically computable proximal operators. The object $\boldsymbol{o}^{(\mathrm{TV})}$ reconstructed with $\mu = 0.01$ and after $1,000$ ADMM iterations is displayed in Figure 3.9(b).

3.11. References

Beck, A. and Teboulle, M. (2009). A fast iterative shrinkage-thresholding algorithm for linear inverse problems. *SIAM Journal on Imaging Sciences*, 2(1), 183–202.

Boyd, S., Parikh, N., Chu, E., Peleato, B., Eckstein, J. (2010). Distributed optimization and statistical learning via the alternating direction method of multipliers. *Foundations and Trends in Machine Learning*, 3, 1 122.

Boykov, Y., Veksler, O., Zabih, R. (2001). Fast approximate energy minimization via graph cuts. *IEEE Transactions on Pattern Analysis and Machine Intelligence*, 23(11), 1222–1239.

Chambolle, A. and Pock, T. (2010). A first-order primal-dual algorithm for convex problems with applications to imaging. *Journal of Mathematical Imaging and Vision*, 40(1), 120–145.

Charbonnier, P., Blanc-Féraud, L., Aubert, G., Barlaud, M. (1997). Deterministic edge-preserving regularization in computed imaging. *IEEE Transactions on Image Processing*, 6(2), 298–311.

Combettes, P.L. and Pesquet, J.-C. (2011). Proximal splitting methods in signal processing. In *Fixed-Point Algorithms for Inverse Problems in Science and Engineering*, Bauschke, H.H., Burachik, R.S., Combettes, P.L., Elser, V., Luke, D.R., Wolkowicz, H. (eds). Springer, Berlin.

Danielyan, A., Katkovnik, V., Egiazarian, K. (2012). BM3D frames and variational image deblurring. *IEEE Transactions on Image Processing*, 21(4), 1715–1728.

Fienup, J.R. (1980). Iterative method applied to image reconstruction and to computer-generated holograms. *Optical Engineering*, 19(3), 193297–193297.

Fienup, J.R. (1982). Phase retrieval algorithms: A comparison. *Applied Optics*, 21(15), 2758–2769.

Fornasier, M. and Rauhut, H. (2008). Recovery algorithms for vector-valued data with joint sparsity constraints. *SIAM Journal on Numerical Analysis*, 46(2), 577–613.

Gerchberg, R.W. and Saxton, W.O. (1972). A practical algorithm for the determination of phase from image and diffraction plane pictures. *Optik*, 35, 237.

Hestenes, M.R. and Stiefel, E. (1952). Methods of conjugate gradients for solving linear systems. *Journal of Research of the National Bureau of Standards*, 49(6), 409–436.

Liu, D.C. and Nocedal, J. (1989). On the limited memory BFGS method for large scale optimization. *Mathematical Programming*, 45(1–3), 503–528.

Matsushima, K. and Shimobaba, T. (2009). Band-limited angular spectrum method for numerical simulation of free-space propagation in far and near fields. *Optics Express*, 17(22), 19662–19673.

Nelder, J. and Mead, R. (1965). A simplex method for function minimization. *Comp. J.*, 7, 308–313.

Nocedal, J. and Wright, S.J. (2006). *Numerical Optimization*. Springer, Berlin.

Noll, D. and Rondepierre, A. (2016). On local convergence of the method of alternating projections. *Foundations of Computational Mathematics*, 16, 425–455.

Press, W.H., Teukolsky, S.A., Vetterling, W.T., Flannery, B.P. (1992). *Numerical Recipes in C*. Cambridge University Press, Cambridge.

Rudin, L.I., Osher, S., Fatemi, E. (1992). Nonlinear total variation based noise removal algorithms. *Physica D: Nonlinear Phenomena*, 60(1–4), 259–268.

Soubies, E., Soulez, F., McCann, M.T., Pham, T., Donati, L., Debarre, T., Sage, D., Unser, M. (2019). Pocket guide to solve inverse problems with GlobalBioIm. *Inverse Problems*, 35(10), 1–20.

Soulez, F. (n.d.). COMCI [Online]. Available at: https://github.com/FerreolS/COMCI.

Soulez, F. (1951). USAF 1951 [Online]. Available at: https://figshare.com/articles/figure/USAF_1951/7998134/1.

Soulez, F. (2021). Gauging diffraction patterns: Field of view and bandwidth estimation in lensless holography. *Applied Optics*, 60(10), B38.

Soulez, F., Thiébaut, É., Schutz, A., Ferrari, A., Courbin, F., Unser, M. (2016). Proximity operators for phase retrieval. *Applied Optics*, 55(26), 7412.

Sun, Y., Wohlberg, B., Kamilov, U.S. (2019). An online plug-and-play algorithm for regularized image reconstruction. *IEEE Transactions on Computational Imaging*, 5(3), 395–408.

Tang, J., Egiazarian, K., Golbabaee, M., Davies, M. (2020). The practicality of stochastic optimization in imaging inverse problems. *IEEE Transactions on Computational Imaging*, 6, 1471–1485.

Thiébaut, E. (2002). Optimization issues in blind deconvolution algorithms. *Proceedings of the International Society for Optics and Photonics: Astronomical Data Analysis II*, 4847, 174–183.

Tikhonov, A.N. (1963). On the solution of ill-posed problems and the method of regularization. *Proceedings of the International Symposium on Figure and Dynamics of the Earth, Moon, and Planets*, Prague.

Trouvé, P., Champagnat, F., Le Besnerais, G., Idier, J. (2014). Theoretical performance model for single image depth from defocus. *JOSA A*, 31, 12.

Venkatakrishnan, S.V., Bouman, C.A., Wohlberg, B. (2013). Plug-and-play priors for model based reconstruction. *Proceedings of the 2013 IEEE Global Conference on Signal and Information Processing*, Austin, Texas, 945–948.

Winick, K.A. (1986). Cramer-Rao lower bounds on the performance of charge-coupled-device optical position estimators. *Journal of the Optical Society of America A*, 3, 1809–1815.

Zhang, K., Li, Y., Zuo, W., Zhang, L., Van Gool, L., Timofte, R. (2021). Plug-and-play image restoration with deep denoiser prior. *IEEE Transactions on Pattern Analysis and Machine Intelligence*, 1–11.

4

In-line Digital Holographic Microscopy Sample Reconstruction

Fabien MOMEY[1], Thomas OLIVIER[2] and Corinne FOURNIER[3]

[1] *Laboratoire Hubert Curien, CNRS, IOGS, IUT de Saint-Étienne, Université Jean Monnet, Saint-Étienne, France*

[2] *Laboratoire Hubert Curien, CNRS, IOGS, Faculté des sciences et techniques, Université Jean Monnet, Saint-Étienne, France*

[3] *Laboratoire Hubert Curien, CNRS, IOGS, Télécom Saint-Étienne, Université Jean Monnet, Saint-Étienne, France*

4.1. Introduction

In this chapter, following some historical and contextual explanations on optical microscopy and digital holography for biomedical purposes (section 4.2), we present (section 4.3) several experimental setups for in-line holographic microscopy, and in particular the specificities and constraints of these setups with or without a lens. We then address the issues underlying the reconstruction, which is an indispensable step in digital holography. We present the main state-of-the-art approaches for digitally reconstructing holographic objects and illustrate them on an experimental example.

For a color version of all the figures in this chapter, see www.iste.co.uk/fournier/unconventional.zip.

Unconventional Optical Imaging for Biology,

Within this context, a model of the objects for defining the physical quantities to be reconstructed is first exposed, followed by a model of the physical phenomenon of hologram image formation (section 4.4.2). Once these models are defined, digital reconstructions based on "alternating projections" and "inverse problems" (IPs) are presented (section 4.4.3.2). We then illustrate the contributions of the IP methodology in the context of the implementation of a digital super-resolution technique (section 4.5). Finally, we conclude by describing more advanced perspectives, made possible by the IP approach-based reconstruction and applicable in holographic microscopy: self-calibration, 3D tomography capabilities (section 4.6).

4.2. From classical microscopy to digital holography in the biomedical field

With the pioneering studies of Hooke et al. (1665), then those of Antoni van Leeuwenhoek on optical microscopy in the 17th century, discoveries in biology were immediately of capital importance. Robert Hooke was the first to observe and describe the organization of living organisms at the microscopic level and introduced the term "cells". For his part, Antoni van Leeuwenhoek observed micro-organisms (bacteria, protozoa, spermatozoa, etc.), which contributed to disrupting the vision of diseases and reproduction and called into question the concept of *spontaneous generation* that was the dominant theory at the time. Thereafter, the microscope has gradually become an essential working tool for biologists and physicians and led to numerous discoveries, including organisms responsible for infectious diseases, but also the description of cell development, for example. However, although the qualities of the components and the optical system improve with time, the samples are mostly very transparent, which makes the observation difficult due to lack of contrast. This problem was first solved by achieving sample staining or labeling. Nowadays, there is a wide variety of stains. Some make it possible, by chemical affinity, to stain particular structures such as cell nuclei or membranes. Others allow objects with similar properties to be differentiated (such as Gram staining, for instance), others use antibodies to bind to proteins of interest (immunolabeling). In any case, for staining to be effective in making structures of a few micrometers or less partially opaque, the concentration of dye must be so high that it is necessary to *fix*, in other words, to dehydrate and kill the living organisms before analysis.

In this context, the invention of the *phase-contrast microscope* in the 1940s by Zernike (1942) made it possible to observe transparent microscopic objects, which would greatly simplify the observation of biological samples in vivo. This discovery earned him the Nobel Prize in 1953. In phase-contrast microscopy, the contrast is obtained by an interference phenomenon between the background light and the light diffracted by the sample. Therefore, the variations of luminosity in the image are not simply generated by variations of absorption in the sample but by the variations in phase of the wave that passed through. In the introduction to his 1942 paper, Zernike (1942) explains where this idea came from: "Every microscopist knows that transparent objects show light or dark contours under the microscope in different ways varying with change of focus and depending on the kind of illumination used".

This quote reminds us that we have long known that contrast can be generated with transparent objects, through adjustments by means of slightly defocusing, as well as by manipulating the illumination. Very shortly afterwards, Dennis Gabor (also awarded a Nobel Prize in 1971) went even further: with the invention of *holography*, he showed that it was possible to record these light distributions and then restore a sample image from the defocused recording. However, the result was not a traditional intensity image of the sample since the complete information of the wave that traveled through was preserved in the recording, giving the impression that it is being looked at directly, particularly with its three-dimensional aspect.

With the numerical computing capabilities available today, these ideas have been recovered to retrieve as much information as possible on a microscopic object of interest from a hologram and digital reconstructions, based on the use of physical models of light propagation. This is the main subject of *digital holography*, and particularly of the configuration known as "Gabor's" or "in-line" setup which is the focus of this chapter. This setup has several advantages, among which is its simplicity, but it does not allow the complex amplitude of the wave perturbed by the sample to be directly measured. This information will be reconstructed by digital means. Under these conditions, this method is one of the *quantitative phase microscopy* methods (Popescu 2011) that makes it possible to find the phase-shift, or the very fine variations of phase-shift induced by a transparent, unlabeled and thus potentially living biological sample. As a result, many applications are possible in biology. For example, some biological models consider this phase-shift information a reflection of the sample dry mass (Aknoun et al. 2015). On the other hand, the resolution in terms of phase-shift and thus optical path (refractive index multiplied by the thickness of the object of interest) can reach a few nanometers, which is not the case for the lateral resolution, limited to a few hundred nanometers (optical microscopy diffraction limit). It is important to properly understand that this resolution on the optical path does not correspond to an axial geometric resolution. As a matter of fact, a change in the optical path can originate from a change in the refractive index, a change in thickness, or both (Popescu 2011). Finally, in the in-line setup, with or without lens, the object of interest is defocused and the reconstruction process will result, by enforcing a priori on the object, in refocusing the object image. Therefore, this type of method, without being a real 3D imaging method, enables an extended depth of field making it possible, for example, for three-dimensional tracking of micrometric objects of interest (Garcia-Sucerquia et al. 2006).

4.3. In-line holographic microscopy setups

4.3.1. *Imaging setup, with or without lens*

Contrary to other digital holography methods, the in-line setup does not require a reference beam (as in off-axis holography), which can lead to building very stable systems, easily adaptable on existing microscopes, but also compact systems, either low cost or adapted to extreme conditions. The in-line or "Gabor's" setup must however satisfy two experimental conditions:

– The sample illumination must be *temporally and spatially coherent* so that the light distribution includes intensity variations that are sufficiently specific to the sample absorption and refraction characteristics. This will be developed in the next section but, as a first approach, we should remember that a monochromatic illumination issuing from a point source has to be used (located at a finite or infinite distance).

– The hologram, that is, the image recorded on the sensor, must correspond to the light intensity distribution diffracted by the sample over a given distance. The hologram thus corresponds to a propagated projection of the object of interest.

Figure 4.1 shows three possible optical in-line holographic microscopy setups. The simplest setup (Figure 4.1(a)) is the one which simply contains a sample illuminated by a point source located at a distance z_s from the sample and a sensor, itself distant from z of the sample. This value z will be referred to as the *defocus* term hereafter because it appears in all setups. This defocus will have to be considered, or rather estimated for the reconstruction of a focused sample projection. As can be seen in the figure, the illumination by a point source creates a homothetic magnification effect of ratio $(z_s + z)/z_s$ between the sample and the sensor, which will have to be taken into account. Most often, for the observation of microscopic objects, the distance z will have to remain small compared to the distance z_S, resulting in a magnification close to 1. Otherwise, we must remain cautious because we are not dealing with a homogeneous magnification on the whole sensor, but with distortion whose tendency will be to deform the holograms. On the other hand, if it is significant, this homothetic effect can be inconvenient, especially when the samples occupy very different axial positions because the magnification depends on the defocus. If this homothetic effect becomes inconvenient or if the source cannot be placed far enough, a collimated illumination will have to be set up with an adapted optic, which is equivalent to making z_s tend toward infinity and the magnification to 1.

The lensless setup can sometimes lack flexibility. Without significant magnification, the pixel size in the reconstructed image will be constrained by the physical size of the sensor pixels. On the other hand, the smallest structures in the sample will form rapidly diverging diffraction patterns, forcing the sample to be placed very close to the sensor, which can become technically challenging. It then proves advantageous to use an objective (microscope objective or not) that allows for significant magnification. Figure 4.1(b) shows this setup. It should then be ensured that the plane conjugated with the sensor is defocused with respect to the object. We will then consider the device equivalent to a lensless device with a virtual sensor whose pixel size is smaller (real pixel size divided by the setup magnification). This last configuration has the advantage of being similar to classical optical microscopy setups, with a simple defocus and coherent illumination. The image in focus is possible, which enables complementary imaging modalities. On the other hand, the introduction of an objective adds slightly more complexity to the setup and requires the use of good quality optics, whose characteristics will have to be adapted to the chosen application (magnification, numerical aperture, quality of aberration correction, etc.). Finally, in digital holography, coherent imaging must be used, which is not the case in traditional microscopy. This raises a number of issues. In particular, the management of stray light becomes problematic and generates speckle noise (Goodman 1996; Bianco et al. 2018) and illumination inhomogeneities. These effects then originate from multiple interference and diffraction patterns from dust on the optics upstream and downstream of the sample or directly from diffraction by out-of-field objects.

The last setup shown in Figure 4.1(c) introduces a second lens, called the *tube lens*. This setup is very common in good quality scientific microscopes. It is used to work with infinity-compensated microscope objectives, that is to say objectives optimized and compensated for aberrations, so that their object plane is located in their object focal plane while the image is located at infinity. Under these conditions, the tube lens reforms this image in its image focal plane. The magnification of the whole setup is then simply equal to the ratio between the tube lens focal length and the objective focal length. This setup has the advantage of being able to change the distance between the two lenses without changing the magnification and to place beam splitters, filters or any other element with parallel faces where the image beam is collimated, that is, without modifying the conjugation of the imaging setup. Finally, in the configuration shown in Figure 4.1(c), the objective image focal plane coincides with the object focal plane of the tube lens, which is a system known as "telecentric", that is, an afocal system. This setup has several advantages. For example, the magnification of such a system does not depend on the sensor position or the object defocus and remains equal to the ratio between the focal lengths of the two elements. In in-line holography, if care has been taken to position a collimated beam at the system input, it will remain collimated at the system output. Although this setup is not always essential, it is the closest to the approximations usually made in reconstructions (plane wave illumination), which can be important in the most demanding quantitative phase microscopy applications (Doblas et al. 2014).

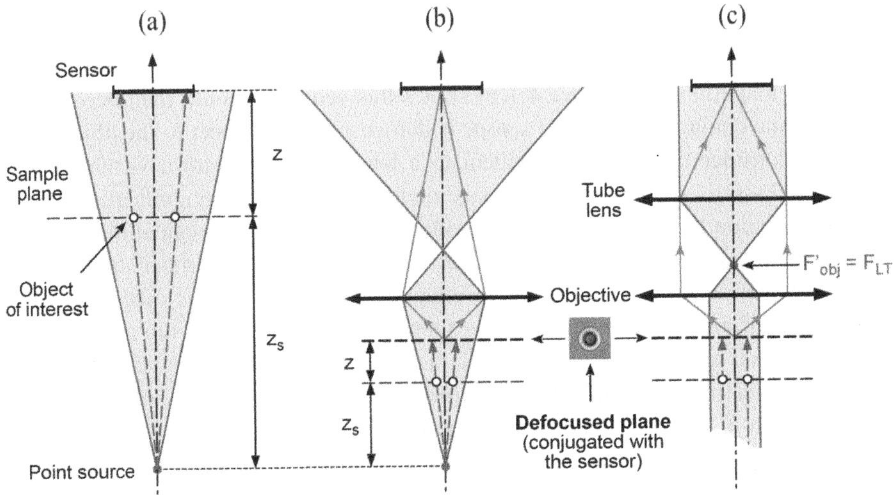

Figure 4.1. *Typical examples of in-line optical microscopy setups*

COMMENTS ON FIGURE 4.1.– *(a) Lensless setup with illumination from a finite distance point source. (b) The addition of an objective lens performs magnification between a plane distant from the sample and the sensor plane. (c) The addition of a tube lens and an infinity-compensated objective in a telecentric system and a collimated illumination (point source at infinity). The red beams represent the illumination path, while the gray arrowed rays formalize the conjugation between the defocused plane and the sensor. F'_{obj}: objective image focus; F_{LT}: tube lens object focus.*

4.3.2. *Coherence and illumination setup*

For the sample illumination, the use of temporally and spatially coherent light is a necessary condition for digital holography. Without going into the details of the physical origin of this phenomenon, we recall that coherence designates the ability of two waves to interfere with one another. In this case, the superposition of two coherent waves is obtained by calculating the intensity of the sum of their complex amplitudes, while the superposition of two incoherent waves will be the sum of their intensities.

Temporal coherence refers to the coherence of two waves in time, that is, the synchronization of their respective phases. This synchronization can be expressed in space by the coherence length, itself related to the spectral width of the source by the relation $\ell_c = \lambda_0^2/\Delta\lambda$, where ℓ_c represents the coherence length, $\Delta\lambda$ is the source spectral width in wavelength and λ_0 is the spectrum central wavelength. The coherence length then represents the maximum optical path difference between two light rays in order for them to interfere significantly. Therefore, with a spectral width of about 20 nm, two rays issuing from an LED at 500 nm will not be able to interfere if their paths differ by more than 12.5 μm. This is a real problem in two-beam digital holography setups because it is necessary to balance and stabilize the optical paths very precisely. On the other hand, in the in-line setup, the interference to be considered occurs between the incident wave, which is the *reference wave* (see Chapter 2) and the wave that was diffracted by the object of interest (*object wave*). Nonetheless, this is not necessarily problematic for microscopic objects with low phase shift. As such, the use of partially temporally coherent sources is possible in this type of setup. The light distributions obtained on the hologram are then the incoherent sum (sum of the intensities) of the various intensities obtained for all the wavelengths in the source spectrum, which creates blurring in the holograms. By adding a bandpass filter with a width less than approximately 10 nm, this spectral coherence can be improved, but at the expense of power losses. According to the reconstruction techniques used, the model can also be corrected to take this spectral blurring into account (Vandewiele et al. 2017), which can add a significant amount of computation time during reconstructions.

Concerning spatial coherence, we should work with a source originating from a reduced spatial extent (point source). Otherwise, two points coming from two spatially incoherent sources will produce the sum of the intensities of two shifted holograms, also causing blurring in the holograms. As mentioned in the introductory section with Zernike's quote, microscopists have long known that changes in illumination and defocus result in highly variable distributions of brightness and contrast within biological samples. Nevertheless, non-experts will find it more difficult to understand what is being referred to. Figure 4.2(b) represents the images of a simple object (here, a silica bead with a diameter of about 1 μm) seen through a conventional laboratory microscope for two defocus conditions (in focus and slightly out-of-focus) and for two illumination settings (coherent and incoherent), achieved here in Köhler illumination with white light[1]. It can be clearly seen that by illuminating with an extended source (spatially incoherent), very strong blurring takes place, to such extent that the visualized object becomes barely visible when defocused. This study with very incoherent light is sought-after in classical microscopy because it makes it possible

1 We will not review this illumination setup, highly conventional in optical microscopy.

to avoid the noise that could originate from diffracting objects located outside the depth of field and thus ensure a very uniform background. This system also makes it possible to eliminate luminosity variations due to interferences and diffraction to solely concentrate on the variations in absorption and color in the samples. However, the use of fairly coherent illumination is sometimes sought for precisely enhancing and adding contrast to transparent objects.

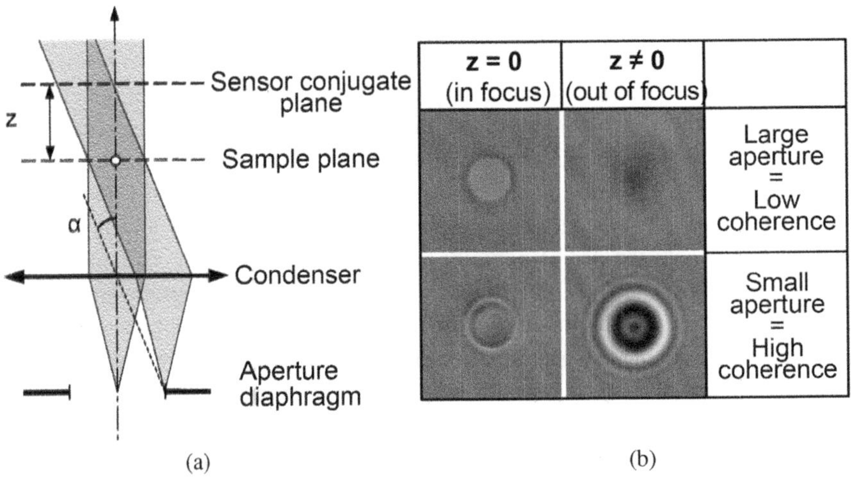

Figure 4.2. *Illumination set up and effect of spatial coherence on holograms. (a) Conventional "Köhler"-type microscopy illumination setup. (b) Effect of illumination beam coherence on focused or defocused images*

On the other hand, in holography, good spatial coherence is essential. As can be seen in Figure 4.2(a), this spatial coherence can be obtained by reducing the illumination aperture, which amounts to working with a smaller point source. In the plane conjugated with the sensor (hologram plane), the origin of the blurring due to partial coherence can be seen because the holograms obtained under various angles of illumination are shifted and are added together in an incoherent way. In the presence of partially coherent light, this blurring can be taken into account by assuming that the partially blurred hologram is a convolution by a disk of radius equal to the tangent of the maximum angle of illumination α by the extended source, multiplied by defocus z. It should be noted that this is an approximation in the case where the coherence is good enough and the maximum illumination angle is not too large. Otherwise, strictly speaking, it would be necessary to consider the projection effect of the holograms on the sensor plane when they are formed by an illumination under too significant an angle.

To conclude, setting up the illumination is an important step in holographic microscopy (as it is in conventional microscopy), especially concerning the introduction of a sufficiently temporally and spatially coherent illumination. This type of microscopy requires good coherence but, depending on the systems, the constraints are not always the same. Despite the fact that partial coherence can be used in an in-line setup, it requires conditioning the initial incoherent source to extract only a coherent part of it, which can significantly reduce the available power. Conversely, the use of laser sources produces very good spatial and temporal coherence while maintaining high illumination power, but this type of source is not always easy to use in imaging because of its tendency to generate significant speckle noise and illumination inhomogeneities which, in addition, can be temporally unstable. Finding a tradeoff adapted to the various constraints is then necessary, depending on the type of sample under study, the chosen configuration (with or without lens), the stability of the setup, the desired acquisition speed, but also the capacity of the numerical reconstructions to take noise or experimental constraints into account in order to limit their influence.

4.4. Typical IP methodology for in-line hologram reconstruction

In this section, we propose, through an experimental example, to apply an IP methodology to the reconstruction of in-line holograms using the approaches and tools presented in Chapter 3 (see section 3.9), and whose key steps are summarized in Figure 4.3.

After recalling the principle behind the usual reconstruction methods and pointing out their drawbacks, we will rely on an IP approach to develop a relevant reconstruction algorithm. It will take into account the specificities of the holographic measurements to be processed, while adapting the desired solution to the characteristics of the observed objects known a priori.

4.4.1. *Test case: in-line holograms of micrometric transparent objects*

Figure 4.4(a) shows a recording of in-line holograms of polystyrene beads placed on a microscope slide, acquired through an experimental setup with the configuration of Figure 4.1(c) presented in section 4.3.1. The diffraction pattern of each bead can be observed. The experimental parameters of interest are summarized in Table 4.1. The characteristics of the objects (size, refractive index) have been selected for mimicking microbiological samples, such as bacteria.

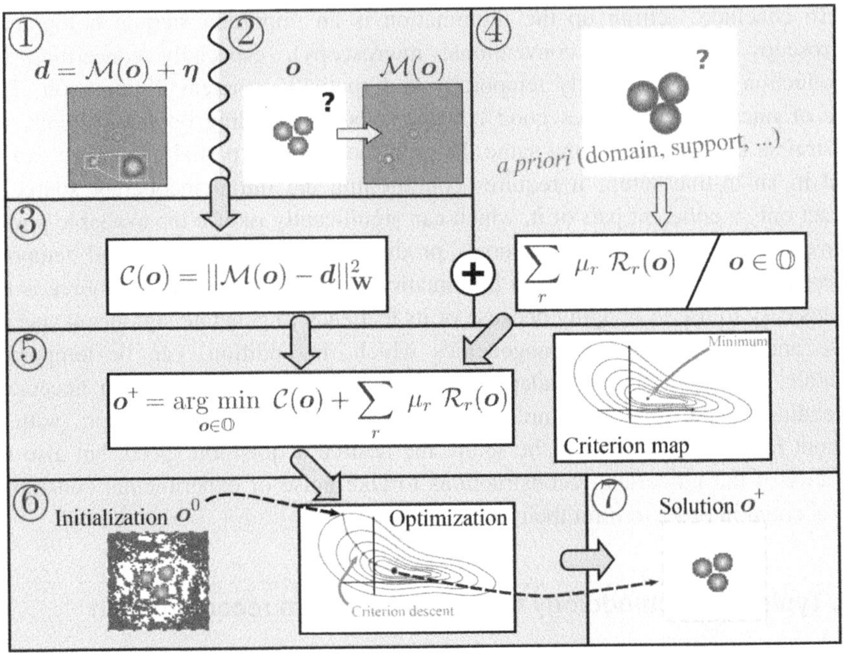

Figure 4.3. *Summary of the inverse problem methodology*

COMMENTS ON FIGURE 4.3.–

① *Expression of the* direct problem*: data formation physical model + noise model. Example: transmittance plane diffraction and propagation of the resulting wave + stationary and independent Gaussian noise.*

② *Development of a numerical* model *for image formation, that is a simulation model for the direct problem* $\mathcal{M}(\mathbf{o})$*. Example: object transmittance discrete convolution* $\underline{o}$ *by a Fresnel or Rayleigh–Sommerfeld propagation kernel* $\boldsymbol{h_z}$*, then computation of the squared modulus* $|\cdot|^2$.

③ *Construction of a data-fidelity criterion* $\mathcal{C}(\mathbf{o})$*. Example: weighted least squares with a matrix* $\mathbf{W}$ *= Gaussian log-likelihood.*

④ *Search for the relevant a priori and representation into appropriate* constraints ($\mathbf{o} \in \mathbb{K}$) and regularizations ($\sum_r \mu_r \mathcal{R}_r(\mathbf{o})$). *Example: positivity constraint +* l_1 *regularization (sparsity) + edge preservation.*

⑤ *Definition of the* IP*: "Find the optimal solution* $\mathbf{o}^+$ *that minimizes the global criterion".*

⑥ *Choice of an* optimization *strategy adapted for solving the IP (*minimize the criterion*). Example: Proximal algorithm (e.g. (F)ISTA) or quasi-Newton algorithm (e.g. VMLM-B).*

⑦ *Algorithm execution (often iterative) and estimation of the* optimal solution $\boldsymbol{o}^+$ *(in the sense of this criterion). Example: the hypothesis of a convex criterion is made (verified hypothesis if the criterion is adapted) making it possible to use optimization methods based on the descent of the criterion along directions computed according to its gradient. For a non-convex criterion, the solution will depend on the starting point (local minimum).*

The observation of the hologram represented in Figure 4.4(a) shows patterns larger than those of the beads (black arrows), which are due to impurities or defects present in the path of the optical system, and located on different planes other than the sample plane. These undesirable patterns are present even in the absence of a sample (microscope slide). They constitute what is called the "background" on the hologram. This background may have an impact on the reconstruction quality. To overcome this problem, the holograms can be divided (pixelwise) by a background image (acquired without a sample). It can then be considered that the background of the hologram is normalized to 1.

Figures 4.4(b–f) show a series of reconstructions using different approaches: usual approaches (backpropagation, alternating projections), and various IP approaches. Indeed, IP approaches provide a rigorous theoretical framework and a methodology that results in utilizing the information contained in the data in a relevant way, while exploiting the a priori knowledge about the observed objects and the noise. Subsequently, we expose in detail the steps that lead to the results in Figures 4.4(e) and 4.4(f).

4.4.2. *In-line hologram formation model*

Before taking a look into the models of in-line hologram formation, it is necessary to define a model of the object, namely its mathematical representation (described by the physical parameters to be measured).

4.4.2.1. *Modeling observed objects*

According to the description of the sample given in section 4.4.1, it is, from a general point of view, a spatial distribution of absorbing and/or phase-shifting objects placed on the plane of a microscope slide, and immersed in a medium with refractive index n_0.

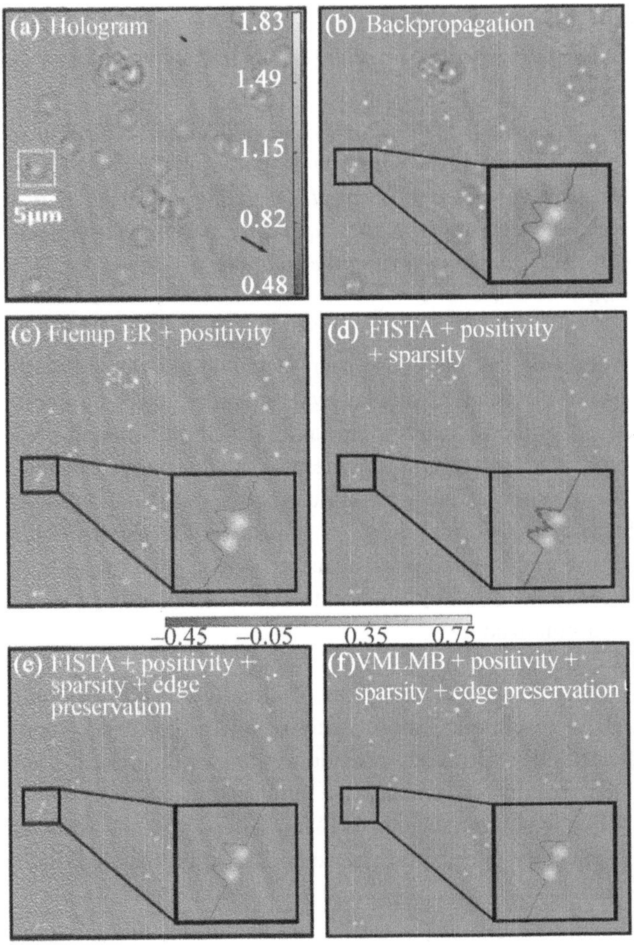

Figure 4.4. *Reconstructions of an in-line hologram of polystyrene beads (experimental parameters given in Table 4.1) using various methods*

COMMENTS ON FIGURE 4.4.– *(a) The black arrows point to background inhomogeneities. (b–f) Reconstructions of the transmittance phase* **o** *at the object plane using various methods. (b) Simple backpropagation reconstruction. The orange arrows point to artifacts related to backpropagation of the intensity called twin images. (c)* Fienup ER *reconstruction with positivity constraints. (d)* Inverse approach *reconstruction using the* FISTA *with positivity constraint and l_1 norm regularization (sparsity). (e)* Inverse approach *reconstruction using the* FISTA *with positivity constraint and l_1 + edge-preserving regularizations. (f) Reconstruction by* inverse approach *using the* VMLM-B *algorithm with positivity constraint and* l_1 + *edge-preserving regularizations.*

Illumination wavelength	λ	532 nm
Propagation distance	z	7.3 μm
Immersion medium refractive index	n_0	1.52
Bead refractive index	n_{bead}	1.59 (manufacturer's data)
Bead diameter	d_{bead}	1 μm (manufacturer's data)
Magnification (microscope objective)	mag	56.7
Image size	$M_x \times M_y$	$1,920 \times 1,080$ pixels
Pixel size	$p_x = p_y$	2.2 μm

Table 4.1. *Experimental parameters of in-line hologram data*

The physical quantities characterizing the interaction of these objects with light in terms of phase shift and absorption are their complex refractive index $\underline{n}(\boldsymbol{r}) = n_{\Re e}(\boldsymbol{r}) + i\, n_{\Im m}(\boldsymbol{r})$[2] and their thickness $e(\boldsymbol{r})$. Conventionally, these objects are considered "optically thin", that is, the phase shift and absorption that they introduce can be modeled by a complex 2D transmittance plane $\underline{t}(\boldsymbol{r})$ such that:

$$\begin{aligned} \underline{t}(\boldsymbol{r}) &= 1 + \underline{o}(\boldsymbol{r}) = \rho(\boldsymbol{r})\mathrm{e}^{i\varphi(\boldsymbol{r})} = \mathrm{e}^{ik(\underline{n}(\boldsymbol{r}) - n_0)e(\boldsymbol{r})} \\ &= \underbrace{\mathrm{e}^{-kn_{\Im m}(\boldsymbol{r})e(\boldsymbol{r})}}_{\rho(\boldsymbol{r})} \mathrm{e}^{ik(n_{\Re e}(\boldsymbol{r}) - n_0)e(\boldsymbol{r})} \end{aligned} \quad [4.1]$$

with $k = \frac{2\pi}{\lambda}$, λ being the illumination wavelength.

Object reconstruction consists of estimating $\underline{t}(\boldsymbol{r})$ and thus the phase shift $\varphi(\boldsymbol{r})$ and absorption $\rho(\boldsymbol{r})$ maps of the sample.

For example, a transparent plane without phase shift is modeled by $\underline{t}(\boldsymbol{r}) = 1$, that is, $\underline{o}(\boldsymbol{r}) = 0$, $\forall \boldsymbol{r}$. The presence of objects will thus be more easily modeled by the quantity $\underline{o}(\boldsymbol{r})$, which represents the transmittance difference with respect to the unit plane. We consider our unknown as being this complex map $\underline{o}(\boldsymbol{r})$ that will be referred to as *object transmittance* (and that is zero at points where there is no object).

2 $\boldsymbol{r} = (x, y)$ corresponding to the 2D spatial coordinates in the object plane.

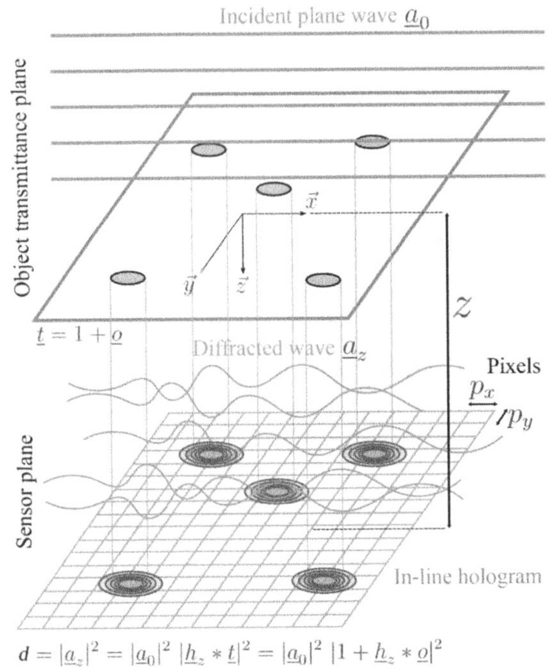

Figure 4.5. *Principle of in-line digital holography: the sample is illuminated by a plane wave $\underline{a}_0$ with a normal incidence to the sensor plane*

COMMENTS ON FIGURE 4.5.– *The spatial distribution of objects existing on the sample plane will perturb the incident wave, generating a diffracted wave $\underline{a}_z$. This distribution of objects, assumed to be "optically thin", is comprehended as an absorbing and phase-shifting plane ⇒ the transmittance plane $\underline{t}$. The intensity d of the diffraction pattern is recorded on the sensor at a distance z from the object plane.*

4.4.2.2. *Modeling image-hologram formation*

Figure 4.5 illustrates the principle of formation and acquisition of an in-line hologram from a plane sample. This hologram comes from a monochromatic incident wave (coherent, typically a plane wave) $\underline{a}_0(\boldsymbol{r})$ passing through the sample (transmittance plane $\underline{t}(\boldsymbol{r})$), generating a complex amplitude $\underline{a}_z(\boldsymbol{r})$ at a distance z from the sample. The sensor (CCD or CMOS) then records the digital image-hologram corresponding to the intensity $d(\boldsymbol{r})$ of the diffracted wave $\underline{a}_z(\boldsymbol{r})$.

It will be assumed that the sample is illuminated by a monochromatic plane wave of amplitude $\underline{a}_0$ (the plane wave at any point is a complex scalar). After traversing the transmittance plane, the wave has the expression $\underline{a}_0\,\underline{t}(\boldsymbol{r})$. According to the

Huygens–Fresnel principle (see Chapter 2), free-space propagation to the sensor, distant of z, is modeled by a convolution with a propagation kernel $\underline{h}_z(\boldsymbol{r})$:

$$\begin{aligned} \underline{a}_z(\boldsymbol{r}) &= \iint_{\mathbb{R}^2} \underline{h}_z(\boldsymbol{r}-\boldsymbol{r}')\,\underline{a}_0\,\underline{t}(\boldsymbol{r}')\,\mathrm{d}\boldsymbol{r}' \\ &= \underline{a}_0\,[\underline{h}_z * \underline{t}]\,(\boldsymbol{r}) \\ &= \underline{a}_0\,[\underline{h}_z * (1+\underline{o})]\,(\boldsymbol{r}) \\ &= \underline{a}_0\,[1 + (\underline{h}_z * \underline{o})]\,(\boldsymbol{r}) \text{ since } (\underline{h}_z * 1) = 1 \end{aligned} \qquad [4.2]$$

where $*$ is the convolution operator.

Depending on the experimental conditions, the propagation kernel may take the form of a Fresnel kernel (given here below) or a Rayleigh–Sommerfeld kernel:

$$\underline{h}_z(\boldsymbol{r}) = \frac{1}{i\lambda z}\exp\left(\frac{i\pi}{\lambda z}||\boldsymbol{r}||^2\right) = \frac{1}{i\lambda z}\exp\left(\frac{i\pi}{\lambda z}(x^2+y^2)\right) \qquad [4.3]$$

Let us notice that it is the intensity $d(\boldsymbol{r})$ of the wave $\underline{a}_z(\boldsymbol{r})$ which is recorded. The complete mathematical model is therefore:

$$\begin{aligned} d(\boldsymbol{r}) &= |\underline{a}_z(\boldsymbol{r})|^2 = |\underline{a}_0|^2\,|1 + (\underline{h}_z * \underline{o})\,(\boldsymbol{r})|^2 \\ &= |\underline{a}_0|^2\,\left(1 + 2\,[\mathfrak{Re}(\underline{h}_z * \underline{o})]\,(\boldsymbol{r}) + |(\underline{h}_z * \underline{o})(\boldsymbol{r})|^2\right) \\ &= |\underline{a}_0|^2\,\mathcal{M}(\underline{o}) \end{aligned} \qquad [4.4]$$

It is very important here to point out that the recorded intensity $d(\boldsymbol{r})$ depends only on the modulus of the wave $\underline{a}_z(\boldsymbol{r})$: *the phase is thus not directly measured on the sensor*. In off-axis holography, the reference wave, tilted with respect to the optical axis, is used as carrier of the object wave, which is modulated in amplitude. Demodulation (filtering in the Fourier space) makes it possible to find the modulus and the phase of $\underline{a}_z(\boldsymbol{r})$. We will see in the following that this loss of phase information on the sensor in in line holography degrades the reconstruction by revealing artifacts called *twin images* (Figure 4.4(b)). The use of advanced signal processing tools and a priori on objects allows us to estimate the wave phase on the sensor plane in the reconstruction step.

It proves advantageous to have a linear model that has useful properties for the problem resolution (for instance, the convexity of the reconstruction criterion, see Chapter 3). This is why we propose a simplification of the model $\mathcal{M}\ (\underline{o})$ of equation [4.4] based on two approximations.

1) From the test case (section 4.4.1), the objects of interest (beads) are transparent (real refractive index n_{bead}), thus essentially phase-shifting ($\rho(\boldsymbol{r}) \approx 1$). Moreover, given their size and the experimental parameters, the theoretical maximum phase-shift that they induce in the medium (linked to the optical path at the maximum thickness locations, $e(\boldsymbol{r}) = d_{\text{bead}}$) can be estimated as:

$$\varphi_{\max} = k(n_{\text{bead}} - n_0)d_{\text{bead}} \approx 0.83\,\text{rad} \qquad [4.5]$$

In this example and in many experimental cases, we can assume that the transmittance $\underline{t}(\boldsymbol{r})$ will induce very small phase shifts. This results in the following approximation:

$$\underline{t}(\boldsymbol{r}) = 1 + \underline{o}(\boldsymbol{r}) = e^{i\varphi(\boldsymbol{r})} \approx 1 + i\varphi(\boldsymbol{r}) = 1 + io(\boldsymbol{r}) \qquad [4.6]$$

2) We overlook, in equation [4.4], the second-order term $|(\underline{h}_z * \underline{o})(\boldsymbol{r})|^2$, corresponding to the intensity diffracted by the object (negligible for small objects). The combination of these two approximations yields the following linear imaging model:

$$\mathcal{M}(o) = 1 - 2\left[\mathfrak{Im}(\underline{h}_z) * o\right](\boldsymbol{r}) = 1 + (g_z * o)(\boldsymbol{r}) \qquad [4.7]$$

Equations [4.4] and [4.7] represent continuous imaging models, which do not take into account the sensor sampling, the sampling of the transmittance plane to be reconstructed or the finite dimensions of these matrices. We must now consider a discrete representation (digital image) of $d(\boldsymbol{r})$ where the spatial coordinates $\boldsymbol{r}$ are constrained to a finite grid of $M_x \times M_y$ pixels, identified by their indexes $(k,\ell)_{\{k=1\ldots M_x|\ell=1\ldots M_y\}}$ giving their respective spatial position $\boldsymbol{r}_{k,\ell} = (x_k, y_\ell) = (k.p_x, l.p_y)$ on the digital image. $p_x \times p_y$ represents the sampling step of the grid (in metric units). A spatially continuous image b is thus, in its discrete version, defined as a matrix (denoted in bold) $\boldsymbol{b} \in \mathbb{K}^{M_x \times M_y}$.

REMARK.– Shifting from continuous to discrete implies, in our equations, that an *image* $\boldsymbol{b} \in \mathbb{K}^{M_x \times M_y}$ has to be considered as a *vector* valued in $\mathbb{K}$ of size $M_x \cdot M_y$ (e.g. by concatenating the image columns). This results in simplifying the notations of the equations while remaining mathematically rigorous. For instance, the discrete convolution product between an image $\boldsymbol{b}$ and a kernel $\boldsymbol{h}$ will be simply written as a matrix-vector product $\mathbf{H}\,\boldsymbol{b}$ where $\mathbf{H}$ is a matrix of size $(M_x \cdot M_y) \times (M_x \cdot M_y)$. In this case, we use the subscript q to refer to an element of the vector $\boldsymbol{b}$, which is therefore denoted by b_q.

In practice, the matrix $\mathbf{H}$ (of prohibitive size) will never be explicitly implemented. The discrete convolution is computed by multiplying "pointwise" the fast discrete

Fourier transforms ($\mathcal{FFT}$) of the kernel $\boldsymbol{h}$ and the image $\boldsymbol{b}$, then applying an inverse transform:

$$\underbrace{\mathbf{H}\,\boldsymbol{b}}_{\substack{\textit{matrix operator}\\ \textit{applied to a vector}}} \quad \leftrightarrow \quad \underbrace{\mathcal{FFT}^{-1}\left(\mathcal{FFT}(\boldsymbol{h})\cdot\mathcal{FFT}(\boldsymbol{b})\right)}_{\substack{\textit{2D convolution product computed in Fourier space}\\ \textit{applied to 2D matrices}}}$$

where the operation $\mathcal{FFT}(\boldsymbol{h})\cdot\mathcal{FFT}(\boldsymbol{b})$ is thus performed pixelwise. The above equation does not take into account the possible need to compute preliminary *zero padding* operations to avoid the phenomena of circular convolution.

We denote by $\boldsymbol{d} \in \mathbb{R}^{M_x \cdot M_y}$ the recorded hologram, by $\underline{\boldsymbol{o}} \in \mathbb{C}^{M_x \cdot M_y}$ the (complex-valued) object transmittance map in the object plane [4.1] and, for the simplified object model [4.6], $\boldsymbol{o} \in \mathbb{R}^{M_x \cdot M_y}$, the (real-valued) transmittance phase map in the object plane. The formation of the hologram $\boldsymbol{d}$ of the sample $\underline{\boldsymbol{o}}$ (respectively, $\boldsymbol{o}$) is, with the notations introduced above, a function $\mathcal{M}(\underline{\boldsymbol{o}})$ (respectively, $\mathcal{M}(\boldsymbol{o})$) of $\mathbb{C}^{M_x \cdot M_y}$ (respectively, $\mathbb{R}^{M_x \cdot M_y}$) in $\mathbb{R}^{M_x \cdot M_y}$. The discrete convolution consists of linearly combining the values $\underline{o}_{k,\ell}$ (respectively, $o_{k,\ell}$) of each pixel of $\underline{\boldsymbol{o}}$ (respectively, $\boldsymbol{o}$) to get the value of each pixel (k,ℓ): $d_{k,\ell} = \mathcal{M}[\underline{o}](\boldsymbol{r}_{k,\ell})$ (respectively, $\mathcal{M}[o](\boldsymbol{r}_{k,\ell})$). We therefore have two possible models of image formation, a nonlinear (equation [4.8]) and a linear one (equation [4.9]):

$$\boldsymbol{d} = c\,\mathcal{M}(\underline{\boldsymbol{o}}) + \boldsymbol{\eta} = c\,|\mathbf{1} + \underline{\mathbf{H}}_z\,\underline{\boldsymbol{o}}|^2 + \boldsymbol{\eta} \qquad [4.8]$$

$$\boldsymbol{d} = c\,\mathcal{M}(\boldsymbol{o}) + \boldsymbol{\eta} = c\,(\mathbf{1} + \mathbf{G}_z\,\boldsymbol{o}) + \boldsymbol{\eta} \qquad [4.9]$$

The operator $|\underline{\cdot}|^2$ is a function of $\mathbb{C}^{M_x \cdot M_y}$ in $\mathbb{R}^{M_x \cdot M_y}$, which computes the squared modulus of each pixel in a vector. The term $\mathbf{1} \in \mathbb{R}^{M_x \cdot M_y}$ corresponds to a vector whose components are all 1, and $\boldsymbol{\eta} \in \mathbb{R}^{M_x \cdot M_y}$ models additional perturbations and errors such as electronic noise from the sensor, and the errors of the model $\mathcal{M}$ (which originate from each model-specific approximation). c is a scaling factor for adjusting the theoretical model to the dynamics of the digital image. It can be observed that in a situation where a background has been taken into account (normalization), this factor is 1. The operator $\underline{\mathbf{H}}_z$ (respectively, $\mathbf{G}_z$) of $\mathbb{C}^{M_x \cdot M_y}$ in $\mathbb{C}^{M_x \cdot M_y}$ (respectively, of $\mathbb{R}^{M_x \cdot M_y}$ in $\mathbb{R}^{M_x \cdot M_y}$) corresponds to the discrete convolution by the propagation kernel $\underline{\boldsymbol{h}}_{\boldsymbol{z}}$ (respectively, $\boldsymbol{g}_{\boldsymbol{z}}$), modeling wave propagation.

The estimation of the object transmittance map $\underline{\boldsymbol{o}}$ or phase map $\boldsymbol{o}$, from the hologram $\boldsymbol{d}$, constitutes the *holographic reconstruction IP*.

In the following, and to address our experimental problem using an IP-based approach, we have chosen to consider the linear model [4.9]. This model allows us to directly reconstruct the map of the transmittance phase o sought, and to exploit the a priori that can be obtained from this transmittance. Finally, based on the assumption that the objects of interest are purely phase-shifting, we only have to reconstruct a purely real image (instead of two images each corresponding, respectively, to the real and imaginary part of the object transmittance $\underline{o}$), thus simplifying how the problem is posed and solved.

4.4.3. *Digital reconstructions*

In this section, we present several digital reconstruction methods applied to the experimental holograms presented in section 4.4.1, starting with commonly used methods and ending up with IP-based resolution methods. All of the results produced by each of these methods are illustrated in Figure 4.4 and we refer to them as we proceed further into our study.

4.4.3.1. *Backpropagation reconstruction and the twin image problem*

The most intuitive approach to reconstruction, already mentioned in Chapter 2, consists of applying the principle of "reversibility of light", that is, hologram backpropagation. This approach imitates the principle of optical reconstruction for a hologram recorded on a holographic plate. This reconstruction is carried out by re-illuminating the plate by the reference wave. The diffraction by the plate generates two images of the object upstream and downstream of the holographic plate. The model corresponding to such an approach consists of applying the backpropagation operator $\underline{\mathbf{H}}_{-z}$ to the measured intensity $\boldsymbol{d}$ (see [4.4]; here we consider $|\underline{a}_0| = 1$ to simplify the equations):

$$\underline{\mathbf{H}}_{-z}\boldsymbol{d} = \underline{\mathbf{H}}_{-z}|1 + \underline{\mathbf{H}}_z\underline{o}|^2$$

By expanding the squared modulus and considering $\underline{\mathbf{H}}_{-z}\mathbf{1} \approx e^{-ikz}\mathbf{1}$ (property of the operator $\underline{\mathbf{H}}_{-z}$[3]) :

$$\underline{\mathbf{H}}_{-z}\boldsymbol{d} = e^{-ikz}\mathbf{1} + \underline{\mathbf{H}}_{-z}\underline{\mathbf{H}}_z\underline{o} + \underline{\mathbf{H}}^2_{-z}\underline{o}^* + \underline{\mathbf{H}}_{-z}|\underline{\mathbf{H}}_z\underline{o}|^2$$

3 This physically corresponds to the fact that plane wave propagation gives a plane wave phase-shifted by $-kz$, this equality is approximately verified in numerical terms.

$\underline{\underline{\mathbf{H}}}_{-z}$ corresponds to the Hermitian transpose operator of $\underline{\underline{\mathbf{H}}}_z$, denoted by $\underline{\underline{\mathbf{H}}}_z^\dagger$. Due to the sensor field truncation, this operator is not the exact inverse of the propagation but an approximation, that is, $\underline{\underline{\mathbf{H}}}_z^\dagger \underline{\underline{\mathbf{H}}}_z \approx \mathbf{I}$:

$$\underline{\underline{\mathbf{H}}}_{-z}\boldsymbol{d} \approx \underbrace{e^{-ikz}\mathbf{1} + \underline{\underline{\mathbf{H}}}_{-z}|\underline{\underline{\mathbf{H}}}_z\underline{\boldsymbol{o}}|^2}_{0} + \underbrace{\underline{\boldsymbol{o}}}_{1} + \underbrace{\underline{\underline{\mathbf{H}}}_{-2z}\underline{\boldsymbol{o}}^*}_{-1}$$

The different terms of this equation can be interpreted as in off-axis holography (Chapter 2):

– a low-frequency zeroth-order term that contains: the backpropagated incident wave along with a term corresponding to the backpropagation of the intensity of the object wave on the sensor (without interference);

– a first-order term corresponding to the object transmittance of the object (called the real image);

– a -1 order term corresponding to the conjugate of the object transmittance propagated by a distance $-2z$. This contribution is that of a virtual image positioned symmetrically to the real image with respect to the hologram plane.

In off-axis holography, the reference wave, tilted relative to the optical axis, acts like a carrier for the object wave. The real image and the virtual image are thus separated in the Fourier space and a simple filtering makes it possible to avoid the virtual image. In in-line holography, the virtual image (–1 order) is superimposed on the real image (+1 order) and makes the analysis of the reconstructed planes difficult. It should be noted that this is intrinsically due to the fact that the diffracted wave phase is lost when recording the hologram intensity (see section 4.4.2). If wave phase recording were possible, backpropagation would be enough to reconstruct the object. Figure 4.4(b) represents a back-propagated image in which the virtual images are visible, also called twin images (orange arrows).

The challenge raised by in-line hologram reconstruction is thus to propose an algorithmic strategy for correctly estimating the missing phase from the measurement $\sqrt{\boldsymbol{d}} \approx |\underline{\boldsymbol{a}}_z|$, so that a simple backpropagation yields the object reconstruction. This is a *phase reconstruction* problem.

4.4.3.2. *Alternating projection reconstructions*

A solution to the *phase reconstruction* problem was proposed in the 1970s, from which a class of methods has been derived that will be called the *alternating projection method* in this chapter. Its most widely known form was introduced by Fienup in 1978 (Fienup 1978) with the *error-reduction (ER)* algorithm. It is an advanced variant of an approach proposed by Gerchberg and Saxton (1972), which is based on alternating propagations and backpropagations between two measured hologram planes.

The *ER* algorithm requires only one hologram $\boldsymbol{d}$ recorded with a defocus z. This hologram must be normalized (see section 4.4.2.2) in order to have a background of intensity 1 (factor $c \approx 1$ in [4.8]), thus ensuring a reconstructed transmittance ranging between 0 and 1, and making sure that the a priori consistent with the scale of transmittance values can be taken into account. If the background image is not known, the normalized hologram, denoted $\bar{\boldsymbol{d}}$, can be obtained by simply dividing the initial hologram $\boldsymbol{d}$ by its median (valid in the case of sparse samples on a uniform background).

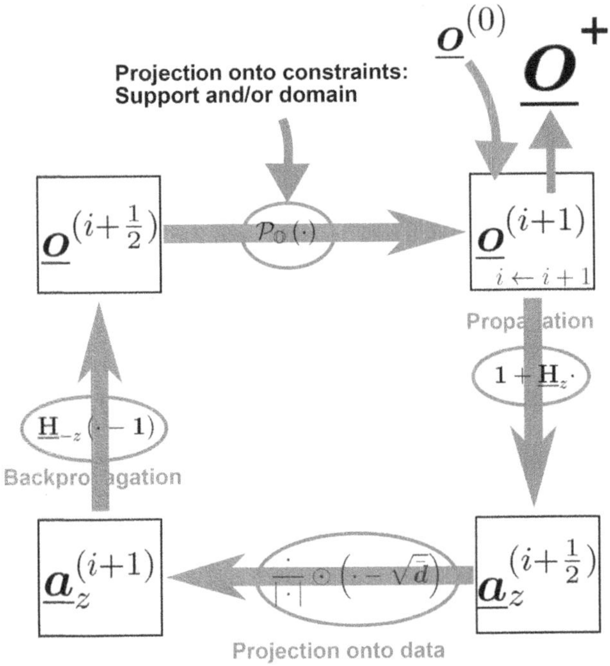

Figure 4.6. *Error-reduction (ER) algorithm iterative scheme*

Figure 4.6 illustrates the operation of the *ER* algorithm: it consists of iteratively applying a succession of four steps. At each iteration (i), the object transmittance $\underline{o}^{(i)}$ is re-estimated in $\underline{o}^{(i+1)}$ in the following manner:

1) a simulated complex hologram (phase and amplitude) $\underline{a}_z^{(i+1/2)} = 1 + \underline{\mathbf{H}}_z \underline{o}^{(i)}$ is computed corresponding to the complex amplitude of the wave diffracted by the object $\underline{o}^{(i)}$;

2) on the sensor plane, a *projection onto data* is applied; in other words, the amplitude of $\underline{a}_z^{(i+1/2)}$ is constrained to be equal to the measured amplitude, thus $\sqrt{\bar{d}}$. The modified wave complex amplitude $\underline{a}_z^{(i+1)}$ is obtained:

$$\underline{a}_z^{(i+1)} = \frac{\underline{a}_z^{(i+1/2)}}{|\underline{a}_z^{(i+1/2)}|} \odot \sqrt{\bar{d}}$$

3) the backpropagation $\underline{o}^{(i+1/2)} = \underline{\mathbf{H}}_{-z}(\underline{a}_z^{(i+1)} - \mathbf{1})$ is computed to obtain a new estimate;

4) on the object plane, a new estimate $\underline{o}^{(i+1)} = \mathcal{P}_{\mathbb{O}}(\underline{o}^{(i+1/2)})$ is computed where $\mathcal{P}_{\mathbb{O}}(\,\cdot\,)$ is a projection step onto a domain of the physically relevant values. This is called *projection onto constraints* (see note below).

In summary, a typical iteration of the *ER* algorithm can be summarized by the following expression:

$$\underline{o}^{(i+1)} = \mathcal{P}_{\mathbb{O}}\left[\underline{\mathbf{H}}_{-z}\left(\frac{\underline{a}_z^{(i+1/2)}}{|\underline{a}_z^{(i+1/2)}|} \odot \sqrt{\bar{d}} - \mathbf{1}\right)\right] \tag{4.10}$$

with $\underline{a}_z^{(i+1/2)} = \mathbf{1} + \underline{\mathbf{H}}_z\,\underline{o}^{(i)}$. The symbol $\odot$ corresponds to the Hadamard product, that is, the termwise product (pixelwise) between two images. The computations of the division $\underline{a}_z^{(i+1/2)}$ by $|\underline{a}_z^{(i+1/2)}|$, of the modulus $|\cdot|$ and the square root $\sqrt{\cdot}$ are also applied in a pixelwise manner.

This strategy of successive back-and-forth propagations between the object plane and the sensor plane, along with the enforcement of object/data constraints on each plane, makes it possible to progressively estimate the missing phase on the sensor and thus to remove the twin image (the data are reinjected at each iteration into the wave modulus as its phase evolves). Figure 4.4(c) illustrates the reconstruction of the phase map of $\underline{o}$ using the *ER* algorithm. The *projection step onto the constraints* $\mathcal{P}_{\mathbb{O}}(\underline{o}^{(i+1/2)})$ consisted here of introducing a zero real part and a strictly positive imaginary part:

$$\mathcal{P}_{\mathbb{O}}(\underline{o}) = \begin{cases} i\mathfrak{Im}(\underline{o}) & \text{if } \mathfrak{Im}(\underline{o}) \geq 0 \\ 0 & \text{otherwise} \end{cases} \tag{4.11}$$

By considering the simplified object model [4.6], we impose a positive phase (corresponding to the imaginary part of $\underline{o}$) on $\underline{o}^{(i+1/2)}$. The objects appear with better contrast than in the backpropagation of Figure 4.4(b), and twin image artifacts have been significantly reduced. The background is not entirely cleaned but it is very low (see the colorbar range) and strictly positive as expected.

REMARK.– *Projection onto constraints.* The operator $\mathcal{P}_{\mathbb{O}}$ can stand for various constraints:

– A commonly used constraint consists of restricting the values of $|\mathbf{1} + \underline{o}| = |\underline{t}|$ between 0 (opacity) and 1 (total transparency). It is in fact considered that values outside this range have no physical meaning. For example, a transmittance greater than 1 would mean that the objects of interest can be light amplifiers. As for the lower limit 0, it naturally translates the constraint that the absorption cannot be negative.

– It is also possible to impose a support constraint on the object $\underline{o}$, that is, a mask imposing non-zero values only in a priori known areas of the image. In the case of biological samples, this type of constraint is feasible because it is possible to determine, at least approximately by way of rudimentary segmentation (e.g. by thresholding on a conventional microscope image), a support for the objects of interest on the sample. Although potentially very efficient, this solution lacks flexibility because it depends on external information and on the quality of the segmentation method. We will see that IP approaches can be employed to fully take advantage of this type of constraint in a more flexible way by means of regularizations imposing a sparsity criterion.

The widespread acceptance of this class of methods is the result of the fact that the approach is very intuitive (successive propagations and backpropagations are "simply" applied, because they are operations that make sense in physical terms) and very simple to implement. The alternating projection approach is therefore still widely used and has a large number of followers due in particular to the work by Latychevskaia and Fink (2007). However, the following section will show that the problem can be approached in a much more rigorous manner by applying the IP-based methodology presented in Chapter 3.

4.4.3.3. *IP approach-based reconstructions*

REMARK.– *Notations.* We recall the definition of the l_2 and l_1 norms applied to a vector $\boldsymbol{b}$: $||\boldsymbol{b}||_2 = \sqrt{\boldsymbol{b}} = \sqrt{\sum_q b_q^2}$ and $||\boldsymbol{b}||_1 = \sum_q |b_q|$. The notation $||\boldsymbol{b}||_{\mathbf{W}}$, where $\mathbf{W}$ is a positive semidefinite matrix (with size $M_x \cdot M_y \times M_x \cdot M_y$), corresponds to: $||\boldsymbol{b}||^2_{\mathbf{W}} = \boldsymbol{b}^{\mathrm{T}}\mathbf{W}\boldsymbol{b}$.

In this section, we present in-line hologram reconstruction using an IP-based approach. Theoretical and methodological aspects having been addressed in more detail in Chapter 3, our presentation will instead be formulated as an application of the approach to the resolution of the reconstruction problem of our experimental example.

To illustrate these approaches, we will first show that the *ER* algorithm (section 4.4.3.2) can be interpreted as an IP algorithm with particular choices of modeling and constraints. We will then show that the IP methodology is much more general. Indeed, it allows for more flexibility in the choice of the a priori on the objects to be reconstructed (constraints and regularizations, for example). It makes it possible to better take into account the image formation model (commonly referred to as the "direct model") and to improve the reconstruction.

Consider again equation [4.10] introducing the computation of an *ER* iteration. Under the assumption that $\underline{\mathbf{H}}_{-z}\,\underline{\mathbf{H}}_{z} = \underline{\mathbf{H}}_{z}^{\dagger}\,\underline{\mathbf{H}}_{z} \approx \mathbf{I}$, the following approximation of this equation can be written as:

$$\underline{o}^{(i+1)} \approx \mathcal{P}_{\mathbb{O}}\left[\underbrace{\underline{o}^{(i)} - \underline{\mathbf{H}}_{-z}\left(\frac{\underline{\boldsymbol{a}}_z^{(i+1/2)}}{|\underline{\boldsymbol{a}}_z^{(i+1/2)}|} \odot \left(|\underline{\boldsymbol{a}}_z^{(i+1/2)}| - \sqrt{\bar{\boldsymbol{d}}}\right)\right)}_{\underline{o}^{(i+1/2)}}\right] \qquad [4.12]$$

The part found between brackets constitutes a gradient descent step $\underline{o}^{(i+1/2)} = \underline{o}^{(i)} - \nabla\mathcal{C}(\underline{o}^{(i)})$ of a criterion $\mathcal{C}$ differentiable ("smooth"):

$$\mathcal{C}(\underline{o}) = \left\| |1 + \underline{\mathbf{H}}_z\,\underline{o}| - \sqrt{\bar{\boldsymbol{d}}} \right\|_2^2 = \left\| \sqrt{\mathcal{M}(\underline{o})} - \sqrt{\bar{\boldsymbol{d}}} \right\|_2^2 \qquad [4.13]$$

We recognize in $\mathcal{C}$ a "least squares" criterion giving a measure of the error between the normalized amplitude data $\sqrt{\bar{\boldsymbol{d}}}$ and the model $\mathcal{M}(\underline{o})$ of the intensity presented in equation [4.8], taken as a modulus (by operation $\sqrt{\cdot}$). We call $\mathcal{C}$ the *data-fidelity term*; minimizing this term is equivalent to fitting the model to the measurements.

The projection step $\mathcal{P}_{\mathbb{O}}(\underline{o}^{(i+1/2)})$ onto the convex domain $\mathbb{O}$ (positivity, negativity, support) represents the proximal operator (see Chapter 3) of the indicator function $\iota_{\mathbb{O}}$ on the domain $\mathbb{O}$:

$$\iota_{\mathbb{O}}(\underline{o}) = \begin{cases} 0 & \text{if } \underline{o} \in \mathbb{O} \\ +\infty & \text{otherwise} \end{cases} \qquad [4.14]$$

The *ER* algorithm is a typical approach of the IP methodology that searches for the optimal solution $\underline{o}^{+}$ minimizing the following criterion:

$$\underline{o}^{+} = \arg\min_{\underline{o}} \underbrace{\left\| \sqrt{\mathcal{M}(\underline{o})} - \sqrt{\bar{\boldsymbol{d}}} \right\|_2^2}_{\mathcal{C}(\underline{o})\text{differentiable}} + \underbrace{\iota_{\mathbb{O}}(\underline{o})}_{\mathcal{H}(\underline{o})\text{non-differentiable}} \qquad [4.15]$$

composed of a smooth function $\mathcal{C}(\underline{o})$ (data-fidelity) and a non-smooth function $\mathcal{H}(\underline{o}) = \iota_{\mathbb{O}}(\underline{o})$ (regularization term). This type of problem is solved by a widely used strategy belonging to the class of *proximal algorithms* (Parikh and Boyd 2014). More specifically, the algorithm in question is the *iterative shrinkage thresholding algorithm* (ISTA).

ER therefore already has a character of optimality with respect to the criterion chosen for the estimation of the solution $\underline{o}^+$. It is however a method that rather lacks flexibility both in terms of the model utilized and the choice of criterion, as well as in terms of solving method, as we show below.

– The correct application of the image formation model $\sqrt{\mathcal{M}(\underline{o})}$ in the iterative resolution [4.12] is constrained by the approximation $\underline{\mathbf{H}}_z^\dagger\,\underline{\mathbf{H}}_z \approx \mathbf{I}$. This approximation is valid due to the simplicity of the initial model. Adding more flexibility and accuracy for modeling could be interesting, making it possible in particular to take into consideration other experimental effects (numerical aperture, field truncation, partial coherence, optical aberrations, etc.). Here is an example:

$$\mathcal{M}(\underline{o}) = \mathbf{T}\,\mathbf{C}\,|1 + \underline{\mathbf{H}}_z\underline{o}|^2 \qquad [4.16]$$

where $\mathbf{C}$ is a convolution operator that takes into account a loss of spatial coherence (according to the model presented in section 6.2.2, illustrated by Figure 4.2), and $\mathbf{T}$ is a field truncation operator.

In our experimental example, we choose a simplifying solution for the propagative part of the model by adopting the linear model of equation [4.9]:

$$\mathcal{M}(\boldsymbol{o}) = \mathbf{1} + \mathbf{G}_z\boldsymbol{o} \qquad [4.17]$$

It would be possible to also take into consideration the partial coherence operator $\mathbf{C}$ and the field truncation operator $\mathbf{T}$ presented in equation [4.16] because these refinements do not modify the linearity property of our new model.

– $\mathcal{C}$ is a least squares criterion that does not take the noise statistics into account. This corresponds to a maximum likelihood criterion (see Chapter 3) for a white Gaussian noise (i.e. independent on each pixel and thus without interpixel spatial correlation) and identically distributed (uniform statistics over the whole field). In this case, the noise variance does not play any role in the criterion minimization. The latter becomes statistically invalid for spatially correlated noise (such as speckle noise, for example) and/or non-stationary noise. Moreover, the normalization step $\bar{\boldsymbol{d}}$ (division by the background) and the fact that we compute the square root of the data modify this noise model established from the raw data. A correct Gaussian maximum likelihood criterion (weighted least squares) is more strictly written as:

$$\mathcal{C}(\boldsymbol{o}, c) = \|c\,\mathcal{M}(\boldsymbol{o}) - \boldsymbol{d}\|_{\mathbf{W}}^2 \qquad [4.18]$$

where $\mathbf{W}$ is the inverse of the noise covariance matrix $\mathbf{C}_{\eta} = \mathrm{E}\left[\eta\,\eta^{\mathrm{T}}\right]$ ($\mathrm{E}\left[\cdot\right]$ represents the expectation) (Flasseur et al. 2019). It should be noted that the case $\mathbf{W} = \mathbf{I}$ corresponds to the previous least squares criterion [4.13]. The criterion [4.18] is thus more general and does not require any data preprocessing. Apart from statistical considerations, the matrix $\mathbf{W}$ is also used to avoid outlier pixels ("dead" or saturated pixels) in the data $\boldsymbol{d}$, or missing data (as out-of-field pixels, for example), by setting their weights to 0 (infinite noise variance). An example is given in section 4.5.

We note that it is now possible to optimally estimate the factor c as a function of $\boldsymbol{o}$:

$$c^{+}(\boldsymbol{o}) = \arg\min_{c} \|c\,\mathcal{M}(\boldsymbol{o}) - \boldsymbol{d}\|^2_{\mathbf{W}} = \frac{\mathcal{M}(\boldsymbol{o})^{\mathrm{T}}\mathbf{W}\boldsymbol{d}}{\mathcal{M}(\boldsymbol{o})^{\mathrm{T}}\mathbf{W}\mathcal{M}(\boldsymbol{o})} \qquad [4.19]$$

This enables the data to be normalized in an optimal way given the object $\boldsymbol{o}$.

The choice of a least squares data fidelity term, combined with the use of a linear image formation model furthermore ensures the convexity of the criterion $\mathcal{C}$. An optimization algorithm will thus converge to a global minimum of this criterion.

– The regularization imposed by the indicator $\iota_{\mathbb{O}}$ is in fact a hard constraint, and therefore not very flexible. Even if a positivity/negativity constraint is in general relevant (or even essential) in an inverse approach, other hard constraints such as imposing a support are, on the other hand, too strict because they require precise knowledge of the support. It is, for example, possible to relax this constraint by using a l_1-norm regularization, that is, a sparsity constraint (see Chapter 3), with the same objective but not imposing a predetermined spatial support:

$$\begin{aligned}\mathcal{R}_{l_1}(\boldsymbol{o}) &= \|\boldsymbol{o}\|_1 = \textstyle\sum_q |o_q| \\ &= \textstyle\sum_q o_q \text{ if } o_q \geq 0\,,\ \forall q \text{ (under positivity constraint)}\end{aligned} \qquad [4.20]$$

As presented in Chapter 3, the l_1-norm regularization introduces a simple proximal operator to compute the soft thresholding $\mathcal{T}_{\alpha}$:

$$\mathcal{T}_{\alpha}(o_q) = \mathrm{prox}_{\alpha\,\mathcal{R}_{l_1}}(o_q) = \mathrm{sign}(o_q)\max\left(0, |o_q| - \alpha\right) \qquad [4.21]$$

The IP methodology thus leads to gains in flexibility and to exploiting the information actually available in the data, while supplementing missing data by means of relevant constraints and regularizations. Bearing these first remarks in mind, we propose hereafter a first reconstruction strategy using an IP-based approach:

$$\boldsymbol{o}^{+} = \arg\min_{\boldsymbol{o}} \left\{ \underbrace{\mathcal{C}\big(\boldsymbol{o}, c^{+}(\boldsymbol{o})\big)}_{\mathcal{G}(\boldsymbol{o})\text{differentiable}} + \underbrace{\mu_{l_1}\mathcal{R}_{l_1}(\boldsymbol{o}) + \iota_{\mathbb{O}}(\boldsymbol{o})}_{\mathcal{H}(\boldsymbol{o})\text{non-differentiable}} \right\} \qquad [4.22]$$

where the differentiable term $\mathcal{G}(\boldsymbol{o})$ comprises the $\mathcal{C}$ data-fidelity term defined in equation [4.18]. $\iota_{\mathbb{O}}(\boldsymbol{o})$ constitutes the indicator on $\mathbb{R}^+$, which is written here as a regularization term. The regularization $\mathcal{R}_{l_1}$ is weighted by a scalar hyperparameter μ_{l_1}, which ensures the compromise between the weight given, on the one hand, to the data-fidelity term and this regularization term, on the other hand. Similarly to *ER* [4.15], this new criterion is a composition of a smooth function $\mathcal{C}$ and a non-smooth function ($\mathcal{H}$). A resolution strategy based on *ISTA* can therefore be used:

$$\boldsymbol{o}^{(i+1)} = \mathcal{P}_{\mathbb{O}}\left(\mathcal{T}_{\mu_{l_1} t}\left(\boldsymbol{o}^{(i)} - t\,\nabla\mathcal{G}(\boldsymbol{o}^{(i)})\right)\right) \qquad [4.23]$$

with:

$$\begin{aligned}\nabla\mathcal{G}(\boldsymbol{o}^{(i)}) &= \frac{\partial\mathcal{C}}{\partial\boldsymbol{o}}(\boldsymbol{o}^{(i)}, c^{(i)}) \\ &= 2\,c^{(i)}\,\mathbf{G}_z^{\mathrm{T}}\mathbf{W}\big(c^{(i)}\,\mathcal{M}(\boldsymbol{o}^{(i)}) - \boldsymbol{d}\big)\end{aligned} \qquad [4.24]$$

with $c^{(i)} = c^{+}(\boldsymbol{o}^{(i)})$. The scalar t is the descent step which should ideally be adjusted according to some theoretical considerations on the model $\mathcal{M}$ (Beck and Teboulle 2009). It includes some of the intuitive steps of an alternating projection approach, and in particular the backpropagation $\mathbf{G}_z^{\mathrm{T}}$ of the "residual" term $(c^{(i)}\,\mathcal{M}(\boldsymbol{o}^{(i)}) - \boldsymbol{d})$ (Figure 4.7).

The reconstruction of the test hologram using this method is shown in Figure 4.4(d). More precisely, we applied the accelerated version of *ISTA* (*FISTA* (Beck and Teboulle 2009)) based on the same solving principle, but that achieves faster convergence (Figure 4.8). As can be observed, the gain brought by the regularization $\mathcal{R}_{l_1}$ on the cleaning of the residual background artifacts is quite spectacular (provided that μ_{l_1} is set correctly). The support of the objects of interest is correctly estimated, allowing for their segmentation in a natural way. On the other hand, the sparsity constraint imposed by this regularization tends to "excavate" the objects (see the thumbnail showing a close-up of two nearby beads in Figure 4.4(d)). This observation shows that they should be considered as spatially extended objects and not point sources. Furthermore, their appearance should have a smooth structure.

To build a solution presenting reconstructed objects with this characteristic, several regularizations can be selected, all involving the spatial gradient of the object (see Chapter 3): (i) quadratic regularization; (ii) edge-preserving smoothing; and (iii) total variation. According to Chapter 3, solution (iii) is to be avoided because it involves piecewise constant solutions whereas we would instead prefer a smooth solution with

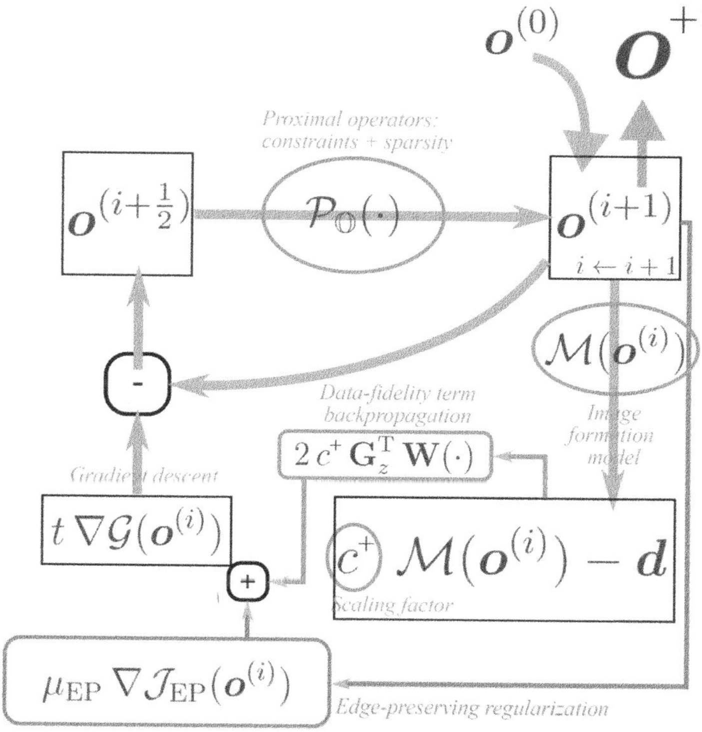

Figure 4.7. *Iterative scheme of the algorithm presented in equations [4.25] and [4.26]*

preserved contrasting edges. In this case, solution (i) is also undesirable because we would lose the sparsity property of the image gradient. Finally, it is solution (ii) that is naturally required. We therefore propose a new strategy involving this additional regularization:

$$o^{+} = \arg\min_{o} \left\{ \underbrace{\mathcal{C}(o, c^{+}(o)) + \mu_{\mathrm{EP}}\, \mathcal{R}_{\mathrm{EP}}(o)}_{\mathcal{G}(o)\text{differentiable}} + \underbrace{\mu_{l_1} \mathcal{R}_{l_1}(o) + \iota_{\mathbb{O}}(o)}_{\mathcal{H}(o)\text{non-differentiable}} \right\} \qquad [4.25]$$

where the differentiable term $\mathcal{G}(o)$ now consists of the data-fidelity term $\mathcal{C}$ and the (differentiable) "edge-preserving smoothing" regularization $\mathcal{R}_{\mathrm{EP}}$ whose definition is given in Chapter 3. The latter is weighted by the scalar hyperparameter μ_{EP}. To solve this new problem, we still use the *FISTA* solving strategy, involving the new computation of the gradient descent term integrating the derivative of the term $\mathcal{R}_{\text{EP}}$:

$$\begin{aligned}\nabla \mathcal{G}(\boldsymbol{o}^{(i)}) &= \tfrac{\partial \mathcal{C}}{\partial \boldsymbol{o}}(\boldsymbol{o}^{(i)}, c^{(i)}) + \mu_{\text{EP}} \tfrac{\partial \mathcal{R}_{\text{EP}}}{\partial \boldsymbol{o}}(\boldsymbol{o}^{(i)}) \\ &= 2\, c^{+}\, \mathbf{G}_z^{\mathrm{T}} \mathbf{W}\big(c^{+}\, \mathcal{M}(\boldsymbol{o}^{(i)}) - \boldsymbol{d}\big) \\ &+\ \mu_{\text{EP}} \textstyle\sum_{k,\ell} \frac{1}{\sqrt{\|\nabla_{k,\ell}\, \boldsymbol{o}^{(i)}\|_2^2 + \epsilon^2}}\, \nabla_{k,\ell}{}^{\mathrm{T}} \nabla_{k,\ell}\, \boldsymbol{o}^{(i)}\end{aligned} \qquad [4.26]$$

where $\nabla_{k,\ell}$ is a finite difference operator computing the gradient components of the object $\boldsymbol{o}$ at pixel (k, ℓ).

The reconstruction of the test hologram from this method is presented in Figure 4.4(e), where the beneficial effect of this new regularization on the smooth structure of the reconstructed objects can be observed; also, the global sparse character of the area occupied by the objects (support) has been preserved relative to the background. It can also be seen that the contrast of objects standing out from the background is also preserved.

At this development stage of our inverse approach, we have validated the various elements that allowed us to construct the criterion to be minimized: the model, the data-fidelity term and the constraints (Figure 4.3). We have nonetheless maintained an *ISTA*-based optimization strategy, which has resulted in highlighting the analogy between an IP approach and an alternating projection approach (*ER*). This optimization strategy is adapted to the minimization of a criterion summing a smooth function with a non-smooth function (proximal algorithms). Problems [4.22] and [4.25], in the form they have been described, therefore justify the relevance of using the *FISTA* optimization algorithm.

However, the constraint imposed by the indicator $\iota_{\mathbb{O}}(\boldsymbol{o})$ can be more appropriately formalized as a hard positivity constraint on $\boldsymbol{o}$. The minimization problem [4.25] can thus be rewritten as follows:

$$\boldsymbol{o}^{+} = \underset{\boldsymbol{o} \geq 0}{\arg\min} \left\{\mathcal{C}\big(\boldsymbol{o}, c^{+}(\boldsymbol{o})\big) + \mu_{\text{EP}}\, \mathcal{R}_{\text{EP}}(\boldsymbol{o}) + \mu_{l_1} \mathcal{R}_{l_1}(\boldsymbol{o})\right\} \qquad [4.27]$$

This problem is strictly equivalent but allows the following observation: according to equation [4.20] for the definition of the regularization in l_1 norm, the term $\mathcal{R}_{l_1}(\boldsymbol{o})$ is differentiable under positivity constraints. As such, problem [4.27] becomes a minimization problem of a differentiable criterion under constraints. According to Chapter 3, other more efficient strategies than proximal methods (first-order methods) can be applied to solve it, such as *conjugate gradients* or *quasi-Newton* methods (second-order methods) based on an estimation of the

Hessian criterion (local curvature). For the latter, we can mention the *Broyden–Fletcher–Goldfarb–Shanno (BFGS)* method and its adaptations, in particular to manage constraints (*L-BFGS-B*, *VMLM-B* (Nocedal 1980; Byrd et al. 1995; Thiébaut 2002)). Unlike *FISTA*, the latter (*VMLM-B*) does not require adjusting the descent step t. The reconstruction of Figure 4.4(f) has been obtained by this method and gives the same reconstruction quality as the solution of problem [4.25] with *FISTA*.

Figure 4.8 illustrates the convergence curves of the various solving methods, in terms of evolution of the criterion to be minimized, according to the number of iterations. A slight advantage for *VMLM-B* can be seen but the convergence of each method remains in the same order of magnitude (around 10 iterations). In this figure, *ISTA* can be considered an *ER*-based alternating projection approach. The main conclusion to be drawn from these curves is that an IP approach does not generate any additional cost in terms of computation time: 10 reconstruction iterations of a 512×512 image on a simple CPU running at 3.2 Ghz take about 10 s. Moreover, an iteration of each algorithm requires approximately the same amount of time since each one approximatively requires the computation of the direct model (propagation) and its adjoint (backpropagation).

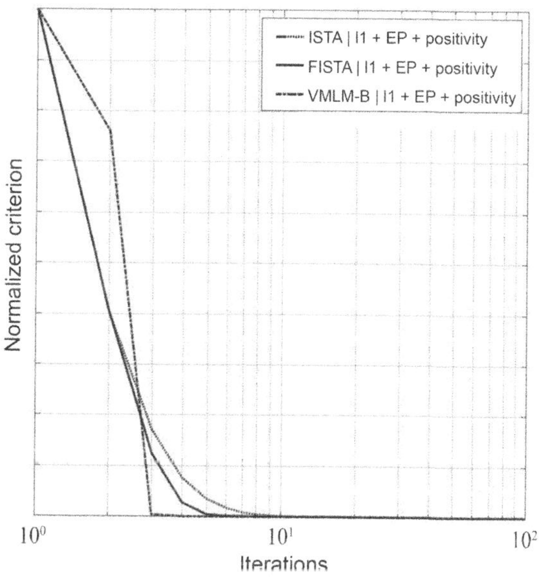

Figure 4.8. *Evolution of the normalized criterion (between 0 and 1) as a function of the number of iterations for three reconstruction criterion minimization methods using an inverse approach with positivity constraint, l_1 + edge-preserving regularizations: ISTA, FISTA and VMLM-B*

According to this case study, the contribution of the IP methodology thus appears very clearly and shows all the interest in addressing reconstruction problems according to this type of approach. Relevant quantitative measurements (for instance, the size of objects of interest) are then facilitated, as are tasks such as automatic object segmentation for statistical object analysis (counting, index value distribution, size, etc.).

4.5. Extended contribution of IP approaches: digital super-resolution and field extension

In [4.18], the distance between data and model is computed by considering the noise covariance matrix. In the case of white noise, the noise covariance matrix is diagonal (coefficients w_q). In this case, it serves to weight the distance between data and model according to the noise variance on each image pixel:

$$\mathcal{C}(\underline{o}) = \sum_q w_q \left| c \left[\mathcal{M}(\underline{o})\right]_q - d_q \right|^2 \qquad [4.28]$$

It can also be used to take missing data into account, in this case the variance tends toward infinity and the weight w_q toward 0. This is the case, for example, for dead or saturated pixels (whose intensities are inaccurate), for pixels in a Bayer matrix, for RGB holograms (Flasseur et al. 2017) or for virtual pixels outside the support of the sensor (Soulez et al. 2007). This methodology can also be employed for reconstructing a digitally super-resolved image, for instance, with a pixel size virtually smaller than the sensor pixel size. An oversampled data grid whose unmeasured values are considered to be missing is then used. These last two cases, reconstruction outside the sensor support (field extension) and digital super-resolution are the ones that we illustrate here.

In conventional imaging, pixel super-resolution consists, from a stack of digital images, acquired with random transverse and subpixel shifts, of reconstructing an image of greater digital resolution. In holography, the first goal of pixel super-resolution is to improve the resolution of the reconstructed object transmittance plane (Figure 4.9).

To address this reconstruction problem using an IP approach, we present below the direct problem, the criterion to be minimized and the proposed algorithm to perform this minimization.

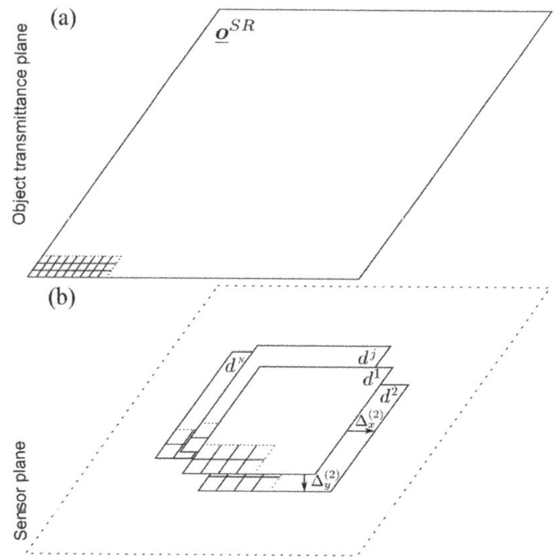

Figure 4.9. *Illustration of the principle of super-resolved and out-of-field holographic reconstruction*

COMMENTS ON FIGURE 4.9.– *(a) Super-resolved object transmittance $\underline{o}^{SR}$ map with extended support (larger than the sensor support). (b) The holograms $\mathbf{d}^j$ transversely shifted by $(\Delta_x^{(j)}, \Delta_y^{(j)})$ with respect to the first hologram are shown in the sensor plane. The pixel and offset size is deliberately enlarged for better visualization.*

4.5.1. *Direct problem*

Consider a stack of N holograms of the same sample acquired with transverse shifts $\vec{\Delta}^{(j)} = (\Delta x^{(j)}, \Delta y^{(j)})$ (relative to the first hologram). For simplicity and without loss of generality, we consider that the sensor is in motion with respect to the object[4]. By considering $|\underline{a}_0|^2$=1, the intensity of the jth hologram of this stack will be modeled mathematically by:

$$\begin{aligned}\mathcal{M}^{(j)}(\underline{o}, \vec{\Delta}^{(j)})(\boldsymbol{r}) &= \left|\underline{\boldsymbol{a}}_{\boldsymbol{z}}{}^{(j)}(\boldsymbol{r})\right|^2 \\ &= \Big[\Big|1 + \underbrace{\underline{o} * \underline{\boldsymbol{h}}_{\boldsymbol{z}}}_{\substack{\text{propagated}\\ \text{complex}\\ \text{amplitude}}} \underbrace{* \delta_{\vec{\Delta}^{(j)}}}_{\substack{\text{transversal}\\ \text{shift}}}\Big|^2 \underbrace{* \boldsymbol{\Pi}_{\kappa p}}_{\substack{\text{integration}\\ \text{on the photosensitive}\\ \text{area}}}\Big](\boldsymbol{r}) \qquad [4.29]\end{aligned}$$

4 A problem with an object in motion with respect to the sensor is similar.

where:

– $\underline{o}$ is the object transmittance.

– $\boldsymbol{\delta}_{\vec{\Delta}^{(j)}}$ is the Dirac distribution centered at $\boldsymbol{r} = \vec{\Delta}^{(j)}$. The convolution by this function models the transversal shift.

– $\boldsymbol{\Pi}_{\kappa p}$ is the bidimensional gate function of width κp. The convolution by this function models the integration on the photosensitive area of a pixel (assumed to be square) with area fill factor κ^2 and width p. It should be underlined that the model can be linearized for purely opaque or weakly phase-shifting objects.

For a reconstruction of the super-resolved object transmittance, the previous model $\mathcal{M}^{(j)}$ is computed over an oversampled grid (which will be denoted by $\mathcal{M}^{SR(j)}$) from a super-resolved object transmittance $\underline{o}^{SR}$ with extended support, if necessary.

4.5.2. *Criterion to be minimized*

The part of the criterion corresponding to the data-fidelity term must not take into account the data artificially added by oversampling and field extension. To this end, the super-resolved model is undersampled and truncated (we will denote by $\mathbf{T}$ the corresponding operator as in [4.16]) in the data-fidelity term:

$$\mathcal{C}(\underline{o}^{SR}, \boldsymbol{\Delta}^{(j)}) = \frac{1}{N} \sum_{j=1}^{N} \left\| c^{+}(\underline{o}^{SR}) \mathbf{T} \left[\mathcal{M}^{SR,(j)}(\underline{o}^{SR}, \boldsymbol{\Delta}^{(j)}) \right] - \boldsymbol{d}^{(j)} \right\|_{\boldsymbol{w}}^{2} \qquad [4.30]$$

where:

– as indicated by equation [4.28], $\boldsymbol{w}$ is a binary weight map of the same size as the model. It acts as a mask: the pixels corresponding to missing or erroneous data are at 0;

– $\|\cdot\|_{\boldsymbol{w}}^2$ is the weighted l_2-norm, defined by: $\|\boldsymbol{b}\|_{\boldsymbol{w}}^2 = \sum_{q=1}^{N} w_q b_q^2$;

– $\boldsymbol{d}^{(j)}$ corresponds to the jth hologram of the stack.

As previously, regularization terms on the object transmittance to be reconstructed can be added to this criterion. They make it possible to enforce sparsity on the object transmittance gradient (minimization of the total variation of $\underline{o}$) or sparsity on the object transmittance (see [4.25]). Similarly, constraints imposed by physically modeling the problem (non-emissive objects, that is $0 < |1 + \underline{o}| < 1$) result in forcing the solution to be physically acceptable.

The criterion to be minimized depends not only on the object transmittance $\underline{o}^{SR}$ to be reconstructed but also on the shifts between holograms $\{\boldsymbol{\Delta}^{(j)}\}_{j=2..N}$:

$$\underline{o}^{SR+} = \underset{\underline{o}^{SR}\in\mathbb{O},\boldsymbol{\Delta}^{(j)}}{\arg\min} \quad \mathcal{C}(\underline{o}^{SR}, \boldsymbol{\Delta}^{(j)}) + \sum_r \mu_r \mathcal{R}_r(\underline{o}^{SR}) \qquad [4.31]$$

by denoting $\mathcal{R}_r$ the rth regularization term and μ_r the associated hyperparameter.

4.5.3. *Alternating reconstruction algorithm*

To solve the digital super-resolution problem [4.31], an alternating minimization strategy can be used. It consists of alternately optimizing the registration between holograms (estimation of $\{\boldsymbol{\Delta}^{(j)}\}_{j=2..N}$) and joint hologram reconstruction ($\underline{o}^{SR}$ estimation). An illustration of an iteration of this algorithm is provided in Figure 4.10.

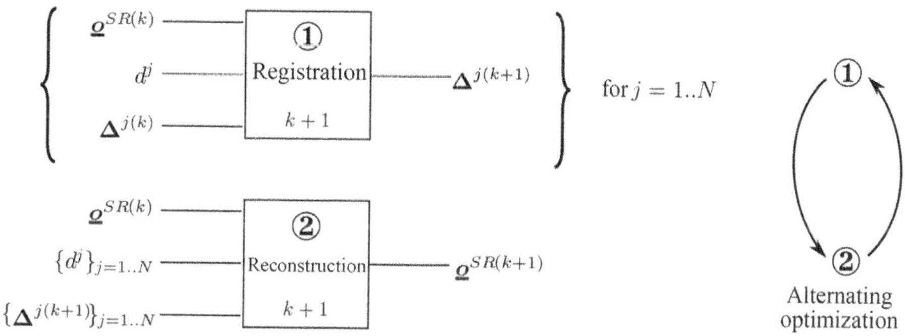

Figure 4.10. *Illustration of the kth iteration of the alternating reconstruction algorithm*

This algorithm has been applied on the experimental holograms of a graduated calibration pattern and compared to a reconstruction using a conventional image super-resolution algorithm, followed by a conventional backpropagation reconstruction (see Figure 4.11). An improvement in the IP reconstruction signal-to-noise ratio and an extension of the reconstructed field can be seen. More details on these results are given in Fournier et al. (2017).

This method improves the conventional super-resolved reconstruction through (1) better hologram subpixel registration and (2) the use of a priori knowledge (sparsity constraints in the presented example) for the IP reconstruction:

– 1) The estimation of shifts between holograms is achieved by searching for the best match, in the sense of (weighted) least squares, between hologram-data and a noise-free model, obtained from the reconstruction of the previous step. However, in the conventional approach, the shifts are estimated by looking for the best match between a digitally registered hologram and a reference hologram, both being noisy.

– 2) The reconstruction methodology by IP approach is based on a hologram formation model including integration on the pixel, for example, and a priori knowledge injected in the regularization terms or constraints.

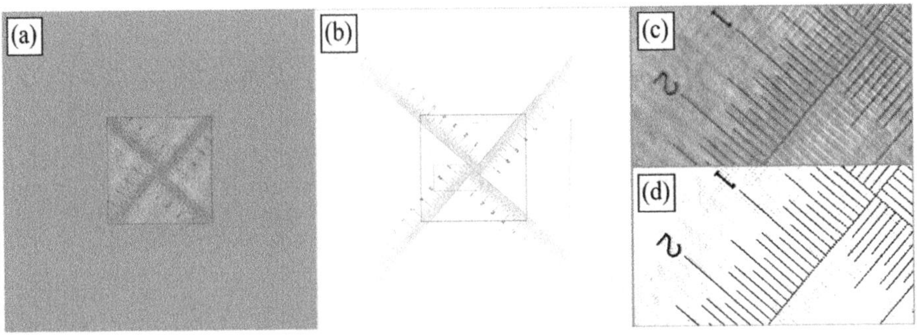

Figure 4.11. *Qualitative comparison of a conventional super-resolved reconstruction (a, c) and an IP approach-based reconstruction (b, d). Subparts (c) and (d) are enlargements of (a) and (b), respectively. The blue frame delineates the sensor support (source: Fournier et al. 2017)*

4.6. Going further

4.6.1. *Model refinement and self-calibration*

Unlike alternating projection methods described in section 4.4.3.2, IP approaches allow for some adaptations or refinement of the model being used. In fact, alternating projection methods are based on a simple backpropagation scheme, followed by applications of constraints on the sample, then by simple propagations. However, further optical phenomena must be considered in the image formation model. This is the case of, for example:

– partial temporal or spatial coherence;

– frequency filtering by the numerical aperture of the lenses;

– optical aberrations of the setup;

– inhomogeneities in the sample illumination, originating when passing through the optical setup, or from stray light.

For instance, for a hologram acquired with an optical setup presenting a partial coherence source, a non-uniform background or even aberrations, it is possible to refine the image formation model to better fit the experiment. Regarding filtering by the numerical aperture, this refinement will simply be a low-pass linear filtering applied on the complex amplitude of the direct model.

Some imaging models require precise knowledge of experimental parameters, such as wavelength, coherence length or magnification. These can be measured during a calibration step of the imaging system using a calibration pattern or calibration objects (Flasseur et al. 2017). For some parameters, it can be appropriate to refine this measurement at the same time as the reconstruction; for example, the magnification, which can vary with the defocusing distance. IP approaches allow for adding to the set of parameters to be reconstructed the parameters of the image formation model. This is called self-calibration.

4.6.2. *Multivariate data reconstruction*

The flexibility of IP approaches also allows for the reconstruction of objects by multivariate or heterogeneous data: a hologram stack acquired at different distances or different transverse shifts (see digital super-resolution in section 4.5), different wavelengths (*multispectral* data), different viewing angles (section 4.6.3), over a time sequence for dynamic tracking of moving objects, etc. Adding information helps to make the reconstruction less sensitive to noise, solution degenerations and thus tend toward a more reliable solution.

In order for this diversity of information to be accounted for, the data-fidelity term will be augmented. For example, for digital super-resolution [4.5], the global data criterion [4.30] consists of summing a least squares criterion per hologram. The same approach would be applied for processing a stack of multi-wavelength holograms. Multivariate data processing is very common in the field of IPs because the formalism easily makes use of this diversity of information.

4.6.3. *Toward 3D reconstruction*

In this chapter, the object model has been simplified and considers only a plane object comprising absorption and phase shift. From the phase-shift information, it is possible to reconstruct an optical thickness (object thickness multiplied by its refractive index), this is thus referred to as 2.5D imaging.

Nevertheless, holography makes it possible to reconstruct, in any plane in the object space, the complex amplitude of the light wave and by way of strong a priori on the objects (spherical or opaque objects, for example), it is possible to reconstruct a distribution of objects in a volume (Denis et al. 2009; Lamadie et al. 2012; Chen et al. 2015).

For thick biological samples composed of various objects, this is no longer possible. The object space must be modeled by a 3D grid of voxels (*volume elements*) forming a set of object transmittance planes. These are also called object space slices. For small and sparse objects, each transmittance plane can be considered to be illuminated by the incident illumination wave (unchanged during propagation in the object space). This corresponds to the first-order Born approximation (Wolf 1969) and the diffracted waves issuing from each plane only interfere with each other at the sensor plane level. The intensity on the sensor is then modeled by the squared modulus of the sum of the complex amplitudes diffracted by each plane. When there are many objects or if there are objects composed of a set of voxels distributed on different slices, it is possible to use a more general model by regarding the wave incident on a plane as the wave diffracted by the plane upstream thereof. This model is called *multi-slice beam-propagation* in the literature (Chowdhury et al. 2019) and makes it possible to take into account the multiple interferences between the waves diffracted by each voxel. In this case, holography is insufficient for capturing the 3D sample structure. It is then necessary to use multiple illumination angles of the sample, following what is done in X-ray scanner imaging (3D reconstruction from hundreds of X-rays acquired from different angles of view); we are now shifting to the field of diffractive tomography which will be covered in Chapter 5. This technique can be seen as an extension of digital holography for 2.5D sample imaging to the observation and reconstruction of 3D samples (whose modeling by a transmittance plane is no longer valid). By means of adapting the image formation model and the data criterion to the sheer number of holograms acquired with different illumination angles, the reconstruction can exploit all the elements of the IP methodology as we have presented them in this chapter.

4.7. References

Aknoun, S., Savatier, J., Bon, P., Galland, F., Abdeladim, L., Wattellier, B.F., Monneret, S. (2015). Living cell dry mass measurement using quantitative phase imaging with quadriwave lateral shearing interferometry: An accuracy and sensitivity discussion. *Journal of Biomedical Optics*, 20(12), 1–15 [Online]. Available at: http://doi.org/10.1117/1.JBO.20.12.126009.

Beck, A. and Teboulle, M. (2009). Fast gradient-based algorithms for constrained total variation image denoising and deblurring problems. *IEEE Transactions on Image Processing*, 18(11), 2419–2434.

Bianco, V., Memmolo, P., Leo, M., Montrésor, S., Distante, C., Paturzo, M., Picart, P., Javidi, B., Ferraro, P. (2018). Strategies for reducing speckle noise in digital holography. *Light, Science & Applications*, 7.

Byrd, R.H., Lu, P., Nocedal, J., Zhu, C. (1995). A limited memory algorithm for bound constrained optimization. *SIAM Journal on Scientific Computing*, 16(5), 1190–1208 [Online]. Available at: http://epubs.siam.org/doi/abs/10.1137/0916069.

Chen, W., Tian, L., Rehman, S., Zhang, Z., Lee, H.P., Barbastathis, G. (2015). Empirical concentration bounds for compressive holographic bubble imaging based on a mie scattering model. *Optics Express*, 23(4), 4715–4725.

Chowdhury, S., Chen, M., Eckert, R., Ren, D., Wu, F., Repina, N., Waller, L. (2019). High-resolution 3D refractive index microscopy of multiple-scattering samples from intensity images. *Optica*, 6(9), 1211–1219.

Denis, L., Lorenz, D., Thiébaut, E., Fournier, C., Trede, D. (2009). Inline hologram reconstruction with sparsity constraints. *Optics Letters*, 34(22), 3475–3477 [Online]. Available at: http://www.osapublishing.org/ol/abs-tract.cfm?uri=ol-34-22-3475.

Doblas, A., Sánchez-Ortiga, E., Martínez-Corral, M., Saavedra, G., Garcia-Sucerquia, J. (2014). Accurate single-shot quantitative phase imaging of biological specimens with telecentric digital holographic microscopy. *Journal of Biomedical Optics*, 19(4), 046022.

Fienup, J.R. (1978). Reconstruction of an object from the modulus of its Fourier transform. *Optics Letters*, 3(1), 27–29 [Online]. Available at: http://www.osapublishing.org/abstract.cfm?uri=ol-3-1-27.

Flasseur, O., Fournier, C., Verrier, N., Denis, L., Jolivet, F., Cazier, A., Lépine, T. (2017). Self-calibration for lensless color microscopy. *Applied Optics*, 56(13), F189–F199.

Flasseur, O., Denis, L., Thiébaut, E., Olivier, T., Fournier, C. (2019). ExPACO: Detection of an extended pattern under nonstationary correlated noise by patch covariance modeling [Online]. Available at: http://hal.archives-ouvertes.fr/hal-02308808.

Fournier, C., Jolivet, F., Denis, L., Verrier, N., Thiébaut, E., Allier, C., Fournel, T. (2017). Pixel super-resolution in digital holography by regularized reconstruction. *Applied Optics*, 56(1), 69–77 [Online]. Available at: http://www.osapublishing.org/abstract.cfm?uri=ao-56-1-69.

Garcia-Sucerquia, J., Xu, W., Jericho, S.K., Klages, P., Jericho, M.H., Kreuzer, H.J. (2006). Digital in-line holographic microscopy. *Appl. Opt.*, 45(5), 836–850 [Online]. Available at: http://ao.osa.org/abstract.cfm?URI=ao-45-5-836.

Gerchberg, R. and Saxton, W. (1972). A practical algorithm for the determination of phase from image and diffraction plane pictures. *Optik*, 35(2), 237–246.

Goodman, J. (1996). *Introduction to Fourier Optics*. McGraw-Hill, New York.

Hooke, R., Allestry, J., Martyn, J. (1665). *Micrographia, or, Some Physiological Descriptions of Minute Bodies Made by Magnifying Glasses: With Observations and Inquiries Thereupon*. Jo. Martyn and Ja. Allestry, London.

Lamadie, F., Bruel, L., Himbert, M. (2012). Digital holographic measurement of liquid–liquid two-phase flows. *Optics and Lasers in Engineering*, 50(12), 1716–1725.

Latychevskaia, T. and Fink, H.-W. (2007). Solution to the twin image problem in holography. *Physical Review Letters*, 98(23), 233901 [Online]. Available at: http://link.aps.org/doi/10.1103/PhysRevLett.98.233901.

Nocedal, J. (1980). Updating quasi-Newton matrices with limited storage. *Mathematics of Computation*, 35(151), 773–782.

Parikh, N. and Boyd, S. (2014). Proximal algorithms. *Foundations and Trends in Optimization*, 1(3), 127–239.

Popescu, G. (2011). *Quantitative Phase Imaging of Cells and Tissues*. McGraw-Hill, New York.

Soulez, F., Denis, L., Thiébaut, E., Fournier, C., Goepfert, C. (2007). Inverse problem approach in particle digital holography: Out-of-field particle detection made possible. *JOSA A*, 24(12), 3708–3716 [Online]. Available at: http://www.osapublishing.org/josaa/abstract.cfm?uri=josaa-24-12-3708.

Thiébaut, E. (2002). Optimization issues in blind deconvolution algorithms [Online]. Available at: http://www.spiedigitallibrary.org/conference-proceedings-of-spie/4847/0000/Optimization-issues-in-blind-deconvolution-algorithms/10.1117/12.461151.short.

Vandewiele, S., Strubbe, F., Schreuer, C., Neyts, K., Beunis, F. (2017). Low coherence digital holography microscopy based on the Lorenz-Mie scattering model. *Opt. Express*, 25(21), 25853–25866 [Online]. Available at: http://www.opticsexpress.org/abstract.cfm?URI=oe-25-21-25853.

Wolf, E. (1969). Three-dimensional structure determination of semi-transparent objects from holographic data. *Optics Communications*, 1(4), 153–156 [Online]. Available at: http://www.sciencedirect.com/science/article/pii/0030401869900522.

Zernike, F. (1942). Phase contrast, a new method for the microscopic observation of transparent objects. *Physica*, 9(7), 686–698 [Online]. Available at: http://www.sciencedirect.com/science/article/pii/S003189144280035X.

5

Transmission Tomographic Diffractive Microscopy

Nicolas VERRIER[1], Matthieu DEBAILLEUL[1], Bertrand SIMON[2] and Olivier HAEBERLÉ[1]

[1] *IRIMAS, Université de Haute-Alsace, Mulhouse, France*

[2] *LP2N, CNRS, IOGS, Université de Bordeaux, Talence, France*

5.1. Introduction

The optical microscope is an irreplaceable tool for biological research, thanks to its unique ability to image living specimens in three dimensions, possibly over long periods of time. Nowadays, fluorescence microscopy is often the reference method, as it allows for specific labeling of structures, and thus of cellular functions, with a sensitivity down to the single molecule. Furthermore, a nanoscopic resolution is possible with the development of STED microscopy techniques or pointillism microscopies, which earned their creators the Nobel Prize in Chemistry in 2014[1]. In some cases, however, the use of fluorescence is to be avoided, which explains the growing interest in the development of new microscopy techniques that do not require sample labeling, such as second or third harmonic generation, or Raman

For a color version of all the figures in this chapter, see www.iste.co.uk/fournier/unconventional.zip.

1 https://www.nobelprize.org/prizes/chemistry/2014/summary/.

microscopies or *coherent anti-stokes Raman scattering* (CARS). These methods have proven their value, but their main disadvantage is that they require complex and expensive instrumentation for image generation.

Many techniques for improving sample visibility in transmission microscopy have been developed: oblique illumination, Rheinberg illumination, dark field microscopy, phase contrast and differential interference contrast microscopies, Dodt gradient contrast microscopy, Huffman modulation, polarized microscopy, etc. Very suitable for dimensional measurements, they remain limited however in that it is difficult to interpret the observed contrast in terms of quantitative measurements of the optical properties.

In fact, the image results from a complex interaction of the specimen with the light illuminating it, and only its intensity is recorded. This contrast makes it possible to detect structures, and is therefore very useful for studying morphological changes, but it does not provide any quantitative information on the optical characteristics of the observed specimen. More particularly, the refractive and absorptive properties mix together to form the final image and, for example, a darker, and therefore apparently more absorbent area may in fact simply result from a destructive interference phenomenon. Coupling modern electronic sensors with the computational capabilities of recent computers has paved the way for new possibilities to reexamine optical microscopy. Phase reconstruction techniques have been developed based on the resolution of the intensity transport equation, DIC image reconstruction or optical ptychography. However, these techniques rely on certain simplifying assumptions, which may restrict their field of application.

5.2. Holographic microscopy: utility and limitations

The utilization of coherent light illumination, with interferometric detection, instead allows the holograms to be recorded directly, encoding the amplitude and phase of the light interacting with the sample. These approaches, known as *digital holographic microscopy* or *phase microscopy*, are very sensitive to small changes in the optical path of the samples due to the unparalleled precision of interferometric measurements. On the other hand, their main drawback probably resides in their low resolution, especially along the optical axis. This limitation is easily understood if we recall that only one illumination direction is used in holographic microscopy. Such a configuration does not meet the classical requirement of transmission microscopy, which consists of using a large numerical aperture (NA) condenser in conjunction with a large NA objective: a Köhler illumination is thus achieved in order to obtain a high resolution image. Holographic microscopy is therefore a very powerful technique when considering integral measurements by projections of accumulated phase changes as light passes through the observed sample. However, in itself it is not a "true" 3D imaging technique effective for imaging transparent samples in transmission mode. It is sometimes referred to as 2.5D imaging, that is, it can be used to image a 2D surface enveloping a 3D volume with high accuracy but not the interior of that volume itself. On the other hand, differences in optical path are measured, resulting from the product of sample thickness by the difference between its optical index and that of its observation medium, but it is not (easily) possible to decouple these two quantities.

In order to compensate for these limitations of holographic microscopy, phase tomography approaches have been proposed. For example, by rotating the sample on itself, a set of 2D phase maps of the sample observed from different angles can be recorded, which are then converted into 3D refractive index maps using a classical Radon transform data back-projection (Barty et al. 2000; Charrière et al. 2006). Nevertheless, this simplified approach disregards the effects of diffraction, and it is no longer suitable when the details sought are of similar size to the observation wavelength. Diffraction limits the quality of the reconstructed data in terms of quantitative refractive index measurements, as well as the final resolution, and can even in some cases lead to misleading reconstructions. In order to obtain the most accurate reconstructions, a diffractive approach must be taken into account, the fundamental ideas of which are recalled in the next section.

5.3. Link between diffracted field and index distribution

5.3.1. *Principle*

Several steps are required to obtain the refractive index map, including the consideration of a direct model describing the diffraction process:

– Establish the direct problem, namely the diffraction model, which will give the link between the refractive index $n(\mathbf{r})$ sought and the measured diffracted field $u_d(\mathbf{r})$. The most common model is based on the Helmholtz equation in a weakly inhomogeneous medium, that is, the index variation is small compared to the surrounding medium.

– Solve the inverse problem, in other words, establish the equations allowing the object to be reconstructed from experimental measurements.

– From an experimental point of view, it is necessary to be able to record the phase and the amplitude of the total electromagnetic field; in optical imaging, this is either ensured by a holographic process coding amplitude and phase, or by digital phase reconstruction (see previous chapters).

– It is necessary to proceed to an aperture synthesis (spectrum extension and data fusion) in order to improve the resolution compared to the simple holography.

5.3.2. *Helmholtz equation in a weakly inhomogeneous medium*

The direct problem is based on the propagation equation in a weakly inhomogeneous medium. For the sake of simplicity, the scalar Helmholtz equation is considered here, that is, possible polarization effects are not taken into account (note that a vector model has also been developed (Lauer 2002)):

$$\nabla^2 u_t(\mathbf{r}) + k^2 u_t(\mathbf{r}) = 0 \qquad [5.1]$$

with $k = k_v n(\mathbf{r})$ and $k_v = \frac{2\pi}{\lambda_v}$, where λ_v is the wavelength in the vacuum, $n(\mathbf{r})$ is the medium index and $u_t(\mathbf{r})$ is the total scalar field (incident field + diffracted field). The positions are marked by the 3D vector $\mathbf{r} = (x\vec{e}_x, y\vec{e}_y, z\vec{e}_z)$.

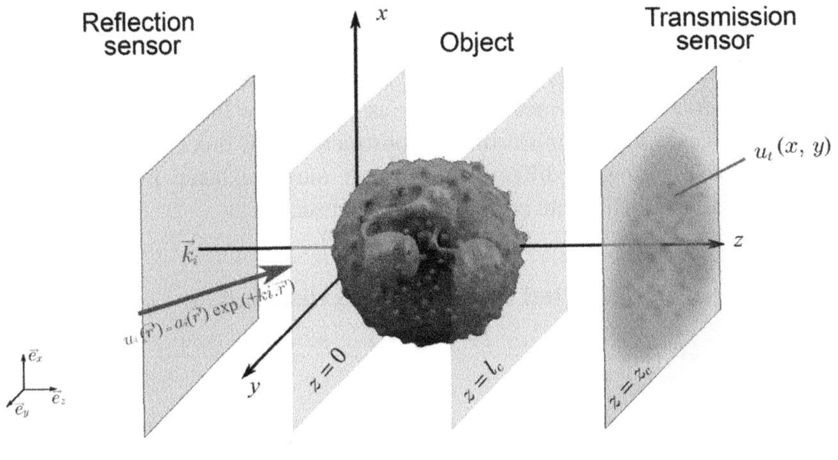

Figure 5.1. *Geometry and notations used for the diffraction problem*

Classically (Born and Wolf 2003), we write the total field $u_t(\mathbf{r})$ as the sum of the incident wave u_i and the diffracted wave u_d:

$$u(\mathbf{r}) = u_i(\mathbf{r}) + u_d(\mathbf{r}) \qquad [5.2]$$

In addition, the plane incident wave u_i ought to satisfy the Helmholtz equation outside the object:

$$\nabla^2 u_i(\mathbf{r}) = -k_0^2 u_i(\mathbf{r})$$

with $k_0 = k_v n_0$ where n_0 is the index of the immersion medium surrounding the object[2].

This allows us to write:

$$(\nabla^2 + k_0^2)u_d(\mathbf{r}) = -k_v^2[n^2(\mathbf{r}) - n_0^2]u_t(\mathbf{r}) \qquad [5.3]$$

$$= -k_0^2(\frac{n^2(\mathbf{r})}{n_0^2} - 1)u_t(\mathbf{r}) \qquad [5.4]$$

$$= -f(\mathbf{r})u_t(\mathbf{r}) \qquad [5.5]$$

So we have:

$$(\nabla^2 + k_0^2)u_d(\mathbf{r}) = -f(\mathbf{r})u_t(\mathbf{r}) \qquad [5.6]$$

where:

$$f(\mathbf{r}) = k_0^2(\frac{n^2(\mathbf{r})}{n_0^2} - 1) = k^2(\mathbf{r}) - k_0^2 \qquad [5.7]$$

is the *diffraction potential*, linked to the object complex index of refraction. This is a real quantity for objects without absorption (purely phase-shifting specimens), and complex in the general case for a phase-shifting and absorbing object.

The differential equation is usually solved using the properties of the Dirac distribution and the Green's function; the latter represents the solution of the wave equation (diffracted field in $\mathbf{r}$) for a Dirac distribution (source point in $\mathbf{r}'$):

$$(\nabla^2 + k_0^2)G(|\mathbf{r} - \mathbf{r}'|) = -\delta(\mathbf{r} - \mathbf{r}') \qquad [5.8]$$

where $G(\mathbf{r} - \mathbf{r}') = \frac{1}{4\pi}\frac{e^{ik_0|\mathbf{r}-\mathbf{r}'|}}{|\mathbf{r}-\mathbf{r}'|}$ (Schmalz et al. 2010) is the Green's function of the 3D Helmholtz equation[3].

2 And thereby approximately equal to the average wave number if δn is small.

3 The constant coefficient may vary, together with that of equation [5.8]. Wolf (1969) recovers the definition used by Baños (1966): $G(\mathbf{r} - \mathbf{r}') = \frac{\exp ik_0|\mathbf{r}-\mathbf{r}'|}{|\mathbf{r}-\mathbf{r}'|}$.

Multiplying by $f(\mathbf{r}')u_t(\mathbf{r}')$ and then integrating on either side of equation [5.8], we obtain the expression:

$$\int (\nabla^2 + k_0^2)G(|\mathbf{r}-\mathbf{r}'|f(\mathbf{r}')u_t(\mathbf{r}'))\mathrm{d}\mathbf{r}' = -\int \delta(\mathbf{r}-\mathbf{r}')f(\mathbf{r}')u_t(\mathbf{r}')\mathrm{d}\mathbf{r}' \quad [5.9]$$

Then, using the property $f(\mathbf{r})u_t(\mathbf{r}) = \int_{-\infty}^{+\infty} f(\mathbf{r}')u_t(\mathbf{r}')\delta(\mathbf{r}-\mathbf{r}')d\mathbf{r}'$ and by identification with equation [5.6], the following solution is obtained:

$$u_d(\mathbf{r}) = \int_V f(\mathbf{r}')u_t(\mathbf{r}')G(|\mathbf{r}-\mathbf{r}'|)\mathrm{d}\mathbf{r}' \quad [5.10]$$

Technically, this integral equation (Lipmann–Schwinger equation) [5.10] is part of the Fredholm second-type homogeneous equations (Zemyan 2012)[4]. The main characteristic of these equations is that they contain the unknown both inside and outside the integral, which makes their solution very difficult, or in general cases even impossible other than numerically (Atkinson 1996).

This integral equation must first be solved in the diffracted field, then we try to evaluate $f(\mathbf{r})$, and thus the complex index, from the measurement of this diffracted field $u_d(\mathbf{r})$.

5.3.3. *Born approximation*

The solution to equation [5.10] is problematic because the integrand contains the diffracted field u_d. The idea then consists of looking for an approximate solution using an approximation on the field. The simplest is the first-order Born approximation, which assumes that the object is weakly diffracting. In this case, the *amplitude* of the diffracted field is small compared to the incident field: $u_d \ll u_i$ and the total field is therefore reduced to the incident field in equation [5.10]:

$$u_d(\mathbf{r}) \simeq u_B^{(1)} = \int_V f(\mathbf{r}')u_i(\mathbf{r}')G(|\mathbf{r}-\mathbf{r}'|)\mathrm{d}\mathbf{r}' \quad [5.11]$$

$u_B^{(1)}$, or more simply u_B, is the first-order diffracted field under the Born approximation.

4 Second-type Fredholm integrals have fixed bounds, and the generic form is $\varphi(x) + \lambda \int_a^b K(x,t)\varphi(t)\mathrm{d}t = f(x)$ where φ is the unknown, λ a real number, f a known function (zero in the homogeneous case). The function K, called the kernel of the integral equation, is a known function, usually set by the system studied in physical problems. Kernels such as $K(x,t) = K(x-t)$ are called *convolution kernels*.

In order to invert equation [5.11], the plane wave decomposition of the Green's function is introduced (Marathay 1975):

$$G(|\mathbf{r}-\mathbf{r}'|)=\frac{i}{4\pi\lambda}\iint_{-\infty}^{\infty}\frac{1}{m}\exp[ik_0(p(x-x') \\ +q(y-y')+m(|z-z'|))]\mathrm{d}p\mathrm{d}q \qquad [5.12]$$

where (p,q,m) are the direction cosines of the diffracted vectors.

This expression is introduced in equation [5.11], and it is assumed that the illumination wave is plane:

$$u_i(\mathbf{r}')=a_i(\mathbf{r}')\exp(i\mathbf{k}_i\mathbf{r}') \qquad [5.13]$$

taking for convention the + sign for waves propagating from left to right (Figure 5.1). Rearranging the terms, and for $z>z'$, it is then obtained that:

$$u_B(\mathbf{r})=\frac{ia_i}{4\pi\lambda}\iint_{-\infty}^{+\infty}\frac{1}{m}\exp[+ik_0(px+qy+mz)]\mathrm{d}p\mathrm{d}q \\ \iiint_V f(\mathbf{r}')\exp\Big[-ik_0\Big((p-p_i)x'+(q-q_i)y'+(m-m_i)z'\Big)\Big]\mathrm{d}^3r' \qquad [5.14]$$

where (p_i,q_i,m_i) are the incident vector director cosines. In the triple integral, the inverse Fourier transform of the ordinary frequency potential is recognizable, defined by:

$$\hat{F}(f_x,f_y,f_z)=\iiint f(x,y,z)\exp\Big[-i2\pi(f_x.x+f_y.y+f_z.z)\Big]\mathrm{d}x\mathrm{d}y\mathrm{d}z \qquad [5.15]$$

This allows the diffracted field to be re-expressed as:

$$u_B(\mathbf{r})=\frac{ia_i}{4\pi\lambda}\iint_{-\infty}^{+\infty}\frac{1}{m}\hat{F}[\frac{2\pi}{\lambda}(p-p_i),\frac{2\pi}{\lambda}(q-q_i)+\frac{2\pi}{\lambda}(m-m_i)] \\ \exp[+ik_0(px+qy+mz)]\mathrm{d}p\mathrm{d}q \qquad [5.16]$$

Equation [5.16] describes the diffracted field according to the formalism used by Wolf (1969). Up to the constant coefficients, we recognize the 2D Fourier transform of:

$$\frac{1}{m}\hat{F}(f_x,f_y,f_z)\exp[+ik_0(+mz)] \qquad [5.17]$$

We simply have to take the inverse Fourier transform (in x, y) of equation [5.16]. This 2D inverse Fourier transform of $\hat{u}_B(\mathbf{r})$ is defined by:

$$\hat{u}_B(f_x, f_y, z) = \iint u_B(x, y, z) \exp[-2i\pi(f_x.x + f_y.y)] \mathrm{d}x\mathrm{d}y \qquad [5.18]$$

The change in variable $f_x = p/\lambda$ and $f_y = q/\lambda$ is then performed in order to express the variables of equation [5.16] in spatial frequencies.

The diffracted spectrum being measured on a 2D sensor (u_d) is then expressed at position z_c in the sensor (Wolf's experimental setup, without image reforming lens (Wolf 1969)). We then obtain the expression:

$$\hat{F}(k_{ox}, k_{oy}, k_{oz}) = \frac{-2ik_{dz}}{a_i} \exp(-ik_{dz}z_c)\hat{u}_B(k_{dx}, k_{dy}; z_c) \qquad [5.19]$$

where $\hat{F}$ and $\hat{u}_d$ are, respectively, the object potential 3D inverse Fourier transform and the 2D inverse Fourier transform of the field diffracted by the object. It should be noted that the division by a_i makes the potential (logically) independent of the illumination wave. Experimentally, the total wave is measured so the input to the reconstruction algorithm requires a method for extracting the incident wave.

Since the problem deals with elastic scattering of light (no energy transfer to matter), the vectors $\mathbf{k_d}$, which are the diffracted wave vectors, and the vectors $\mathbf{k_o}$, which are the object vectors, are related by the relation:

$$\mathbf{k_o} = \mathbf{k_d} - \mathbf{k_i} \qquad [5.20]$$

with $\mathbf{k_i}$ the incident wave vector.

Equation [5.19] shows that the diffracted field spectrum measured in 2D can be used to obtain the object 3D Fourier transform. The 3D reconstruction is performed based on these geometrical properties on the frequency coordinates (see section 5.3.4).

The term $\exp(-ik_{dz}z_c)$ is a backpropagation term (in $z = z_c$). It should be noted that this term is applied to each hologram; given that the object is then reconstructed in a 3D volume, this backpropagation term is a *global* shifting term of the 3D volume under observation. In the case of the experimental setup assumed by Wolf in his original paper (Wolf 1969), this term is used to refocus the 3D object in the volume reconstructed from the out-of-focus diffracted waves. In a setup making use of an optical microscope type configuration, a tube lens reforms the image on the camera and this term can then simply be ignored. The central plane ($z = 0$) of the reconstructed 3D volume will then be the focus plane set during hologram acquisition.

Equation [5.19] differs from that obtained by Wolf (1969) by the constant coefficient, which depends on the convention used for the Fourier transform and the minus sign resulting from the difference in the definition of the object potential. Fourier transforms are expressed by Wolf in wave vectors. The convention adopted here corresponds to the one used for the discrete Fourier transforms (DFT), which are calculated in spatial frequencies, necessary to be able to write computer code for image reconstruction.

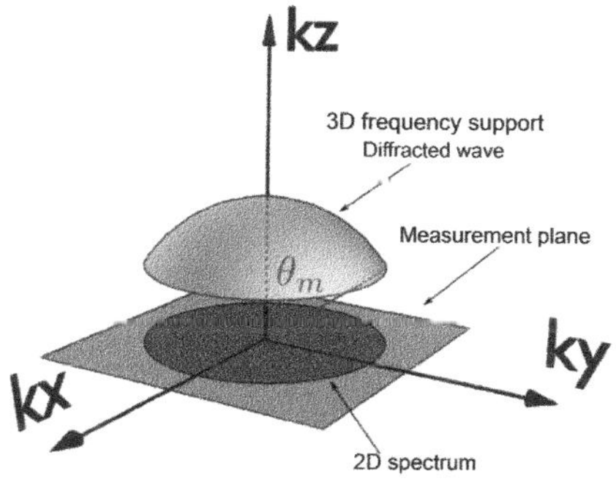

Figure 5.2. *The set of diffracted vectors defines a portion of the Ewald sphere limited by the numerical aperture of the lens. The 2D spectrum is thus also limited by the total numerical aperture of the system, thus defining the maximum collection angle θ_m. It should be noted that the representation is perfect here (continuous surface), which is not the case for the experimental data*

5.3.4. *Spectral support in 3D Fourier space*

Equation [5.20] shows that to each vector $\mathbf{k_d}$ measured in 2D (lateral coordinates k_{dx}, k_{dy}) corresponds an object wave vector $\mathbf{k_o}$ in 3D.

The lateral coordinates of vectors k_d and k_i are obtained from the measurement on the sensor (the original illumination beam, or specular, represents vector k_i), while the longitudinal coordinates (k_{dz} and k_{iz}) are obtained based on the elasticity relation:

$$k_x^2 + k_y^2 + k_z^2 = k_0^2 \qquad [5.21]$$

Applied to the vectors k_d, this reflects the fact that only the elastic diffraction regime is considered (no energy deposition in the specimen, and thus no variation in wavelength of the diffracted photons with respect to the incident photons).

With a fixed incident vector $\mathbf{k_i}$, the coefficients of the object spectrum are thus distributed on a sphere (Ewald's sphere) of radius k_0. However, the limited NA of microscopy objectives makes it impossible to entirely record this sphere. Only a portion thereof is collected, delimited by the maximum collection angle θ_m linked to the numerical objective aperture, which gives the maximum frequency that can be recorded on the camera (Figure 5.2).

To obtain the spectral support of the object, the set of diffracted wave vectors must finally be shifted by subtracting the incident vector $\mathbf{k_i}$ (Figure 5.3). An object image can then be obtained by simple inverse 3D Fourier transform.

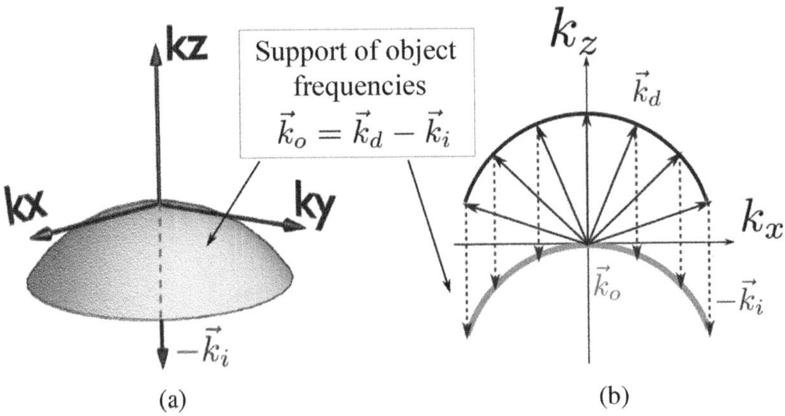

Figure 5.3. *(a) Support of the object spatial frequencies obtained in transmission for an illumination along the optical axis and according to equation [5.20]. (b) Detail of the operation in a 2D central cross-section*

5.3.5. Holographic algorithm

A basic 3D reconstruction algorithm with a single hologram can therefore finally be written as follows:

– from a recorded hologram, reconstruct the phase and amplitude of the measured field;

– compute the 2DFT (2D Fourier Transform) of the diffracted field;

– identify the specular coordinates of the diffracted field, which is the pixel of maximum intensity, in order to obtain $k_{i\perp} = (k_{ix}, k_{iy})$;

– compute the coordinate k_{iz} with the elasticity relation: $k_{ix}^2 + k_{iy}^2 + k_{iz}^2 = k_0^2$;

– extract the values $k_{d\perp} = (k_{dx}, k_{dy})$ and compute k_{dz} with the relation:

$$(k_{dx} - k_{ix})^2 + (k_{dy} - k_{iy})^2 + (k_{dz} - k_{iz})^2 = k_0^2 \qquad [5.22]$$

– project the coefficients onto the Ewald sphere cap;

– compute the inverse 3DFT (3D Fourier Transform).

This simple approach already anticipates some limitations of holographic microscopy. From Figure 5.3, it is understood that the extension along $k_x - k_y$ of the set of object vectors k_o will provide a good lateral resolution in the image space. In contrast, the small extension along the k_z axis (a sphere cap having zero thickness in mathematical terms) will be represented by very poor longitudinal resolution.

In fact, without additional assumptions about the sample, holographic imaging is not true 3D imaging. It is sometimes referred to as 2.5D imaging; we can easily identify 2D surfaces folded into 3D, such as the outer surface of a reflective object (reflection holography) or reconstruct the thickness profile of a transparent object with uniform index (transmission holography).

5.4. From holography to tomography

In order to improve the 3D reconstructions, it is therefore necessary, before the final 3D Fourier transform, to increase filling with object vectors k_o in the Fourier space, which is what the various diffractive tomography techniques developed in recent years thus aim to do.

Figure 5.4 resumes the information acquisition process with a holographic microscope, considering the reconstruction of the 3D image of a transparent specimen according to the Born approach described in the previous section (Figure 5.4(a)). It also describes the principle of filling the Fourier space to extend the optical transfer function (OTF) in diffractive tomographic microscopy with illumination rotation or TDM-IR (Figures 5.4(b–d)), TDM-SR specimen rotation (Figures 5.4(e–g)) and a combination of these two TDM-IRSR techniques (Figure 5.4(h–k)).

The following sections describe these three techniques developed for TDM systems in transmission.

5.4.1. *Illumination rotation*

In TDM with illumination rotation, this illumination can be inclined (Figure 5.4(b)). This is achieved by adding in a holographic microscope an optical system making it possible to control the incidence angle of the illumination on the specimen, an angle which is conventionally zero; in other words, with an illumination that is colinear to the optical axis of the hologram recording system. It should be noted that the position of the detected frequencies k_d is the same as previously, which reflects the fact that the detection system is fixed with respect to the observed object. On the other hand, the application of the vector construction of the diffraction (Figure 5.3) shows that another sphere cap of the object frequencies k_o can now be recorded (Figure 5.4(b)).

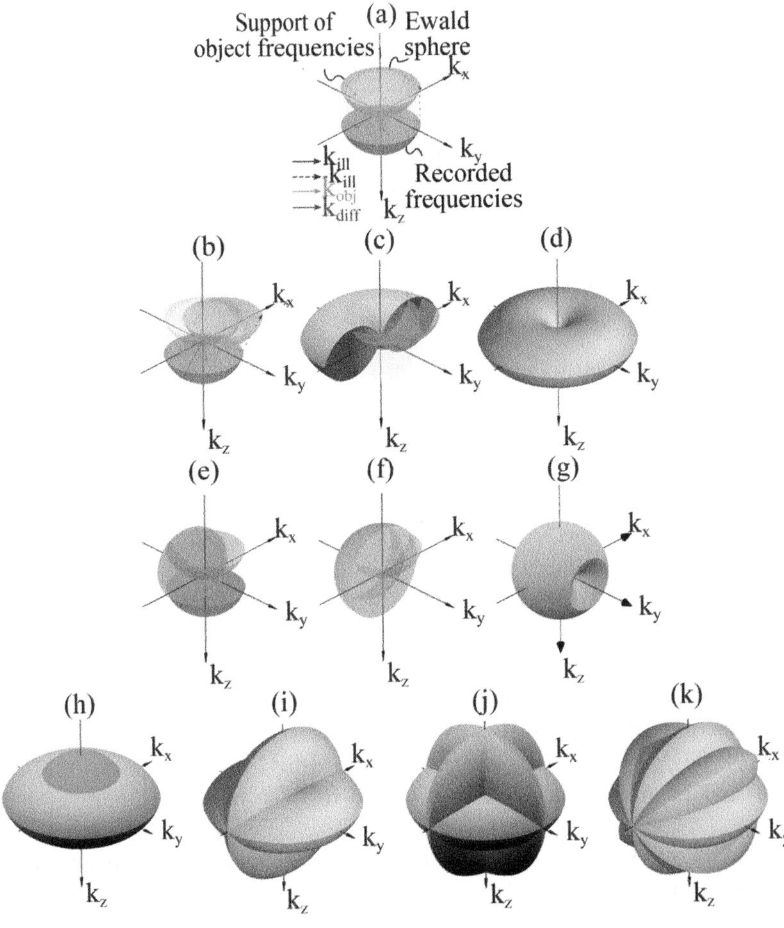

Figure 5.4. *Geometric construction of theoretical frequency supports in TDM*

COMMENTS ON FIGURE 5.4.– *(a) Holographic microscopy with a single illumination parallel to the optical axis. (b) With an inclined illumination, another set of object frequencies is recorded. (c) With a large number of illuminations, an extended support is reconstructed (only half is drawn here). (d) Full support for a large number of illuminations. (e) TDM with sample rotation, a change in the sample* *angle corresponds to a rotation of the recorded frequency set around the same axis. (f) Similarly, for a large number of illuminations, an extended support is obtained (here again, only half is shown). (g) Full support for a large number of object orientations. (h) TDM combining the two approaches by successive acquisitions (one illumination rotation acquisition and then one specimen rotation acquisition); as such, the supports shown in (d) and (f) are added. (i, j, k) If the specimen rotation is implemented, it is also possible to make an acquisition in illumination rotation for each object position: with two positions corresponding to a 90° rotation around the x axis (i), with three positions corresponding to a 90° rotation around the x axis and a 90° rotation around the y axis (j), for four sample positions (four 45° rotations around the x axis) for which a nearly spherical support is obtained (k).*

It is also important to note that the angular extension of the spherical cap of the detected frequencies k_d is a function of the NA of the detection lens. Similarly, the translation of this sphere cap to obtain the object frequencies k_o is limited by the NA of the illumination system, which determines the maximum inclination angle of the incident wave.

For a large number of illuminations, an aperture synthesis-based approach, by accumulating the object frequencies k_o captured for each illumination inclination, then provides an expanded and filled frequency support (Figures 5.4(c) and (d)). For simplification, only the case where the NA of the illumination is identical to the NA of the detection is considered here.

In this configuration, the final optical transfer function is symmetric about the origin. In addition, the characteristic "wedge" shape of the optical transfer function of transmission optical microscopy is clearly recognizable. This shape explains the better resolution and optical sectioning capabilities of TDM compared to holographic microscopy (conversely, a holographic microscope can be thought of as a simplified, single-illumination tomographic microscope).

This transfer function has several remarkable characteristics:

– Its lateral extension is doubled compared to that of a holographic microscope (Lauer 2002). The lateral resolution can thus be theoretically improved by a factor 2, a little less in practice (Debailleul et al. 2009; Cotte et al. 2013).

– The longitudinal extension is also doubled compared to holographic microscopy, but mainly the fact of having an extended and filled support allows for true 3D imaging, that is, the possibility of reconstructing an object in 3D, and not simply of reconstructing a complex 2D surface in a 3D volume. On the other hand, since the longitudinal extension is much less than the lateral extension, the longitudinal resolution will be worse than the lateral resolution.

– It is important to note the presence of a (*missing cone*) along the optical axis (Streibl 1985). This is reflected by low optical sectioning capabilities along this axis (compared to a confocal microscope, for example).

Diffractive tomographic microscopy with rotational illumination has proven itself, and it is now even available in commercial form; so it can be used by any interested biologist without having to wait for specific experimental developments. However, the obtained measurements can suffer from two limitations: the non-isotropic resolution means that measurements of shapes, volumes and concentrations can be affected by systematic errors (e.g. a small bead (a few μm) will appear elongated along the optical axis, and thus the measurement of its volume will be overestimated). In addition, image quality can be affected by the so-called "missing cone" problem along the optical axis (Figure 5.4(d)): this is reflected, for example, by the fact that the interfaces perpendicular to the optical axis are not detected, which makes the observation of cell membranes difficult.

Things can be improved if advanced reconstruction methods and/or a priori knowledge about the sample are employed; these will result in digitally filling in the missing cone, leading to improved optical slices, but the final images will still be characterized by strong resolution anisotropy, resulting from the shape of the OTF.

In particular, methods based on inverse problems for reconstruction (see Chapters 3 and 4) and approaches making use of artificial intelligence are very promising for extracting physical parameters very accurately and/or for improving the quality of reconstructed images (Kamilov et al. 2015, 2016; Berdeu et al. 2017; Pham et al. 2018).

5.4.2. *Sample rotation*

At the macroscopic scale (X-ray medical imaging, X- or gamma-ray industrial quality control), the common procedure consists of performing a tomography by rotating the sample on itself, or by rotating the source-sensor assembly around the sample, as in a medical scanner.

The adaption of the technique to the microscopic scale therefore seems natural. It is however important to stress the high accuracy requirements for the rotation of the sample and/or the lighting/detection device; not only are the specimens small, and the aim is a micrometric resolution, but moreover the holographic measurements are very sensitive, and thus any parasitic movement at the time of the rotation results in errors in phase measurements. The holograms can nevertheless also be reajusted to compensate for these errors.

The first experiments in this field were done with relatively large specimens, and therefore with objectives with large working distance and relatively small NA. In such a setup, it is then usual to disregard the effects of diffraction if high resolution is not the main objective. This is equivalent to disregarding the sphere cap curvature of the detected frequencies. The support of the set of captured frequencies is therefore a disk in Fourier space. When the specimen is rotated by an angle α, each recorded disk is therefore shifted in Fourier space by an angle $-\alpha$, which describes a full sphere. After reconstruction, a final isotropic resolution image will be obtained.

If the diffraction is taken into consideration, the situation becomes more complex. The curvature of the whole frequency range cannot be ignored (especially at large NAs). Rotating a sphere cap along an axis constructs an OTF, which is no longer a complete sphere. Figures 5.4(e–g) describe the object frequency support thus obtained.

This transfer function has the following characteristics:

– its lateral extension is smaller than for illumination rotation but the longitudinal frequency coverage is much better, which is more favorable for accurate morphological measurements;

– on the other hand, due to the curvature of the initial sphere cap, a hole remains along the axis of rotation of the sample (Figure 5.4(g)), known as the "apple-core" of missing frequencies (*missing apple-core*) (Vertu et al. 2009).

Therefore, stricto sensu, this approach does not provide isotropic resolution images. There remains a small, but nevertheless noticeable, residual elongation along the axis of rotation of the sample (Lin and Cheng 2014). A solution to completely fill the OTF would be to perform a second acquisition via a rotation of the sample around another axis, perpendicular to the first one (vertically or horizontally).

5.4.3. *Sample and illumination rotation*

In TDM with illumination rotation, the lateral and axial resolutions are improved compared to holography, and true 3D imaging is possible. Nonetheless, from Figure 5.4(d), it can be deduced that the smaller extension of the OTF along the direction k_z (corresponding to the optical axis) and the presence of the "missing cone" of uncaptured frequencies along the same axis result in lower axial resolution than lateral resolution, and poor optical sectioning capabilities for 3D samples.

If a sample rotation technique is used (Figure 5.4(g)), the resulting OTF is spherical and almost completely full. However, a small set of missing frequencies remains along the sample rotation axis, slightly degrading the resolution in this direction. In addition, the diameter of this nearly spherical OTF is smaller than the lateral extension of the OTF obtained with illumination rotation.

In practice, sample rotation is carried out along an axis perpendicular to the optical axis. The axes along which frequencies are missing in both techniques (optical axis in Figure 5.4(d) and sample rotation axis in Figure 5.4(g)) are therefore perpendicular. It has therefore been proposed to combine the two methods in order to obtain OTFs with no "hole" (Vertu et al. 2011). Three approaches are possible:

– Combining the data obtained by illumination rotation acquisition with those obtained via a sample rotation acquisition yields the OTF described in Figure 5.4(h). It can be seen that the cone of the missing frequencies in Figure 5.4(d) is filled by the quasi-sphere of Figure 5.4(g). The resulting OTF has been referred to as the "flying saucer" in the literature (Vertu et al. 2011). On the other hand, the disadvantage of this approach is that it requires a large number of sample rotations (Vinoth et al. 2018).

– A more efficient approach is to merge several TDM "doughnuts" with illumination rotation, which requires only a few sample rotations (Vertu et al. 2011; Simon et al. 2017). Figures 5.4(i-k) show the OTF support obtained for two, three and four acquisitions by rotating the sample after the first acquisition by 90°, or twice 90° along two different axes, or still by 45°, 90° and then 135°, respectively. Extended and quasi-spherical OTFs are obtained (Figure 5.4(k)), which will yield images with twice the resolution of holography, but mainly with isotropic resolution, without any specific direction affected by an effect of missing frequencies (Vertu et al. 2011; Simon et al. 2017; Ziemczonok et al. 2019; Lee et al. 2021).

– The variant with only three acquisitions (Figure 5.4(j)) also results in obtaining a quasi-spherical OTF (Vertu et al. 2011). It consists of performing a TDM acquisition by illumination rotation, and then rotating the sample by 90°, first along the x axis, then along the y axis. It should be noted that there are still eight directions less well covered in terms of recorded frequencies. This approach has not yet been implemented in practice.

REMARK.– Starting from Figure 5.4 which is in 3D, we can easily draw in 2D, in the k_x-k_y plane and in the k_x-k_z plane, the OTFs of a holographic microscope, a tomographic diffractive microscope with illumination rotation, and a tomographic diffractive microscope with sample rotation. We simply consider Ewald circles instead of Ewald spheres (see Figure 5.3).

For the sake of simplicity, we consider that the NA of the illumination is identical to the detection NA, with respect to the observation wavelength λ and the observation medium index n, the lateral and longitudinal extensions of the optical transfer functions (resolution as Nyquist defines it) are then written for the setups being examined as:

$$R_{x,y}^{Holo} = \lambda/(2nsin\theta) \text{ and } R_z^{Holo} = \lambda/(n(1-cos\theta)) \quad [5.23]$$

$$R_{x,y}^{MTD-RI} = \lambda/(4nsin\theta) \text{ and } R_z^{MTD-RI} = \lambda/(2n(1-cos\theta)) \quad [5.24]$$

$$R_{x,z}^{MTD-RS} = \lambda/(4nsin(\theta/2)) \text{ and } R_y^{MTD-RS} = \lambda/(2nsin\theta) \quad [5.25]$$

$$R_{x,y,z}^{MTD-RIRS} = \lambda/(4nsin\theta) \quad [5.26]$$

It can therefore be seen that only an approach combining sample and illumination rotation is able to deliver isotropic resolution images, as can be seen in Figure 5.5, which shows the type of image that can be obtained with these different methods.

5.5. Practical implementations

5.5.1. *Sample rotation techniques*

The main advantage of this approach is that a standard holographic microscope can be used since the interferometric acquisition system is static. The difficulty lies in achieving high-accuracy sample rotations, compatible with interferometric measurements for reconstructions, whereas a large number of acquisitions is required if the Fourier space is to be filled correctly.

To this end, samples can be encapsulated in a microcapillary (Kuś et al. 2014; Lin and Cheng 2014), which is then used as a mechanical support for the rotation. This approach simplifies sample handling but may require some care in the image reconstruction process given the microcapillary may act as a cylindrical lens, distorting the observed sample (Kostencka et al. 2015). It also requires lenses with larger working distance, thus having a smaller NA, limiting the final resolution. Although this technique has proven its worth, sample handling remains sensitive, which has limited its acceptance.

In some cases, the sample itself can be directly rotated, such as when observing optical fibers or microtips (Simon et al. 2017; Gorski and Osten 2007; Dragomir et al. 2008; Kostencka et al. 2017), but this does not generally apply to biological samples, for which handling approaches need to be developed (it may work for particular samples such as textile fibers (Malek et al. 2016)).

The manipulation of microscopic objects by light is an active research topic and recently, optical tweezers have indeed been successfully used to perform TDM observations (Habaza et al. 2015, Kim et al. 2015; Lin et al. 2017). Conversely, it has been shown that accurate knowledge through TDM measurements of the sample 3D refractive index distribution can be used to optimize trapping with optical tweezers of any arbitrarily shaped microscopic samples (Kim and Park 2017; Lee et al. 2021).

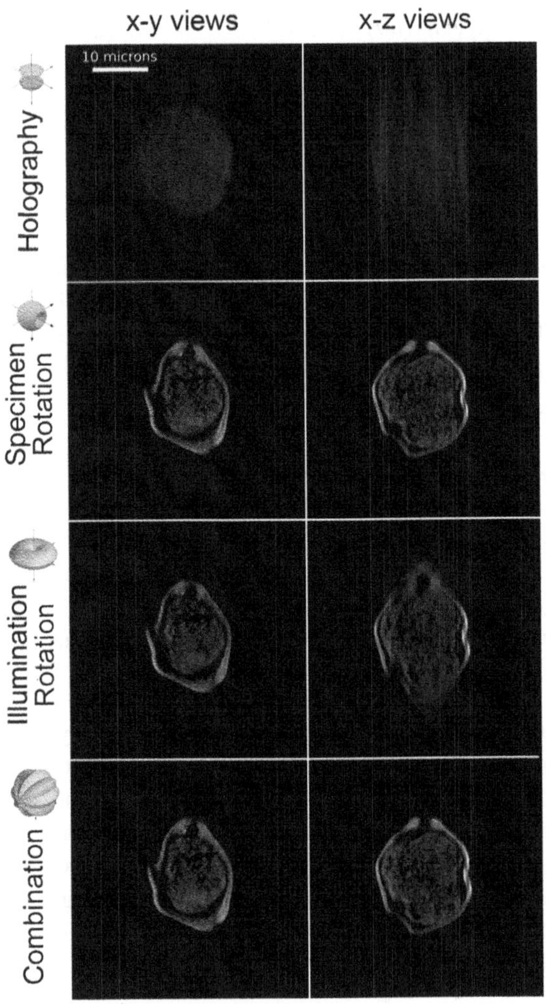

Figure 5.5. *Birch pollen grain (Betula pendula) views for different TDM setups: holographic microscopy with a single illumination parallel to the optical axis, in TDM by specimen rotation, TDM by illumination rotation and in TDM combining specimen and illumination rotation*

In some cases, since the sample has electrical potential variations, use of an electric field induces sample motion. Cell rotation by dielectrophoresis has therefore also been used in tomography (Habaza et al. 2017). Rotation induced by cells passing through microfluidic channels has also been used successfully (Merola et al. 2017; Villone et al. 2018). Sample rotation has also been utilized in combination with in-line holographic microscopy to simplify the setup used (Remacha et al. 2014).

5.5.2. *Scanning illumination techniques*

Specimen rotation techniques imply that the specimen has to be handled, which raises specific problems and also limits the class of observable specimens, which must be isolable (single cells, pollens, natural or artificial fibers, microcrystals). For these reasons, TDM with illumination rotation is often preferred, as it allows the samples to be studied with the usual preparation protocols.

As discussed in section 5.4.1, the optimal set of illuminations, the one that by aperture synthesis will provide the greatest extension of frequency support and thus the best resolution, must meet two requirements:

– cover the largest possible angular aperture;

– fill in the object frequency support as best as possible.

The technical implementation of these two requirements can be complex because of the need to control illumination angles over large apertures in a constrained optical system and the need to obtain an optimal sampling of object frequencies through the acquisition of data sets that will increase with the aperture angle. They impact both the acquisition time and the amount of data to process. On the other hand, the possible use of moving parts (scanning mirrors for instance) can degrade system stability and therefore image quality.

5.5.2.1. *Opto-mechanical scanning*

In order to perform the angular scan on the specimen, an optical assembly is devised that is capable of scanning the rear aperture of a condenser or a microscope objective utilized as a condenser with a focused beam. For this purpose, an opto-mechanical system can be used based on stepper mirrors (Lauer 2002; Simon et al. 2008; Debailleul et al. 2009; Simon et al. 2010), fast tip-tilt mirrors (Liu et al. 2014; Simon et al. 2017; Foucault et al. 2019; Taddese et al. 2021), galvanometric mirrors (Choi et al. 2007; Sung et al. 2012; Kostencka et al. 2016) or rotating prisms (Kawata et al. 1990; Cotte et al. 2013).

Stepper mirrors are simple to use and their main advantage is that they allow for large angular deflections, which makes them suitable for use with conventional microscope condensers but they are slow and sensitive to vibrations. This is why faster devices are now preferred. Galvanometric mirror-based systems are the fastest, resulting in TDM data acquisitions at the rate of about 10 3D images per second, through the use of an ultrafast camera recording about 4,500 holograms per second and with post-reconstruction (Kim et al. 2011). Membrane tip-tilt mirrors are also very fast but are limited by the fact that they are merely able to provide small angular deviations, making it so that high magnification lenses must be used as condensers, which limits the possible working distances.

In some cases, the use of a simple rotating arm (Berdeu et al. 2018; Zdańkowski et al. 2021) makes it possible to achieve an angular scanning with fixed angle (annular scanning), often satisfactory enough in practice (Krauze et al. 2015); the microscope manufactured by Nanolive is also based on this principle.

5.5.2.2. *Optical scan*

By acting directly on the phase of the light beam illuminating them, spatial light modulators (SLMs) are ideal candidates for deflecting a wave without involving any mechanical motion. They have therefore also been used in TDM, advantageously replacing galvanometric or tip-tilt mirrors (Kuś et al. 2015; Chowdhury et al. 2017; Lin et al. 2018; Vinoth et al. 2018; Balasubramani et al. 2019; Deng et al. 2020). However, the speed of these systems, with repetition rates of a few tens of Hertz at best is slower than that of resonant galvanometric mirrors (repetition rate in kHz). SLMs based on ferroelectric crystals are much faster but have not yet been used in this field. On the other hand, these SLMs can also be used to correct the aberrations induced by the various optics present on the path of the illumination beam (active optics), in contrast to an a posteriori correction on the recorded holograms, which also measure these aberrations (Liu et al. 2014).

Another approach is based on the use of a matrix of micromirrors (*digital micromirror device* (DMD)). Initially developed for applications such as digital projectors, DMDs work by reflection on micromirrors that can switch between two different positions: deflecting (pixel ON) or not deflecting (pixel OFF) the incident beam. DMDs are fast but, acting as diffraction gratings, they imply specific constraints: it is necessary to filter out unwanted diffraction orders to produce the plane waves necessary for illumination, the illumination directions have discretized positions and are not continuous as with tip-tilt or galvanometric mirrors. Several groups have nevertheless used DMDs successfully in TDMs (Shin et al. 2015, 2016; Lee et al. 2017; Jin et al. 2018), and form the basis of the systems sold by Tomocube, Inc.

5.5.2.3. *Electronic scanning*

A method that would combine, at least in theory, the advantages of the two previous approaches (speed and no mechanical motion) would be to use a fully electronically-performed scan, with a set of light sources (pixels) corresponding to the desired illumination directions. The first implementation of this concept was made using a set of LEDs (Isikman et al. 2011), but with a 1D scan (in azimuth only), and according to a lensless imaging principle, in Gabor holography.

This technique has been successfully used in ptychography applications (Tian et al. 2014; Sen et al. 2016; Pan et al. 2018), in which phase and amplitude are not measured but digitally reconstructed. A complete implementation of this type of illumination in TDM still remains to be done, but should benefit from the approaches developed in ptychography.

5.6. Reconstruction under the Born hypothesis

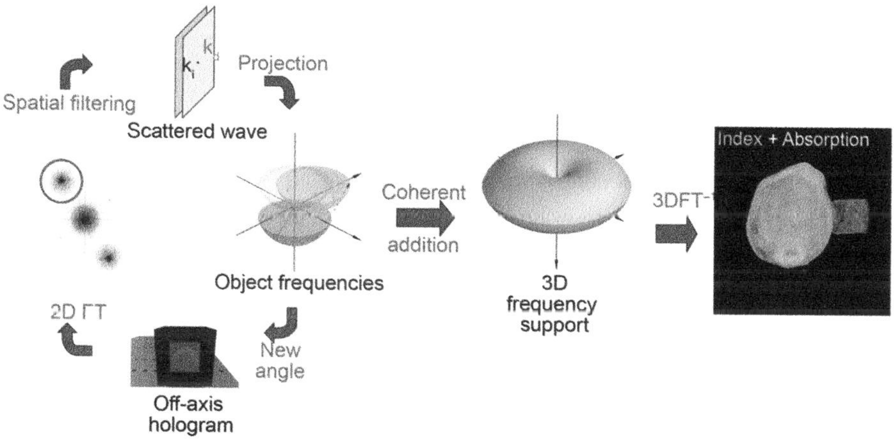

Figure 5.6. *Acquisition/reconstruction principle in TDM: following the acquisition of an off-axis hologram for a given illumination, a 2D Fourier transform is carried out, which, following a spatial filtering of order 1, makes it possible to obtain the Fourier coefficients of the diffused wave*

COMMENTS ON FIGURE 5.6.– *These coefficients are projected onto a sphere cap whose position is defined by the illumination angle. These steps are repeated for each illumination angle and the caps are accumulated by coherent addition. For a sufficient number of angles and covering the entire NA of the condenser, an extended and filled frequency support is obtained. A 3D Fourier transform is then performed to obtain, in the end, a three-dimensional image of the object according to the real and imaginary components of the complex index (refractive and absorption index).*

This approach is the simplest to implement since it is just based on Fourier transforms. A basic algorithm for 3D tomographic reconstruction with a succession of holograms acquired by varying the illumination conditions of the specimen can be deduced from the algorithm described previously for holography, and is described by Figure 5.6:

– from the first recorded hologram, reconstruct the phase and amplitude of the measured field;

– compute the 2DFT of the diffracted field. Measure the specular amplitude and phase, which is the maximum intensity pixel. To normalize the measurements between them, divide by this value;

– identify the coordinates of the diffracted field specular in order to obtain $k_{i\perp} = (k_{ix}, k_{iy})$;

– compute the coordinate k_{iz} with the elasticity relation: $k_{ix}^2 + k_{iy}^2 + k_{iz}^2 = k_0^2$;

– extract the values $k_{d\perp} = (k_{dx}, k_{dy})$ and compute k_{dz} with the relation:

$$(k_{dx} - k_{ix})^2 + (k_{dy} - k_{iy})^2 + (k_{dz} - k_{iz})^2 = k_0^2 \qquad [5.27]$$

– project the coefficients onto the Ewald sphere cap;

– either vary the illumination or rotate the specimen on itself, or both, and repeat the process to fill the Fourier space;

– when it is considered that enough data have been taken, and thus that the Fourier space has been correctly filled, compute the inverse 3DFT.

5.6.1. *Examples of commercial systems*

TDM systems are currently developed in optical and instrumentation laboratories, and the technique continues to be developed for the purpose of optimizing it (Taddese et al. 2021) or simplifying it (Foucault et al. 2019), accelerating the acquisitions (Sung 2019) or developing new modalities (hyperspectral TDM (Jung et al. 2016; Sung 2018) or polarized TDM (van Rooij and Kalkman 2020; Saba et al. 2021)). However, for end-users who do not want to develop such an instrument, there are several commercial variations.

The company Nanolive[5] was created in 2013 and emerged from the research carried out by Christian Depeursinge's group at the *Ecole polytechnique federale de Lausanne*, Switzerland. It proposes an instrument based on the illumination scanning technique, with 532 nm illumination, and uses an air objective (NA 0.8) for a lateral resolution advertised to be better than 200 nm. An originality of this instrument is that it performs the angular scan by means of a rotating arm, which allows a large free space above the sample. Therefore, the sample can be prepared between slide and coverslip, or in Petri dishes, and also in an incubator, or with 96-well plates, which makes it a rather versatile instrument.

5 https://www.nanolive.ch.

Tomocube, Inc.[6] started as a company in 2016 following the research of JongKeun Park's group at the Korea Advanced Institute of Science and Technology (KAIST, Daejeon, South Korea) by commercializing an instrument that is instead dedicated to high resolution, based on a water-immersion lens (NA 1.2) with 570 nm or 532 nm illumination, and lateral and longitudinal resolutions advertised at 110 nm and 356 nm, respectively. One of the strong advantages of this instrument is its fast data acquisition, based on the use of a DMD to perform the illumination angular scanning, making it possible to image up to 2.5 3D images per second (or 150 2D images per second).

Phi Optics, Inc. was founded in 2009 and transfers the studies carried out by Gabriel Popescu's group at the University of Illinois Urbana-Champaign in the US. The approach is different, based on white light illumination and a modulation of the detected interferometric signal, using a phase modulator. The technique can be seen as a generalization of phase contrast microscopy, the phase ring having a controllable phase shift, with a digital reconstruction. The advantage of this technique is that it does not require any specific microscope. On the other hand, the achieved resolution is lower and to carry out a tomography, a z-scan of the specimen is necessary.

In a similar vein, by using a wavefront analyzer, such as those supplied by Phasics S.A. (Saint-Aubin, France) and based on the four-wave lateral interferometry technology, it is also possible, with the same advantages and disadvantages, to achieve an index tomography at the microscopic scale.

5.7. Conclusion

In this chapter on TDM, we have described the most common data acquisition principles and the simplest image reconstruction method, based on the first Born approximation, thus allowing fast image reconstructions given that they are based on simple Fourier transforms. This limits the class of objects that can be analyzed with this technique but a large volume of literature has been dedicated to developing inversion approaches bypassing this limitation. These involve deconvolution, techniques that enable a reduction in the number of images to be taken and approaches that take into account large phase changes, in thick and/or absorbing samples.

This imaging method is capable of providing high-resolution images of unlabeled samples and is generating increasing interest. This is due to its performance (better resolution than holography or conventional unlabeled microscopies; possibility of very fast imaging as it is not limited by weak signals as in fluorescence) and to the

6 http://www.tomocube.com.

fact that commercial systems are now available. Nevertheless, certain limitations still affect the technique, which has led to a great deal of research to broaden its field of application and simplify its use.

Its sequential nature limits the final acquisition speed, a single 3D image requiring a few tens to a few hundred holograms to be recorded. Moreover, the image must be recomputed after the acquisitions. This drives developments to increase the data acquisition speed, as well as to accelerate image computations and rendering. By combining acquisitions, camera-computer transfer rates and fast GPU reconstructions, the display in real time of 3D images would be achievable (Bailleul et al. 2018).

Another active area of research focuses on multimodal imaging. Commercial TDM systems offer complements in fluorescence imaging, but not yet in confocal microscopy and/or with associated imaging modes such as fluorescence lifetime imaging, or fluorescence recovery after photobleaching, or modern super-resolution methods. It is likely that by providing additional information, more imaging modalities will be included in the systems in the future. An all-in-one polarized hyperspectral tomographic microscopy system would make it possible to obtain all recordable optical information from a specimen, leading to greater specificity; absorption is often highly variable according to the wavelength and polarization provides specific information about birefringent samples.

Finally, unlike systems operating in intensity only, TDM records all the physical information resulting from the interaction between the illumination wave and the specimen. This makes it possible to reconstruct images that would be obtained by other transmission optical microscopes (Meyrueis et al. 2017, Chapter 18).

Figure 5.7 illustrates these remarks with the images, recomputed from the same holograms acquired in TDM, giving the index and absorption (TDM reconstruction), the image in intensity only (Meyrueis et al. 2017), which would be obtained in a bright-field microscope (computed by taking the squared high norms of the different measured fields, and finally summed), as well as the image that would be obtained in a dark-field microscope[7] (Meyrueis et al. 2017; Chang et al. 2020), obtained by the same procedure, but after digital specular extinction, whose position is identified according to the procedure described in Figure 5.6.

Similarly, rigorous modeling of the image formation process can result in simulating an oblique illumination microscope, or a Rheinberg illumination

7 A dark-field microscope requires the use of a condenser whose numerical aperture is larger than that of the collection objective. The condenser is coupled to a ring filter for keeping only the contribution at the maximum numerical aperture. Therefore, only the contribution scattered by the object on a dark background is collected (hence the name of the technique).

microscope (Fan et al. 2019), a phase-contrast microscope, a differential phase contrast microscope (Vishnyakov et al. 2016), etc. This approach could also be recombined with polarized imaging techniques (van Rooij and Kalkman 2020; Saba et al. 2021).

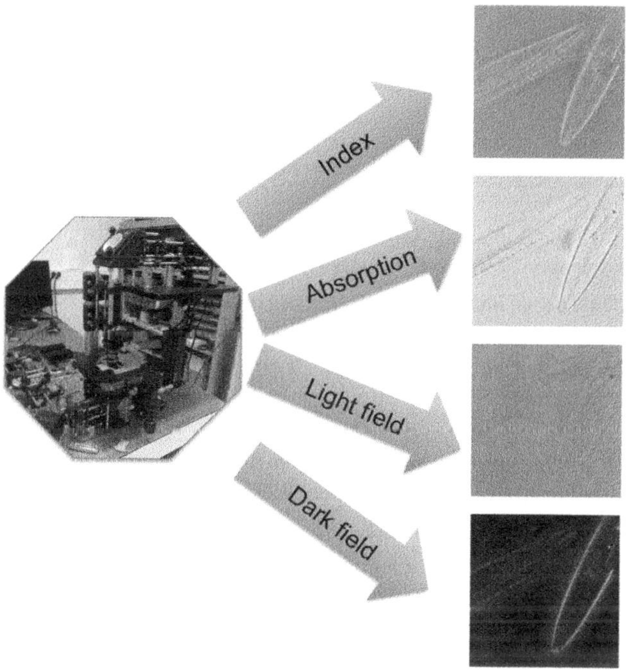

Figure 5.7. *Examples of diatom image reconstructions, computed from the same diffractive tomographic microscopy data, simulating a multimodal microscope: index and absorption imaging (diffractive tomography), bright-field imaging and dark-field imaging*

Finally, specific and purely numerical configurations can be conceivable, whose physical equivalent would be impossible or very difficult to realize experimentally, for example a dark-field microscope whose detection NA is higher than that of the illumination or a confocal transmission microscope, by adapting the approach already proposed in reflection (Rasedujjaman et al. 2020)

This technique of unlabeled microscopy is therefore certainly destined to evolve further. In particular, the coupling of fast, high-sensitivity, high-resolution sensors with the ever-increasing power and memory capabilities of computers paves the way for a complete redesign of how transmission optical microscopy will be able to provide high-resolution, content-enhanced images.

5.8. References

Atkinson, K.E. (1996). *The Numerical Solution of Integral Equations of the Second Kind*. Cambridge University Press, Cambridge.

Bailleul, J., Simon, B., Debailleul, M., Foucault, L., Verrier, N., Haeberlé, O. (2018). Tomographic diffractive microscopy: Towards high-resolution 3-D real-time data acquisition, image reconstruction and display of unlabeled samples. *Optics Communications*, 422, 28–37.

Balasubramani, V., Tu, H.-Y., Lai, X.-J., Cheng, C.-J. (2019). Adaptive wavefront correction structured illumination holographic tomography. *Scientific Reports*, 9(1), 1–7.

Baños, A. (1966). *Dipole Radiation in the Presence of a Conducting Halfspace*. Pergamon Press, Oxford.

Barty, A., Nugent, K., Roberts, A., Paganin, D. (2000). Quantitative phase tomography. *Optics Communications*, 175(4), 329–336.

Berdeu, A., Momey, F., Laperrousaz, B., Bordy, T., Gidrol, X., Dinten, J.-M., Picollet-D'hahan, N., Allier, C. (2017). Comparative study of fully three-dimensional reconstruction algorithms for lens-free microscopy. *Applied Optics*, 56(13), 3939–3951.

Berdeu, A., Laperrousaz, B., Bordy, T., Morales, S., Gidrol, X., Picollet-D'hahan, N., Allier, C. (2018). 3D+ time acquisitions of 3D cell culture by means of lens-free tomographic microscopy. In *Three-Dimensional and Multidimensional Microscopy: Image Acquisition and Processing XXV*. International Society for Optics and Photonics, Bellingham.

Born, M. and Wolf, E. (2003). *Principles of Optics: Electromagnetic Theory of Propagation, Interference and Diffraction of Light*, 7th edition. Elsevier, Amsterdam.

Chang, T., Shin, S., Lee, M., Park, Y. (2020). Computational approach to dark-field optical diffraction tomography. *APL Photonics*, 5(4), 040804.

Charrière, F., Marian, A., Montfort, F., Kuehn, J., Colomb, T., Cuche, E., Marquet, P., Depeursinge, C. (2006). Cell refractive index tomography by digital holographic microscopy. *Optics Letters*, 31(2), 178–180.

Choi, W., Fang-Yen, C., Badizadegan, K., Oh, S., Lue, N., Dasari, R.R., Feld, M.S. (2007). Tomographic phase microscopy. *Nature Methods*, 4(9), 717–719.

Chowdhury, S., Eldridge, W.J., Wax, A., Izatt, J. (2017). Refractive index tomography with structured illumination. *Optica*, 4(5), 537–545.

Cotte, Y., Toy, F., Jourdain, P., Pavillon, N., Boss, D., Magistretti, P., Marquet, P., Depeursinge, C. (2013). Marker-free phase nanoscopy. *Nature Photonics*, 7(2), 113.

Debailleul, M., Georges, V., Simon, B., Morin, R., Haeberlé, O. (2009). High-resolution three-dimensional tomographic diffractive microscopy of transparent inorganic and biological samples. *Optics Letters*, 34(1), 79–81.

Deng, Y., Huang, C.-H., Vinoth, B., Chu, D., Lai, X.-J., Cheng, C.-J. (2020). A compact synthetic aperture digital holographic microscope with mechanical movement-free beam scanning and optimized active aberration compensation for isotropic resolution enhancement. *Optics and Lasers in Engineering*, 134, 106251.

Dragomir, N., Goh, X.M., Roberts, A. (2008). Three-dimensional refractive index reconstruction with quantitative phase tomography. *Microscopy Research and Technique*, 71(1), 5–10.

Fan, X., Healy, J.J., O'Dwyer, K., Hennelly, B.M. (2019). Label-free color staining of quantitative phase images of biological cells by simulated Rheinberg illumination. *Applied Optics*, 58(12), 3104–3114.

Foucault, L., Verrier, N., Debailleul, M., Courbot, J.-B., Colicchio, B., Simon, B., Vonna, L., Haeberlé, O. (2019). Versatile transmission/reflection tomographic diffractive microscopy approach. *JOSA A*, 36(11), C18–C27.

Gorski, W. and Osten, W. (2007). Tomographic imaging of photonic crystal fibers. *Optics Letters*, 32(14), 1977–1979.

Habaza, M., Gilboa, B., Roichman, Y., Shaked, N.T. (2015). Tomographic phase microscopy with 180 rotation of live cells in suspension by holographic optical tweezers. *Optics Letters*, 40(8), 1881–1884.

Habaza, M., Kirschbaum, M., Guernth-Marschner, C., Dardikman, G., Barnea, I., Korenstein, R., Duschl, C., Shaked, N.T. (2017). Rapid 3D refractive-index imaging of live cells in suspension without labeling using dielectrophoretic cell rotation. *Advanced Science*, 4(2), 1600205.

Isikman, S.O., Bishara, W., Mavandadi, S., Frank, W.Y., Feng, S., Lau, R., Ozcan, A. (2011). Lens-free optical tomographic microscope with a large imaging volume on a chip. *Proceedings of the National Academy of Sciences*, 108(18), 7296–7301.

Jin, D., Zhou, R., Yaqoob, Z., So, P.T. (2018). Dynamic spatial filtering using a digital micromirror device for high-speed optical diffraction tomography. *Optics Express*, 26(1), 428–437.

Jung, J., Kim, K., Yoon, J., Park, Y. (2016). Hyperspectral optical diffraction tomography. *Optics Express*, 24(3), 2006–2012.

Kamilov, U.S., Papadopoulos, I.N., Shoreh, M.H., Goy, A., Vonesch, C., Unser, M., Psaltis, D. (2015). Learning approach to optical tomography. *Optica*, 2(6), 517–522.

Kamilov, U.S., Papadopoulos, I.N., Shoreh, M.H., Goy, A., Vonesch, C., Unser, M., Psaltis, D. (2016). Optical tomographic image reconstruction based on beam propagation and sparse regularization. *IEEE Transactions on Computational Imaging*, 2(1), 59–70.

Kawata, S., Nakamura, O., Noda, T., Ooki, H., Ogino, K., Kuroiwa, Y., Minami, S. (1990). Laser computed-tomography microscope. *Applied Optics*, 29(26), 3805–3809.

Kim, K. and Park, Y. (2017). Tomographic active optical trapping of arbitrarily shaped objects by exploiting 3D refractive index maps. *Nature Communications*, 8(1), 1–8.

Kim, M., Choi, Y., Fang Yen, C., Sung, Y., Dasari, R.R., Feld, M.S., Choi, W. (2011). High-speed synthetic aperture microscopy for live cell imaging. *Optics Letters*, 36(2), 148–150.

Kim, K., Yoon, J., Park, Y. (2015). Simultaneous 3D visualization and position tracking of optically trapped particles using optical diffraction tomography. *Optica*, 2(4), 343–346.

Kostencka, J., Kozacki, T., Kuś, A., Kujawińska, M. (2015). Accurate approach to capillary-supported optical diffraction tomography. *Optics Express*, 23(6), 7908–7923.

Kostencka, J., Kozacki, T., Kuś, A., Kemper, B., Kujawińska, M. (2016). Holographic tomography with scanning of illumination: Space-domain reconstruction for spatially invariant accuracy. *Biomedical Optics Express*, 7(10), 4086–4101.

Kostencka, J., Kozacki, T., Józwik, M. (2017). Holographic tomography with object rotation and two-directional off-axis illumination. *Optics Express*, 25(20), 23920–23934.

Krauze, W., Makowski, P., Kujawińska, M. (2015). Total variation iterative constraint algorithm for limited-angle tomographic reconstruction of non-piecewise-constant structures. In *Modeling Aspects in Optical Metrology V*. International Society for Optics and Photonics, Bellingham.

Kuś, A., Dudek, M., Kemper, B., Kujawińska, M., Vollmer, A. (2014). Tomographic phase microscopy of living three-dimensional cell cultures. *Journal of Biomedical Optics*, 19(4), 046009.

Kuś, A., Krauze, W., Kujawińska, M. (2015). Active limited-angle tomographic phase microscope. *Journal of Biomedical Optics*, 20(11), 111216.

Lauer, V. (2002). New approach to optical diffraction tomography yielding a vector equation of diffraction tomography and a novel tomographic microscope. *Journal of Microscopy*, 205(2), 165–176.

Lee, K., Kim, K., Kim, G., Shin, S., Park, Y. (2017). Time-multiplexed structured illumination using a DMD for optical diffraction tomography. *Optics Letters*, 42(5), 999.

Lee, M., Kim, K., Oh, J., Park, Y. (2021). Isotropically resolved label-free tomographic imaging based on tomographic moulds for optical trapping. *Light: Science & Applications*, 10(1), 1–9.

Lin, Y.-C. and Cheng, C.-J. (2014). Sectional imaging of spatially refractive index distribution using coaxial rotation digital holographic microtomography. *Journal of Optics*, 16(6), 065401.

Lin, Y.-C., Chen, H.-C., Tu, H.-Y., Liu, C.-Y., Cheng, C.-J. (2017). Optically driven full-angle sample rotation for tomographic imaging in digital holographic microscopy. *Optics Letters*, 42(7), 1321–1324.

Lin, Y.-C., Vinoth, B., Lai, X.-J., Tu, H.-Y., Cheng, C.-J. (2018). Integrated dual-mode tomography for unlabeled free-floating single cell imaging. In *Digital Holography and Three-Dimensional Imaging*. Optical Society of America, Cambridge.

Liu, H., Bailleul, J., Simon, B., Debailleul, M., Colicchio, B., Haeberlé, O. (2014). Tomographic diffractive microscopy and multiview profilometry with flexible aberration correction. *Applied Optics*, 53(4), 748–755.

Malek, M., Khelfa, H., Picart, P., Mounier, D., Poilâne, C. (2016). Microtomography imaging of an isolated plant fiber: A digital holographic approach. *Applied Optics*, 55(3), A111–A121.

Marathay, A.S. (1975). Fourier transform of the Green's function for the Helmholtz equation. *JOSA*, 65(8), 964–965.

Merola, F., Memmolo, P., Miccio, L., Savoia, R., Mugnano, M., Fontana, A., D'Ippolito, G., Sardo, A., Iolascon, A., Gambale, A. et al. (2017). Tomographic flow cytometry by digital holography. *Light: Science & Applications*, 6(4), e16241–e16241.

Meyrueis, P., Sakoda, K., Van de Voorde, M. (2017). *Micro- and Nanophotonic Technologies*. John Wiley & Sons, New York.

Pan, A., Zhang, Y., Wen, K., Zhou, M., Min, J., Lei, M., Yao, B. (2018). Subwavelength resolution Fourier ptychography with hemispherical digital condensers. *Optics Express*, 26(18), 23119–23131.

Pham, T.-A., Soubies, E., Goy, A., Lim, J., Soulez, F., Psaltis, D., Unser, M. (2018). Versatile reconstruction framework for diffraction tomography with intensity measurements and multiple scattering. *Optics Express*, 26(3), 2749–2763.

Rasedujjaman, M., Affannoukoué, K., Garcia-Seyda, N., Robert, P., Giovannini, H., Chaumet, P.C., Theodoly, O., Valignat, M.-P., Belkebir, K., Sentenac, A. et al. (2020). Three-dimensional imaging with reflection synthetic confocal microscopy. *Optics Letters*, 45(13), 3721–3724.

Remacha, C., Nickerson, B.S., Kreuzer, H.J. (2014). Tomography by point source digital holographic microscopy. *Applied Optics*, 53(16), 3520–3527.

Saba, A., Lim, J., Ayoub, A.B., Antoine, E.E., Psaltis, D. (2021). Polarization-sensitive optical diffraction tomography. *Optica*, 8(3), 402–408.

Schmalz, J.A., Schmalz, G., Gureyev, T.E., Pavlov, K.M. (2010). On the derivation of the Green's function for the Helmholtz equation using generalized functions. *American Journal of Physics*, 78(2), 181–186.

Sen, S., Ahmed, I., Aljubran, B., Bernussi, A.A., de Peralta, L.G. (2016). Fourier ptychographic microscopy using an infrared-emitting hemispherical digital condenser. *Applied Optics*, 55(23), 6421–6427.

Shin, S., Kim, K., Yoon, J., Park, Y. (2015). Active illumination using a digital micromirror device for quantitative phase imaging. *Optics Letters*, 40(22), 5407–5410.

Shin, S., Kim, K., Kim, T., Yoon, J., Hong, K., Park, J., Park, Y. (2016). Optical diffraction tomography using a digital micromirror device for stable measurements of 4D refractive index tomography of cells. In *Quantitative Phase Imaging II*. International Society for Optics and Photonics, Bellingham.

Simon, B., Debailleul, M., Georges, V., Lauer, V., Haeberlé, O. (2008). Tomographic diffractive microscopy of transparent samples. *The European Physical Journal – Applied Physics*, 44(1), 29–35.

Simon, B., Debailleul, M., Beghin, A., Tourneur, Y., Haeberlé, O. (2010). High resolution tomographic diffractive microscopy of biological samples. *Journal of Biophotonics*, 3(7), 462–467.

Simon, B., Debailleul, M., Houkal, M., Ecoffet, C., Bailleul, J., Lambert, J., Spangenberg, A., Liu, H., Soppera, O., Haeberlé, O. (2017). Tomographic diffractive microscopy with isotropic resolution. *Optica*, 4(4), 460–463.

Streibl, N. (1985). Three-dimensional imaging by a microscope. *J. Opt. Soc. Am. A*, 2(2), 121–127.

Sung, Y. (2018). Spectroscopic microtomography in the visible wavelength range. *Phys. Rev. Applied*, 10, 054041.

Sung, Y. (2019). Snapshot holographic optical tomography. *Physical Review Applied*, 11(1), 014039.

Sung, Y., Choi, W., Lue, N., Dasari, R.R., Yaqoob, Z. (2012). Stain-free quantification of chromosomes in live cells using regularized tomographic phase microscopy. *PLoS One*, 7(11), e49502.

Taddese, A.M., Verrier, N., Debailleul, M., Courbot, J.-B., Haeberlé, O. (2021). Optimizing sample illumination scanning in transmission tomographic diffractive microscopy. *Applied Optics*, 60(6), 1694–1704.

Tian, L., Li, X., Ramchandran, K., Waller, L. (2014). Multiplexed coded illumination for Fourier ptychography with an LED array microscope. *Biomedical Optics Express*, 5(7), 2376–2389.

Van Rooij, J. and Kalkman, J. (2020). Polarization contrast optical diffraction tomography. *Biomedical Optics Express*, 11(4), 2109–2121.

Vertu, S., Delaunay, J.-J., Yamada, I., Haeberlé, O. (2009). Diffraction microtomography with sample rotation: Influence of a missing apple core in the recorded frequency space. *Central European Journal of Physics*, 7(1), 22–31.

Vertu, S., Flügge, J., Delaunay, J.-J., Haeberlé, O. (2011). Improved and isotropic resolution in tomographic diffractive microscopy combining sample and illumination rotation. *Central European Journal of Physics*, 9(4), 969–974.

Villone, M.M., Memmolo, P., Merola, F., Mugnano, M., Miccio, L., Maffettone, P.L., Ferraro, P. (2018). Full-angle tomographic phase microscopy of flowing quasi-spherical cells. *Lab on a Chip*, 18(1), 126–131.

Vinoth, B., Lai, X.-J., Lin, Y.-C., Tu, H.-Y., Cheng, C.-J. (2018). Integrated dual-tomography for refractive index analysis of free-floating single living cell with isotropic superresolution. *Scientific Reports*, 8, 5943.

Vishnyakov, G., Levin, G., Minaev, V., Latushko, M., Nekrasov, N., Pickalov, V. (2016). Differential interference contrast tomography. *Optics Letters*, 41(13), 3037–3040.

Wolf, E. (1969). Three-dimensional structure determination of semi-transparent objects from holographic data. *Optics Communications*, 1(4), 153–156.

Zdańkowski, P., Winnik, J., Patorski, K., Gocowski, P., Ziemczonok, M., Józwik, M., Kujawińska, M., Trusiak, M. (2021). Common-path intrinsically achromatic optical diffraction tomography. *Biomedical Optics Express*, 12(7), 4219–4234.

Zemyan, S.M. (2012). *The Classical Theory of Integral Equations: A Concise Treatment*. Springer Science & Business Media, Berlin.

Ziemczonok, M., Kuś, A., Wasylczyk, P., Kujawińska, M. (2019). 3D-printed biological cell phantom for testing 3D quantitative phase imaging systems. *Scientific Reports*, 9(1), 18872.

6

Interference Microscopy

Rémy CLAVEAU, Sébastien MARBACH, Stéphane PERRIN, Amir NAHAS, Manuel FLURY and Paul MONTGOMERY

ICube, CNRS, Université de Strasbourg, Illkirch, France

6.1. Introduction

The emergence of micro- and nanotechnologies (in optics, electronics and mechanics) and their recent progress, in terms of performance, miniaturization and quality, are largely due to increasingly accurate and reliable surface characterization techniques. Indeed, the surface metrology of an element leads not only to finding its macroscopic shape but also its characteristics, such as roughness or surface condition, in order to deduce its functional parameters.

Before the 1990s, the measurement of surface topography relied mainly on the use of mechanical tips (commonly called styli) that, through contact, scanned large object areas and derived a mapping of heights with very high axial resolution. However, the use of mechanical tips yields significant mechanical noise or surface abrasion (scratches). With the appearance of atomic force microscopy, considerable gains in spatial resolution have been achieved (see Figure 6.1). In recent years, local-probe microscopes have been able to reconstruct in near real time the surface

For a color version of all the figures in this chapter, see www.iste.co.uk/fournier/unconventional.zip.

Unconventional Optical Imaging for Biology,
coordinated by Corinne FOURNIER and Olivier HAEBERLÉ.

topography at the nanometric scale (Leach 2011). Electron microscopy has also established itself as a pioneering technique for the observation and characterization of micro- and nanometric structures due to its high resolution. In contrast, quantitative depth measurements remain limited without damaging the sample. In parallel, optical devices offering quantitative, non-destructive and contactless measurements have been developed. Techniques such as fringe projection, confocal microscopy and interference microscopy (Leach 2011; de Groot 2015) remain the most common in research and industry (see Figure 6.2). This last technique is the subject of this chapter.

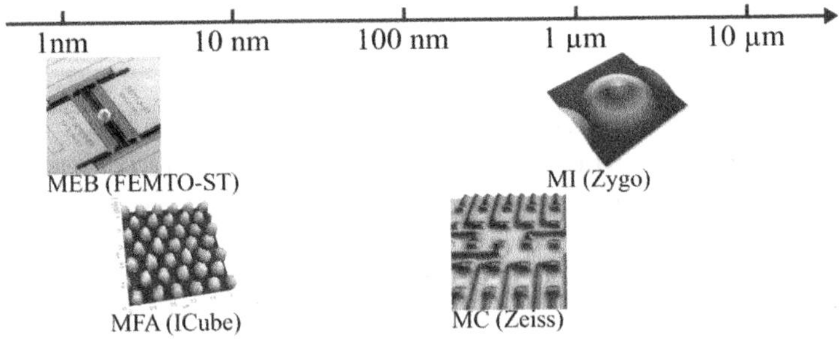

Figure 6.1. *Lateral resolution of contactless microscopes commonly used for surface characterization. SEM: scanning electron microscopy. AFM: atomic force microscopy. IM: interference microscopy. CM: confocal microscopy*

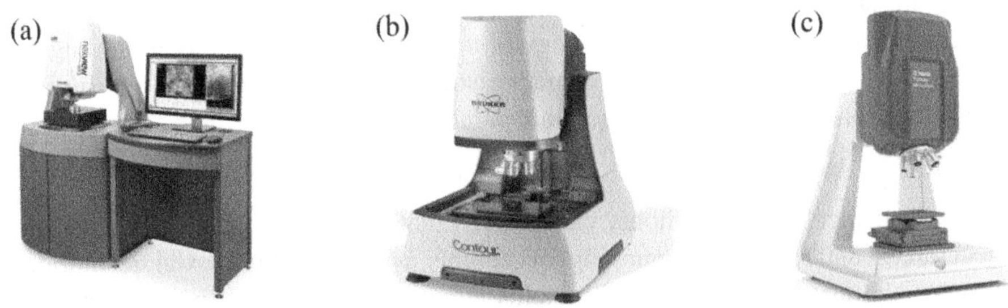

Figure 6.2. *Commercial interference microscopes based on white light interferometry. (a) Nexview^{TM} NX2, Zygo. (b) ContourX-500, Bruker. (c) TopMap MicroView, Polytec*

6.2. Principle and theory

6.2.1. *Interference*

Interference microscopy uses the phenomenon of interference between two waves to indirectly recover depth information. In order to create interference fringes, the incident beam originating from a light source is split in two by a beam splitter, as illustrated in Figure 6.3(a). The beam transmitted by the splitter is then reflected by a known surface, usually a plane mirror, at an axial position z_{ref}. This is called the reference beam. The reflected beam, called the object beam, interacts with the object. The object is a circularly textured silicon surface with different heights h_n. The splitter then recombines the two beams to direct them toward the detector, generally a camera, where they will interfere. At a given transverse position (x,y), the optical path difference δ_n between the two beams is the axial position difference of the planes $(z_s ref - h_n)$. When this difference is smaller than the coherence length (see section 6.2.2), the camera records an interference pattern.

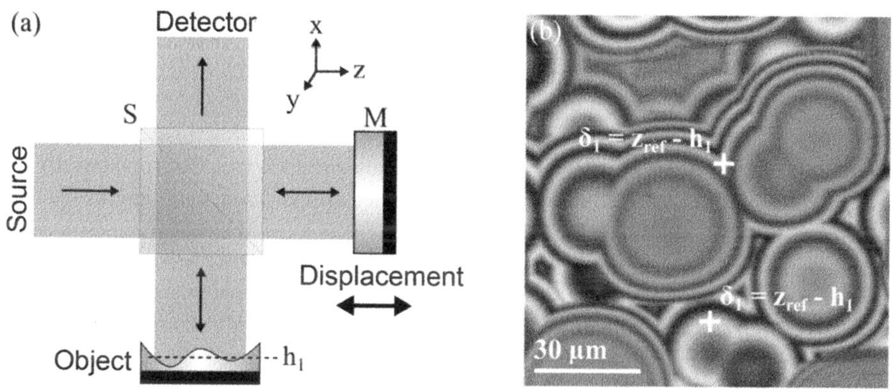

Figure 6.3. *Principle of interference microscopy. (a) Schematic diagram of the technique. M: mirror. S: separator. (b) Interferogram recorded in gray levels showing the variations in height of a circularly textured silicon surface. Its maximum intensity corresponds to a zero optical path difference* δ_1 $(z_{ref} = h_1)$

At every sensor point (x,y), the intensity varies and the interference fringes are then distorted according to the variations in height of the object (see Figure 6.3(b)). In order to recover this height distribution, a series of interferograms must be recorded by moving the reference mirror (or the object plane) along the optical axis z, for example, via a piezoelectric actuator. The number of interferograms, the increment and the total displacement depend on the coherence of light, as well as on the algorithm used (see section 6.3).

6.2.2. *Coherence of light*

The coherence of light defines the ability of two waves to interfere with each other. It is determined by two coherence phenomena (sometimes three if polarization is taken into consideration), which are temporal coherence when the two waves are temporally separated (on the longitudinal axis) and spatial coherence when they are spatially separated (on the transverse axis).

Temporal coherence is related to the propagation of the wave along the optical axis, and thus to its spectrum. It is possible to quantify it by the Fourier transform of the wave power spectral density (according to the Wiener–Khinchin theorem). Wave coherence duration τ (or coherence length l_c) is defined as the ratio between the square of the spectrum average wavelength λ_0^2 and its spectral width ($\Delta\lambda = \lambda_M - \lambda_m$) up to a factor. This factor depends on the shape of the spectrum (Saleh and Teich 1991). When the spectral distribution is Gaussian, the coherence length is defined by:

$$l_c = c\,\tau = \frac{4\sqrt{\ln 2}}{\pi}\frac{\lambda_M \lambda_m}{\Delta\lambda} \approx \frac{4\sqrt{\ln 2}}{\pi}\frac{\lambda_0^2}{\Delta\lambda} \qquad [6.1]$$

where c is the celerity. When the time delay between two waves (or the optical path difference δ) is less than l_c, then an interference signal is generated (see Figure 6.4). Beyond the coherence length, the contrast of the interference fringes drops rapidly to reach a zero value. A laser source offers interference fringes over long lengths (l_c is a few meters), while a light emitting diode allows these fringes to be obtained only over short lengths (l_c is a few micrometers).

Spatial coherence is related to the transverse spatial intensity distribution ΔS of the light source and the distance D along the optical axis between the source and the observation plane. This is then referred to as the spatial coherence width L_c. In the case of Young's slit experiment, the following expression can be written as

$$L_c \approx \frac{\lambda D}{\Delta S} \qquad [6.2]$$

Similarly to the coherence length, it has an influence on the contrast of the interference fringes (according to the Van Cittert–Zernike theorem). A point source (such as a single-mode fiber or a pinhole) generates a very contrasted interference signal as opposed to an extended source (such as a lamp or a light emitting diode, for instance). Moreover, by moving the source (D » λ) away, the wave becomes more and more spatially coherent.

Light polarization is also to be considered in interferometry. Two waves presenting the same polarization will provide a contrasted interference pattern. On the other hand, if the polarizations are oriented differently, the contrast of the interference figure decreases until reaching a zero value when they are perpendicular to each other.

Coherent light interferometry (e.g. digital holography and phase-shifting interferometry) relies on the use of spatially and temporally coherent sources. In contrast, for white light interferometry, weakly or partially coherent illumination is sufficient. Equation [6.3] gives the theoretical expression of the interference signal represented in Figure 6.4:

$$I(x, y, \delta) = 2I_0(x, y)\left[1 + |\gamma(\delta(x, y))| \cos\left(2\pi\delta(x, y)/\lambda_0\right)\right] \quad [6.3]$$

The object relative height distribution (i.e. the optical path difference) is then established by considering either the temporal coherence function $|\gamma(\delta)|$ (sometimes called the fringe envelope) as in coherence scanning interferometry or the phase term $\cos(k\delta)$ as in phase-shifting interferometry.

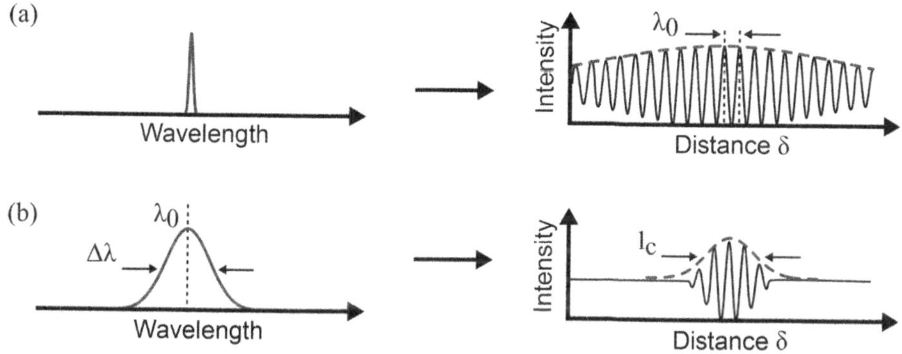

Figure 6.4. *Spectral densities of two light waves and intensity of the resulting interferograms. Black solid line: the longitudinal distribution of the intensity of the interferogram. Red dotted line: the coherence function $|\gamma(\delta)|$ (or fringe envelope)*

6.3. Algorithms

Interferometry is useful for metrology because the height information is contained in the fringe intensity distribution. The interference signal appears only when the optical path difference is smaller than the temporal coherence length of the light source (see section 6.2.2). The fringes superimposed on a structure in relief make it possible to find its three dimensional shape by measuring the phase information or the optical path difference. There are two main families of algorithms to quantify the fringes: phase-shifting microscopy and coherence scanning interferometry.

6.3.1. *Phase-shifting microscopy*

Phase-shifting interferometry consists of extracting the phase term $\phi = k\delta$ from relation [6.3]. In phase-shifting microscopy, microscope objectives are used for increasing the resolution power. This consists of applying an additional known phase-shifting ψ between the object and reference arms, for example by axially moving the reference mirror over a known short distance (see Figure 6.5(b)). Mathematically, the intensity distribution of the interferogram $I(\delta, \psi)$ per pixel then becomes:

$$I(\delta, \psi) = 2I_0 \left[1 + |\gamma(\delta)| \cos\left(2\pi\delta/\lambda_0 + \psi\right)\right] \qquad [6.4]$$

Repeated at least three times, the series of interferograms is used to find the phase distribution ϕ between the object and the reference mirror. The most commonly used algorithms are based on three-, four- or five-phase shifts:

$$\phi = \arctan\left\{\frac{I(5\pi/4) - I(3\pi/4)}{I(\pi/4) - I(3\pi/4)}\right\} \qquad \text{3 interferograms}$$

$$\phi = \arctan\left\{\frac{2I(\pi) - I(\pi/2)}{I(0) - I(\pi/2) - I(\pi) + I(3\pi/2)}\right\} \qquad \text{4 interferograms}$$

$$\phi = \arctan\left\{\frac{2I(-\pi/2) - I(\pi/2)}{I(\pi) + I(-\pi) - 2I(0)}\right\} \qquad \text{5 interferograms}$$

These algorithms, proposed in the mid-1980s (Creath 1988), have popularized the measurement of roughness by way of interferometry. Other more robust algorithms, such as that of Carré (Malacara 2007), make it possible to increase the signal-to-noise ratio of the measurement. Increasing the number of acquisitions also reduces the noise component but simultaneously increases the acquisition and phase reconstruction time.

Finally, the surface topography of the object $h(x, y)$ is extracted from the computed phase distribution $\phi(x, y)$ through the relation:

$$\phi(x, y) = 2\pi\frac{\delta(x, y)}{\lambda} = 4\pi\frac{h(x, y)\, n(x, y)}{\lambda} \qquad [6.5]$$

with $n(x, y)$ the refractive index of the ambient medium. Generally, the index of the surrounding environment is unitary (n = 1.0), because the characterization of non-organic objects does not require working in immersion. The factor 4 is due to the reflection measurement of the topography.

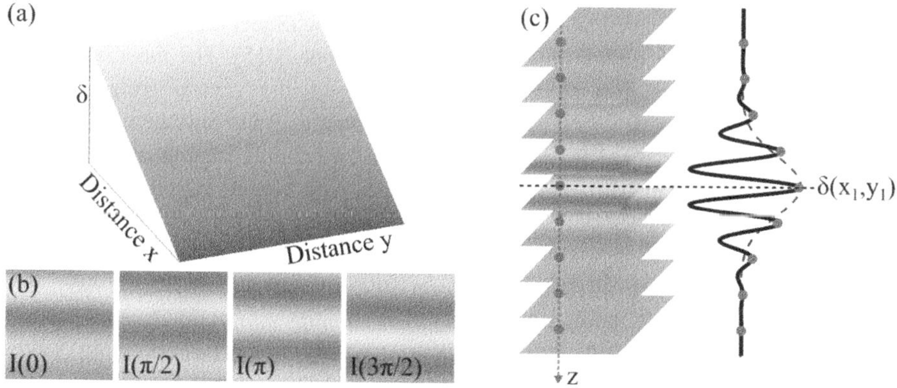

Figure 6.5. *Algorithms for quantifying the interference fringes*

COMMENTS ON FIGURE 6.5.– *(a) Reconstruction of the relative height distribution of an inclined surface. (b) Four interferograms for phase-shifting interferometry. (c) Stack of interferograms for coherence scanning interferometry. The black solid line represents the longitudinal intensity distribution of the interferogram at a transverse position* (x_1, y_1)*. The blue dashed line represents the fringe envelope.*

Although phase-shifting interferometry gives a nanometer axial resolution for roughness measurements, the measurement of straight steps is limited by the periodicity of fringes. For these reasons, coherence scanning interferometry has been developed.

6.3.2. *Coherence scanning interferometry*

Coherence scanning interferometry uses the fringe envelope term $|\gamma(\delta)|$ to map the object height distribution. When the optical path difference is zero ($\delta = 0$), the contrast (or visibility) of the interference fringes is at its maximum (Leach 2011). Therefore, the position of the envelope peak of the interference signal provides direct information on the position of the object with respect to the reference mirror. The detection of the envelope is performed after having built the interferometric signal, as shown in Figure 6.5(c). The object is axially moved with respect to the reference mirror in order to record the signal over a large distance (from a few micrometers to several hundred micrometers depending on the sample) with a sampling (displacement step) of the order of $\lambda_0/10$. Compared to phase-shifting microscopy, techniques based on fringe envelope detection require that a larger number of images be acquired.

Several algorithms have been developed to extract the object topography from the interferometric signal acquisition (Leach 2011; de Groot 2015). The most basic one is based on the estimation of the axial position of the central fringe of the interferogram (when the interference contrast is at its maximum and the optical path difference is zero) per pixel (Montgomery and Fillard 1992; Sandoz and Tribillon 1993). Other more powerful algorithms have been developed based on different signal processing techniques: the centroid (Balasubramanian 1982), the variance (Davidson et al. 1987), demodulation and filtering (Lee and Strand 1990; Caber 1993), the Fourier transform (Kino and Chim 1990; de Groot and Deck 1995), the interference signal local derivative method (*five sample adaptive*) (Larkin 1996), wavelet decomposition (Sandoz 1997), Hilbert approximation (Harasaki et al. 2000) or the Teager Kaiser energy operator (TKEO) (Salzenstein et al. 2014).

The sensitivity, accuracy and speed of white light interferometry measurements depend on the algorithm, the nature of the surface and the presence of photon or mechanical noise (see section 6.5).

As an example, the Hilbert transform technique is described here for finding the analytic signal formed from the interferometric signal and whose modulus corresponds to the instantaneous amplitude (the envelope) of the interferogram. Mathematically, the analytic signal can be found by removing the "negative" frequencies from the interferometric signal. After removing the mean value, the interference signal given in equation [6.3] is rewritten as

$$I(\delta) = 2I_0 \left|\gamma(\delta)\right| \cos\left(2\pi\delta/\lambda_0\right) \qquad [6.6]$$

Its Fourier transform is simply written as

$$\mathcal{F}_\sigma[I] = 2I_0 \mathcal{F}_\sigma[|\gamma(\delta)|] * \left[\frac{\delta_D(\sigma - 1/\lambda_0) + \delta_D(\sigma + 1/\lambda_0)}{2}\right] \qquad [6.7]$$

with σ the wave number, the symbol $\mathcal{F}$ representing the Fourier transform and δ_D the Dirac distribution. By removing the part of the negative frequencies, that is, the Dirac distribution centered on $-1/\lambda_0$, the analytic signal $\tilde{I}$ is found after an inverse Fourier transform, which is written as

$$\tilde{I}(\delta) = I_0 \left|\gamma(\delta)\right| \exp\left(-i2\pi\delta/\lambda_0\right) \qquad [6.8]$$

This signal modulus is equal to $I_0\left|\gamma(\delta)\right|$: it thus allows for the extraction of the envelope of the interference fringes. The surface position at point (x, y) is then simply obtained by computing the position of the maximum of $\left|\gamma(\delta)\right|$.

6.4. Instrumentation

In interferometric profilometry, three types of interference objectives are mainly used (see Figure 6.6). These three configurations are based on the same principle of interference generation and collection. The Michelson objective consists of a reference mirror placed laterally with respect to the optical axis, which reflects part of the incident beam by way of a splitter. Due to the limitation of their working distance, Michelson objectives offer numerical apertures and small magnifications (ON $\sim$ 0.1 and $\leq \times 10$).

The Mirau objective is based on a more compact vertical architecture by introducing the reference mirror and the separator along the optical axis. With this type of interference objective, magnifications can reach $\times 100$ (de Groot and Biegen 2016). Enabling medium numerical apertures (ON $\leq$ 0.6) and easier alignment, Mirau objectives are often used for characterization in materials science, such as semiconductors, for example.

For topography measurements with numerical apertures greater than 0.6 and better lateral resolutions, the Linnik configuration is required. This configuration is based on the use of two ideally identical microscope objectives in the object arm and the reference arm but is nonetheless larger. And in addition, it is more prone to mechanical noise and misalignment.

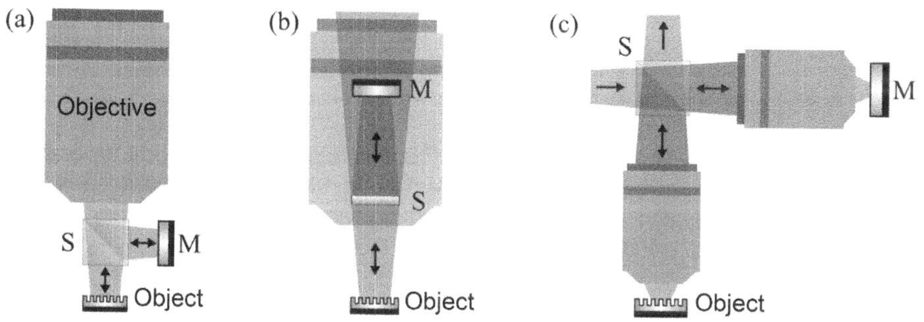

Figure 6.6. *Objectives for interference microscopes in: (a) Michelson, (b) Mirau and (c) Linnik setups. S: separator. M: mirror*

In order to apply a temporal coherence function scan or a phase shift, a motorized stage, or more often a piezoelectric actuator, is integrated into the system. Its function is to move the reference mirror or the object to be visualized, along the optical axis over large distances with nanometric accuracy (Lehmann et al. 2016). When the objective depth of field is less than the axial displacement distance (sometimes the case in a Linnik configuration), all of the optical components of the arm must be moved. In the Mirau configuration, it is often impossible to move the reference mirror.

The control of the piezoelectric system, as well as the acquisition and processing of the interference patterns, are achieved by means of proprietary software for commercial systems (see Figure 6.7), in-house software developed in laboratories or free software.

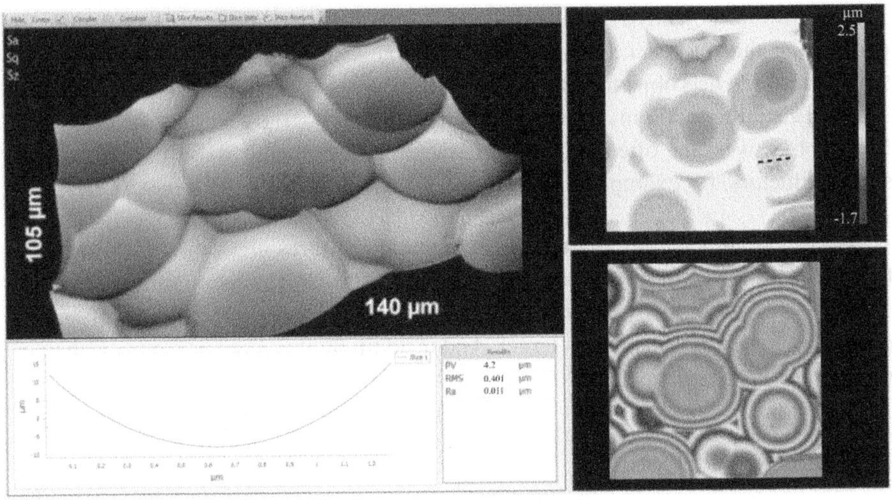

Figure 6.7. *Man-machine interface of the Mx^{TM} software program by Zygo Corporation. The software allows for control of the system instruments, interferogram analysis, topography reconstruction and quantification of surface parameters. Reconstruction of a circularly textured silicon surface (see Figure 6.3)*

6.5. Physical performance and limitations

As with any measurement system, interference microscopy has its own limitations. These are lateral resolution and axial resolution, field of view and measurement dynamics. There are also several possible sources of error in topography measurements.

6.5.1. *Lateral resolution*

In conventional microscopy, the microscope objective determines the lateral resolution capacity of the system. Depending on the coherence of light, the lateral resolution is limited in air to λ, the wavelength of the collected light, for strongly coherent illumination or $\lambda/2$ for weakly coherent illumination (Latychevskaia 2019). This assumes that the system has no optical aberrations or undersampling problems during acquisition. Figures 6.8(a) and 6.8(b) schematically illustrate the performance of an ideal system using the Fourier optics-based approach. The lateral resolution is said to be limited by the phenomenon of diffraction.

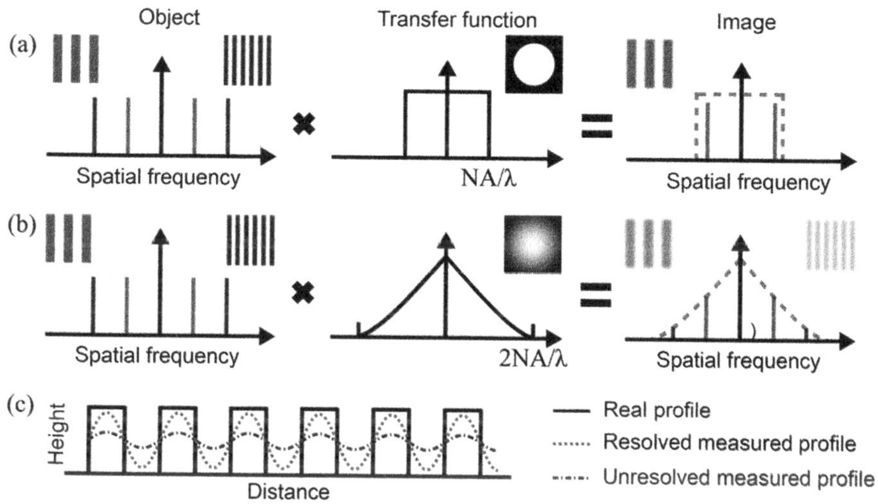

Figure 6.8. *Interference microscopy performance. Lateral resolution of an optical microscope when the light is: (a) coherent and (b) incoherent. (c) Lateral resolution of an interference microscope*

There are other resolution criteria in microscopy such as Abbe, Rayleigh and Sparrow, widely discussed in the literature as a means of analyzing lateral resolution (Heintzmann and Ficz 2006; Leong-Hoi et al. 2016; Latychevskaia 2019; Masters 2020). The Abbe criterion equation is written as

$$\Delta x_{Abbe} = \frac{\lambda}{2n\sin\theta} = \frac{\lambda}{2ON} \quad [6.9]$$

where λ is the working wavelength (central wavelength for a broad spectrum source) and n is the refractive index of the surrounding medium between the objective and the object. θ is the half angle at the apex of the cone of light collected by the microscope objective. The product of n and $\sin\theta$ defines the numerical aperture of the objective, denoted by ON. Δx_{Abbe} represents the smallest discernible pattern within this criterion.

In interferometry, the resolving power depends not only on the diffraction of light but also on the ability of the system to reconstruct the surface topography (Giusca and Leach 2013). The lateral resolution of an interferometer, often defined as its ability to reconstruct at least 50% of the height of a topographic modulation (de Groot 2015; ISO 2019), as illustrated in Figure 6.8(c), typically reaches the micrometer in the visible range. When the object material to be measured allows it, reducing the illumination wavelength of the system increases the spatial resolution of the interference microscope (Montgomery and Montaner 1999). Increasing the system numerical aperture also contributes to improving the lateral resolution at the expense of the field of view.

6.5.2. *Axial resolution*

Interference microscopy enables the reconstruction of surface topographies with high axial sensitivity, ranging from a fraction of a nanometer in phase-shifting microscopy on smooth surfaces to a few tens of nanometers in coherence scanning interferometry on rough surfaces (Malacara 2007; Montgomery et al. 2012; Guellil et al. 2014; de Groot 2015). This axial sensitivity implies errors in topography measurements, mostly due to mechanical system vibrations or photon noise.

In contrast, phase detection interferometry (e.g. phase-shift and digital holography) proves unable to recover height information from an abrupt pattern (a step, for instance) with a greater height than half a wavelength. In fact, a steep wall whose angle is greater than the system numerical aperture cannot be clearly resolved. A rounded shape of the wall will then be reconstructed resulting from the convolution of the pattern by the system impulse response (Lehmann et al. 2016). Furthermore, the phase reconstruction algorithm requires a 2D arc-tangent function that operates in the interval $]-\pi, \pi[$. This mathematical constraint limits the measurable phase jump to 2π, corresponding to an optical path difference of λ ($\delta = 2\,h = \lambda$). When the surface to be measured has a continuous height distribution over an interval greater than $\lambda/2$, a phase unwrapping algorithm is required (Ghiglia and Pritt 1998). This limitation explains why white light interferometry has become the preferred technique for measuring surface roughness and 3D structures (Schmit et al. 2008; Liu et al. 2014).

6.5.3. *Spatial sampling*

In interference microscopy, as in classical microscopy, micrometric lateral resolutions are achievable if and only if the spatial sampling of the object and the interference fringes are correctly taken into consideration. Indeed, when the size of the detector elements is larger than the optical resolution or the fringe period, the resolution will be truncated or the fringe contrast reduced. The size of the pixels Δx must be at least twice as small as the lateral resolution and the fringe period (interfringe $i = \lambda / [2 \sin(\alpha/2)]$, with α the angle between the two beams incident to the detector) due to the Shannon criterion.

6.5.4. *Sources of measurement error*

In interferometry, measuring the topography of an object made of several materials, one of which has a complex refractive index, may be incorrect. This is because the wavelength dispersion of the refractive index causes a variation in the phase term ϕ and the envelope of the fringes (Dubois 2004). Table 6.1 lists the values of the offset provided by some materials. Other height measurement errors may occur, such as nonlinearity in the axial movement system of the reference mirror and the signal-to-noise ratio. To overcome these problems, a closed-loop piezoelectric system for control (capacitive sensor, inductive sensor, etc.) and digital processing of interferograms (median filter, averaging, etc.) are employed.

Material	Envelope shift [nm]	Phase shift [nm]
Glass	0	0
Copper	–1	–31
Silicon	–3	0
Aluminium	–9	–13
Chrome	–15	–13

Table 6.1. *Fringe and phase envelope position errors according to the observed material (source: Leach (2011))*

In addition, the use of large numerical apertures can lead to different types of reconstruction errors (Schulz and Elssner 1991). Lateral and axial calibration of the interferometer is then necessary by calibrated measurement standards. In coherence scanning interferometry, an interpolation step yields an axial resolution greater than the axial displacement step.

6.6. Applications

6.6.1. *Roughness measurement*

As mentioned previously, one of the main applications of interference microscopy is the measurement of statistical indicators of the condition of a surface, such as roughness. To quantify the roughness, geometric parameters are computed from a profile extracted from a surface (see Figure 6.9). The arithmetic mean roughness R_a, the root mean square roughness R_q and the total profile height R_t can be calculated. The ISO 1302:2002 standard describes these tools for calculating statistical indicators of the condition of a surface (ISO 2012) with:

$$R_a = \frac{1}{l_x}\int_0^{l_x} |h(x)|dx \qquad R_q = \sqrt{\frac{1}{l_x}\int_0^{l_x} h(x)^2dx} \qquad [6.10]$$

where l_x is the profile length and $h(x)$ is the profile height at a position x. In order to compute surface roughness parameters, the double integral operator must be considered. Moreover, the names of the parameters vary and become, for example, S_a and S_q for the surface arithmetic and quadratic mean. Interference microscopy not only allows for contactless characterization of roughness, but also of surface topography for an object with high axial sensitivity and micrometric lateral resolution. The results in Figure 6.10 show the characterization of silicon crystals after excimer laser annealing of an amorphous silicon layer used in flat panel display manufacturing technology. The three-dimensional view from phase-shifting interferometry measurements (Figure 6.10(a)) makes it possible to visualize the distribution of different crystal sizes, while the measurement of R_q provides quantification of the roughness according to the position. Typical values of polysilicon roughness in this case are R_a = 4 nm, R_q = 5 nm and R_t = 120 nm (with a 10 nm sensitivity). The high nanometric sensitivity of the phase-shifting interferometry is clearly visible in this example.

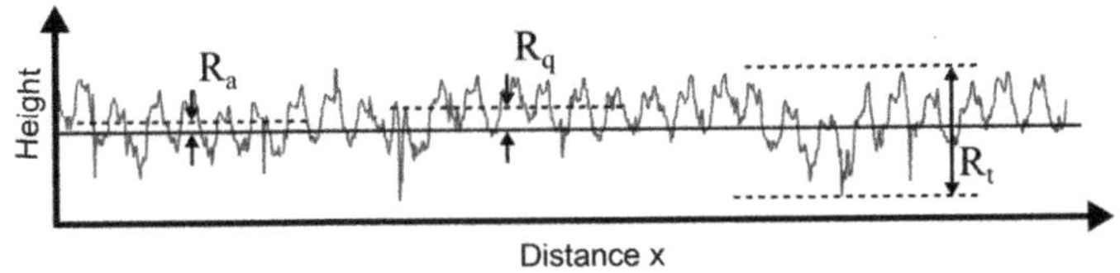

Figure 6.9. *Extraction of the parameters commonly used to quantify the roughness of a surface profile. R_a is the arithmetic mean height, R_q is the quadratic mean height and R_t is the total height of the profile*

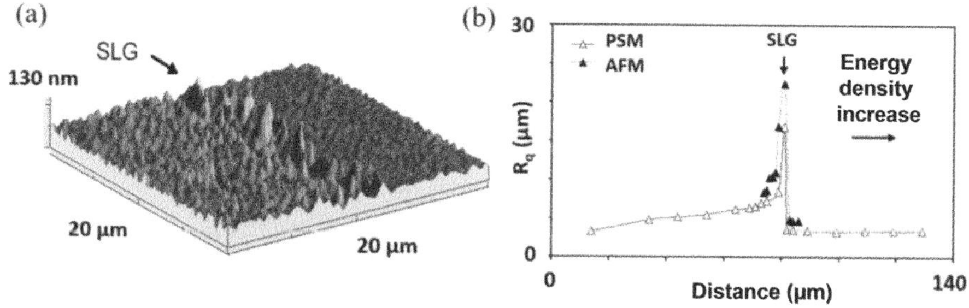

Figure 6.10. *Measurement of roughness variation in polysilicon crystals after laser annealing of amorphous silicon in a heterogeneous fluence zone (application: flat screens)*

COMMENTS ON FIGURE 6.10.– *(a) Region measured by phase-shifting interferometry near the area of the largest crystals. (b) Comparison of measurements between phase-shifting interferometry and atomic force microscopy near this region, Linnik,* ×*50 (source: Benatmane et al. 2003).*

6.6.2. *The measurement of static surfaces*

For measuring the deeper shape of microelectronic components, MOEMS systems or structured or rocky surfaces (Leong-Hoi et al. 2018), coherence scanning interferometry provides high accuracy (see Figure 6.11).

Topography analysis then results not only in tracing geometrical parameters such as surface roughness (De Chiffre et al. 2000; DigitalSurfé 2021), inclination (Harris et al. 2012) or planarity, but also in quantifying optical parameters such as the curvature radius of a microlens, as well as its taper constant and numerical aperture. By using wide field of view interference objectives and area acquisition techniques (*stitching*), analysis of large surfaces is also accessible. Furthermore, in addition to the many applications in topography, coherence scanning interferometry inherently makes it possible to perform optical coherence tomography for the observation of high-resolution defects in transparent homogeneous media (Leong-Hoi et al. 2016).

6.6.3. *The measurement of moving surfaces*

Through the synchronization of the different elements in the interference microscope, it is possible to measure moving surfaces. If the motion is periodic, for example, a mirror or a resonating membrane, stroboscopic illumination can be used to freeze the motion and to measure the shape at different oscillation phases (Petitgrand 2006). For surfaces evolving non-periodically in time, measurement of the evolution of the surface topography is possible in near real-time by continuously scanning the interference fringes and an acquisition using a fast synchronized camera.

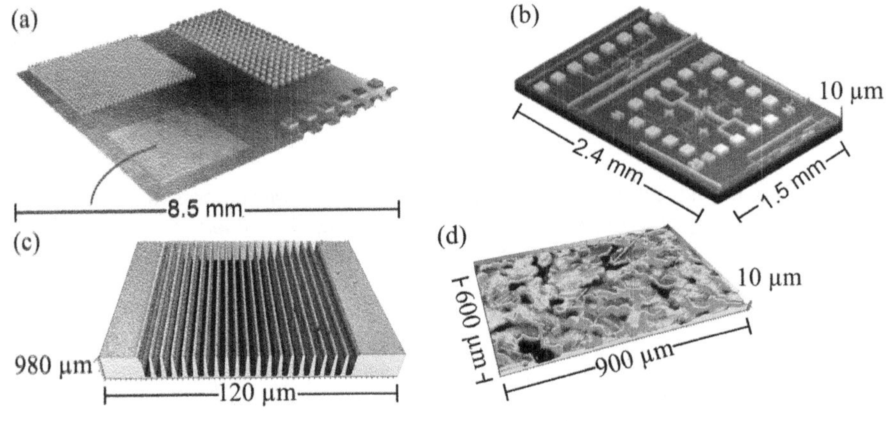

Figure 6.11. *Topographies of static surfaces. (a) Standard grids, Fizeau, ×1.4 (de Groot and Biegen 2016). (b) Magnetic probe, Michelson, ×5 (Montgomery et al. 2016). (c) Standard array and (d) microstructures, Mirau, ×100 GBS GmbH*

While phase-shifting microscopy allows for real-time nanoscale measurement of roughness, for micron depths by coherence scanning interferometry, much faster parallel processing is required, for example, on an *field programmable gate array* (FPGA) (Dubois et al. 2002). Figure 6.12(b) shows the real-time measurement (acquisition and processing) of a magnetic probe in CMOS technology moving laterally at a speed of 200 µm/s and reconstructed with a rate of 20 topographic reconstructions per second (256 × 320 px) following an acquisition at 1,320 i/s and processing in FPGA at the same rate using the local derivative algorithm (Montgomery et al. 2016). Finally, the combination of interferometry with an environmental chamber makes it possible to study the behavior of materials under different conditions, such as the change of glass transition temperature in ultrathin polymer films (Chapuis et al. 2017).

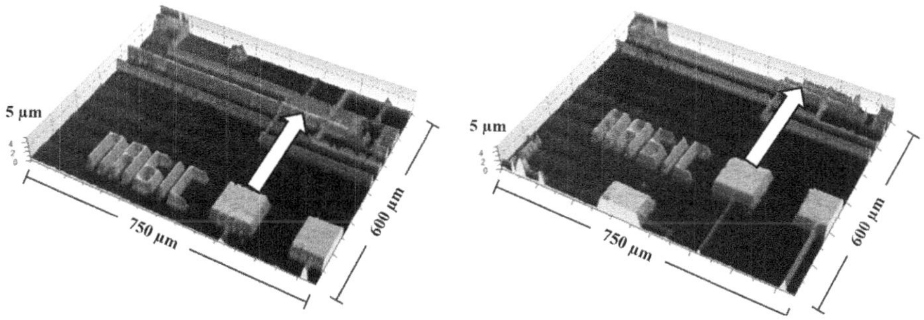

Figure 6.12. *Two topographies of a CMOS magnetic probe moving laterally at a speed of 200 μm/s, measured in real time by white-light interferometry at a rate of 20 topographic frames/s (256 x 320 px) following FPGA acquisition and processing at 1,320 fps, with a 0.4 s inter-frame gap, Michelson, ×5 (source: Montgomery et al. 2016)*

6.7. Recent findings

6.7.1. *Full-field optical coherence tomography*

Based on the principle of coherence scanning interferometry, optical coherence tomography (OCT) is an imaging technique adapted to turbid media (Huang et al. 1991). The zero path difference only detects ballistic photons that have thus been backscattered by a sample interface (organic tissue, for instance) and to the reconstruction of its volumetric information. This technique is similar to medical ultrasound but requires interferometry to measure very short flight times. Currently, OCT is known to the general public for in vivo retina analysis in ophthalmology.

Numerous variants and improvements have been developed, including spectral-domain optical coherence tomography (Leitgeb et al. 2003; Perrin 2016) and full-field optical coherence tomography (Beaurepaire et al. 1998; Dubois et al. 2004). Unlike conventional OCT techniques, a particular feature of full-field OCT is that it utilizes a 2D detector (such as camera CCD or CMOS, etc.) for the acquisition, in a series of acquisitions, of a full-field OCT image. In full-field optical coherence tomography, a simple algorithm based on scanning the coherence function is not optimal, because the assumption of single reflectors or scatterers no longer applies in scattering, absorbing and moving media. Indeed, speckles appear as a result of interferences between scatterers spaced less than the coherence length. Implementation of a specific phase-shifting algorithm is therefore preferred in order to extract an amplitude image at a given axial position. The imaging contrast is then largely explained by refractive index heterogeneities within the scattering medium.

The axial resolution of optical coherence tomography is defined as the coherence length of the source in the medium to be observed (see equation [6.1]). This can typically reach the micrometer when the illumination is a halogen lamp or an arc lamp and 5 μm when the illumination is an LED. The lateral resolution and field of view depend on the performance of the microscope objective (see section 6.5). Ballistic signal extinction, multiple scattering and sample-induced aberrations mainly influence the imaging depth. This is about 200 μm in dermatological or brain imaging (in the visible range, ON $\sim$ 0.3).

In recent years, full-field optical coherence tomography has had a flagship application: in vivo diagnosis during tumor surgery. Previously, the surgeon would remove a piece of tissue and have it analyzed in anatomopathology to determine whether the tumor tissue was benign or malignant in order to determine the margins of the tumor. This invasive step was relatively long (from 20 min when performed live on cryogenic sections to 1–2 weeks when performed post-op). Full-field optical coherence tomography provides images comparable to those obtained in conventional histology while being non-invasive and fast (Jain et al. 2011; Assayag et al. 2014).

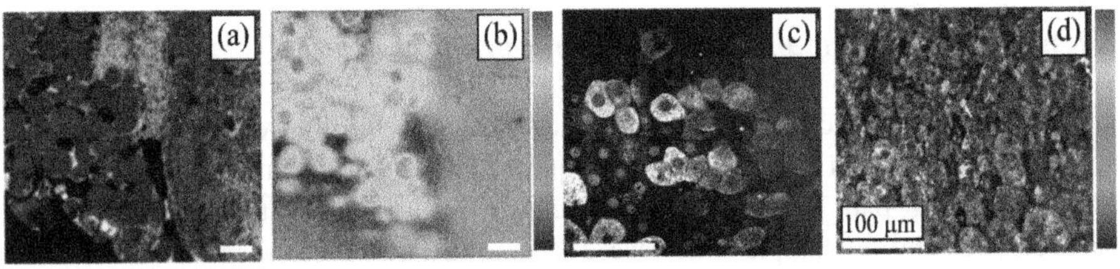

Figure 6.13. *Optical coherence tomography images*

COMMENTS ON FIGURE 6.13.– *(a) Full-field optical coherence tomography image (ON $\sim$ 0.3 and $\times$10) and (b) its stress mapping obtained by the tactile approach. The color code corresponds to stress ranging from 0.5 kPa (blue) to 0.4 kPa (red). (c, d) Dynamic full-field optical coherence tomography images of fresh rat liver tissue with (c) a $\times$40 (On $\sim$ 0.8) objective and (d) a $\times$10 (ON $\sim$ 0.3) objective. In (d), the color code corresponds to the period of the temporal variation of the signal ranging from 5 s (in blue) to 25 ms (in red). The white scale bars correspond to 100 μm (source: Thouvenin et al. 2017a).*

In some cases, however, morphological contrast alone is not sufficient to achieve the diagnosis. To this end, many efforts have recently been undertaken to add new contrasts to the full-field tomographic images (Thouvenin et al. 2017a). More particularly, elastography contrast enables the addition of mechanical stiffness information to full-field tomographic images (Nahas et al. 2013a,b; Leroux et al. 2015; Chatelin et al. 2014). This contrast is relevant for histopathology because organs, tissues and cells that make up biological organisms have intrinsic mechanical properties related to their structure and functions. A change in their mechanical properties can reflect their health condition. Alternatively, dynamic contrast, based on the temporal fluctuation of the full-field OCT signal, makes use of intracellular motility as a new contrast. As illustrated in Figure 6.13, this approach is a means to reveal cell nuclei; they are usually difficult to observe in full-field optical coherence tomography. Their detection is essential for diagnosis (Apelian et al. 2016; Leroux et al. 2016; Thouvenin et al. 2017b; Scholler et al. 2019, 2020).

6.7.2. *Local spectroscopy*

In interference microscopy, some properties of the observed object are encoded in the recorded interferogram. Therefore, the fringes contain information on the object topography as well as its spectral signature. The spectrum describes the sample behavior in the frequency domain, for example its ability to reflect or absorb light within a certain range of wavelengths. Interference microscopy enables quantitative spectral measurements to be made, in particular for finding the reflectance spectrum of a sample. The spectral information is "encoded" in the shape and amplitude of the interference fringes; it is obtained by applying a Fourier transform to the interferogram. We use the theoretical expansion of the interference signal $I(\delta)$ (see equation [6.3]) to show that the modulus of its Fourier transform is given by (Latour et al. 2010; Claveau et al. 2016)

$$\left|\mathcal{F}_k\left[I(\delta)\right]\right| = \frac{1}{4}S(k)\sqrt{R_{ref}(k)}\sqrt{R_e(k)} \qquad [6.11]$$

where $k = 2\pi/\lambda$ is the wave vector, $R_{ref}(k)$ and $R_e(k)$ are the intensity reflection coefficients of the reference mirror and of the sample, and $S(k)$ designates the source spectral density.

In practice, the measured spectrum takes into account the sensor spectral sensitivity and the optical system spectral response. This is called the uncalibrated spectral response (USR): $USR(k) = S(k)R_{sys}(k)\sqrt{R_{ref}(k)}\sqrt{R_e(k)}$ with $R_{sys}(k)$ which includes the camera and the optical system response. It is therefore necessary that the spectral properties of the whole system be known to be able to find the sample spectral reflectance by way of a preliminary calibration step. A known reflectance surface $R_e(k) = R_{cal}(k)$ is measured, from which the spectral transfer function $STF(k) = USR(k)/\sqrt{R_{cal}(k)} = S(k)R_{sys}(k)\sqrt{R_{ref}(k)}$ is deduced. To obtain the specular spectral reflectance of the object in question, the second measurement is carried out under the same experimental conditions:

$$R_e(k) = \left|\frac{\mathcal{F}_k[I(\delta)]}{STF(k)}\right|^2 \qquad [6.12]$$

Several advantages related to the properties of the interferometric system can be obtained with this approach. In the case of Marbach et al. (2021), a single sample axial scan is enough to acquire spectral information over a wide band (~500–900 nm) and a large volume (~200 × 200 × 20 μm³, for example). The measurement produced is resolved in the three spatial directions (Claveau et al. 2017). This performance obviously depends on the instrument. Spatial resolutions are linked to the properties of the source and the optical system (see sections 6.2.2 and 6.5). In spite of an acquisition carried out in the far-field, this technique leads to a localized analysis with an area of micrometric dimension. By repeating the processing applied to the interferometric signal on the whole image, a reflectance map of the object at different wavelengths is obtained (see Figure 6.14). This representation in the form of a "spectral cube" makes it possible to study locally the composition of the sample by extracting the spectrum at a given pixel in the image. The spectral resolution obtained is limited by the spatial length of the interferometric signal (Marbach et al. 2021). This spectral characterization method can be applied to different types of samples, from simple surfaces up to transparent layers comprising randomly distributed structures in the medium (Montgomery et al. 2021). As such, several applications can be derived from this analysis technique: namely the measurement of a material thickness and dispersion (Li et al. 2012; Claveau et al. 2018), the correction of topographic measurements (see Figure 6.15) through the identification of the materials (Leach 2011; Marbach et al. 2021) or even the morphological and optical characterization of micrometric particles (Claveau et al. 2020).

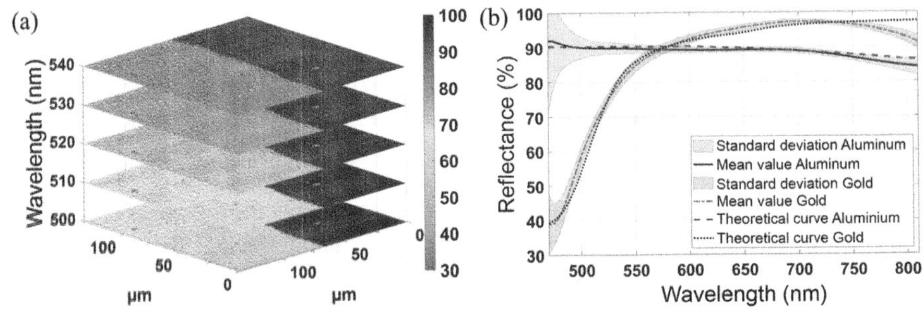

Figure 6.14. *(a) Spectral reflectance mapping of a gold layer deposited on aluminum for different wavelengths (spectral cube). (b) Spectra extracted in two regions of 10 x 10 pixels² = 3.25 x 3.25 μm². The first one is located at the level of the gold layer, the second one is located at the aluminum substrate level*

In the last case, it is possible to demonstrate that white light interference microscopy is a promising tool for the study of deposited or buried spherical particles. Being spatially resolved in 3D, it is capable of resolving microparticles and sub-microparticles buried in the depths of a transparent sample, but also of distinguishing them, with an axial resolution of about 0.8 μm and a lateral resolution of 2.8 μm in the above-mentioned study. Although this is not its primary strong point, the method does not require excessively long acquisition times since only one scan in z is performed. Thanks to it giving single-point measurements and because it employs digital signal processing, this method takes only a few seconds.

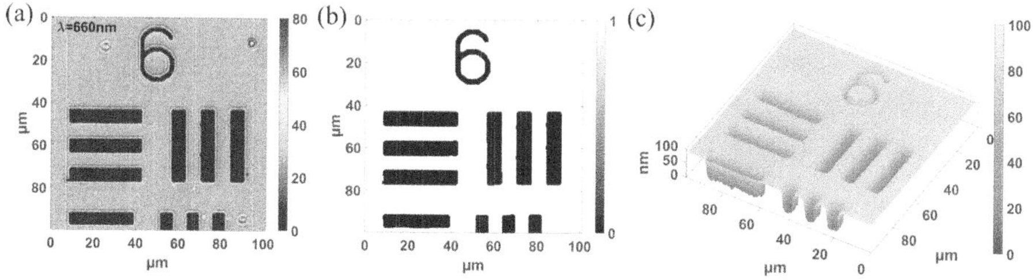

Figure 6.15. *(a) Spectral map at λ = 660 nm of a USAF resolution test pattern. (b) Material classification map: chromium is shown in white (pixel value 1) and glass in black (pixel value 0). (c) Topography measured after correction of reflection phase-shift introduced by chromium*

6.7.3. *Microsphere-assisted microscopic interferometry*

Spatial resolution in conventional interference microscopy is non-homogeneous and limited by diffraction (see section 6.5). Recently, the addition of microspheres in the system object arm has resulted in increasing the lateral resolution of the technique. The method consists of introducing a glass microsphere between the interference objective and the object to be viewed (Figure 6.16(a)). The microsphere diameter D generally ranges between 5 and 60 μm for the super-resolution phenomenon to operate (Boudoukha et al. 2021) and for the lateral field of view to be acceptable ($\sim \sqrt{D/2}$ (Lin et al. 2016)).

The refractive index contrast between the microsphere and the ambient medium is about 1.5, making it possible to work not only in air (Wang et al. 2011) but also in liquid (Darafsheh et al. 2012). A virtual (under the object plane) or real (above the object plane) magnified image is then generated by the microsphere (Perrin et al. 2019; Lecler et al. 2019) and collected by the objective. Microsphere-assisted interference microscopes with Linnik (Wang et al. 2016; Perrin et al. 2017) and Mirau setups (Kassamakov et al. 2017) have been achieved and have facilitated the reconstruction of topographies with a lateral resolution of 200 nm and an axial sensitivity of 10 nm in air (Figure 6.16(b) and (c)).

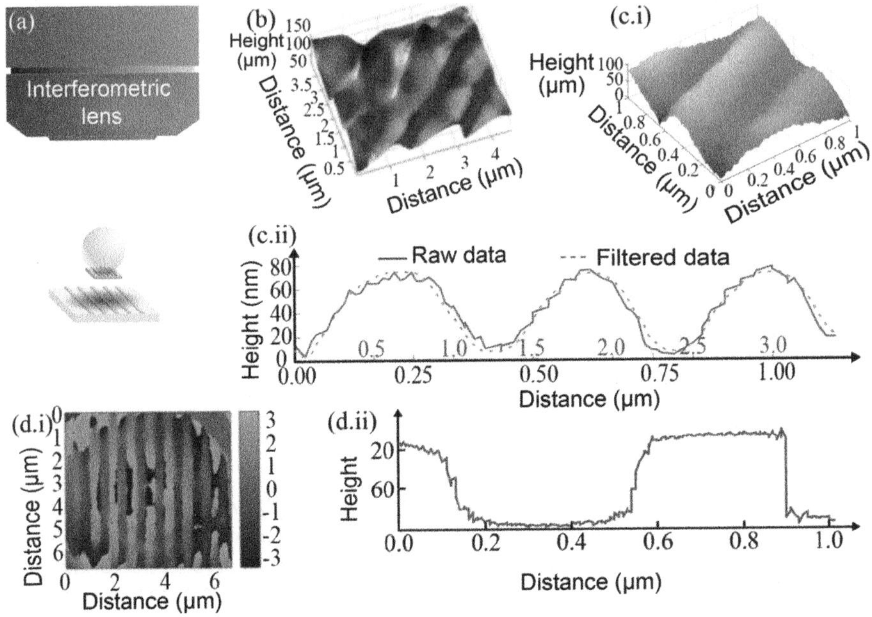

Figure 6.16. *Microsphere-assisted interference microscopy. (a) Technique principle. Topographic reconstructions (b) of laser nano-ripples, (c.i) of a 200 nm linewidth grating with (c.ii) the profile and (d.i) a 400 nm linewidth grating with (d.ii) the profile*

By introducing a similar microsphere into the interferometer reference arm, optical aberrations (mainly spherical and chromatic), as well as dispersion, are then compensated for (Perrin et al. 2020) and the topographic reconstructions obtained are considerably closer to reality (Figure 6.16(d)). Measurement mismatch appears in the phase reconstruction in Figure 6.16(d.i), likely originating from a defect in the quality of the microspheres. Improvements such as increasing the quality of microspheres, as well as contactlessly positioning the microspheres or their displacement, thus offer many opportunities.

6.8. Conclusion

As a metrology technique, interference microscopy has many advantages such as high resolution as well as being fast and contactless. After a general introduction, this chapter has summarized the principles and underlying theory, algorithms, required instrumentation and performance. Current developments in the technique are also described. These systems utilize interference objectives, automated microscopy platforms and electronic cameras, and can be controlled from a computer. The scope of the systems comprises laboratory research and development tools up to large-scale systems for the semiconductor industry, for instance. In surface metrology, interference microscopy plays, and will continue to play, an important role in the transition from tactile to contactless methods. Currently, data acquisition and analysis methods most often use fringe scanning and phase-shifting information to achieve sub-nanometer noise levels over large height ranges. Software and data processing have undergone significant development but the fundamental principles are still the same.

There is continuous refinement of the flexibility, speed and robustness of these methods, as well as improvement in the range of accessible surfaces, from machined materials to multilayer semi-transparent film stacks. In parallel with these advances, new specification standards for surface metrology that facilitate access to structural information lead to easier comparisons of methods and regular technology improvements. There is a large number of existing applications that are frequently updated; in this chapter, we have only cited the most common and best documented ones, but the technique evolves through the contribution of new challenges at the interface of micro- and nano-technology, materials science and life sciences.

White light interference microscopy remains an active area of research, in light of the examples given in this chapter. It aims at miniaturization, very high-speed data acquisition, working in controlled environments, improved performance on complex surfaces and system automation. As camera, light source and computing platform technologies advance, future microscopes are also developed into multimodal instruments that combine different contactless measurement techniques.

6.9. Acknowledgments

The authors would like to thank the members of the IPP team of the ICube Laboratory for their contributions, and especially J. Schiffler, F. Anstotz, F. Salzenstein and S. Lecler for their input and discussions on unconventional imaging. We also thank all partners who directly or indirectly contributed to the research projects.

6.10. References

Apelian, C., Harms, F., Thouvenin, O., Boccara, C. (2016). Dynamic full field optical coherence tomography: Subcellular metabolic contrast revealed in tissues by interferometric signals temporal analysis. *Biomedical Optics Express*, 7(4), 1511–1524.

Assayag, O., Antoine, M., Sigal-Zafrani, B., Riben, M., Harms, F., Burcheri, A., Grieve, K., Dalimier, E., Le Conte de Poly, B., Boccara, C. (2014). Large field, high resolution full-field optical coherence tomography: A pre-clinical study of human breast tissue and cancer assessment. *Technology in Cancer Research & Treatment*, 13(5), 455–468.

Balasubramanian, N. (1982). Optical system for surface topography measurement. Patent US4340306A.

Beaurepaire, E., Boccara, C., Lebec, M., Blanchot, L., Saint-Jalmes, H. (1998). Full-field optical coherence microscopy. *Optics Letters*, 23(4), 244–246.

Benatmane, A., Montgomery, P., Fogarassy, E. (2003). Phase stepping microscopy for rapid control of laser crystallization of Si for flat panel display applications. In *Proc. SPIE Poly-silicon Thin Film Transistor Technology and Applications in Displays and Other Novel Technology Areas*. International Society for Optics and Photonics, Bellingham.

Boudoukha, R., Perrin, S., Demagh, A., Montgomery, P., Demagh, N.-E., Lecler, S. (2021). Near- to far-field coupling of evanescent waves by glass microspheres. *Photonics*, 8(3), 73.

Caber, P. (1993). Interferometric profiler for rough surfaces. *Applied Optics*, 32(19), 3438–3441.

Chapuis, P., Montgomery, P., Anstotz, F., Leong-Hoï, A., Gauthier, C., Baschnagel, J., Reiter, G., McKenna, G., Rubin, A. (2017). A novel interferometric method for the study of the viscoelastic properties of ultra-thin polymer films determined from nanobubble inflation. *Review of Scientific Instruments*, 88(11), 1818–1827.

Chatelin, S., Bernal, M., Deffieux, T., Papadacci, C., Flaud, P., Nahas, A., Boccara, C., Gennisson, J.-L., Tanter, M., Pernot, M. (2014). Anisotropic polyvinyl alcohol hydrogel phantom for shear wave elastography in fibrous biological soft tissue: A multimodality characterization. *Physics in Medicine & Biology*, 59(22), 6923.

Claveau, R., Montgomery, P., Flury, M., Montaner, D. (2016). Local reflectance spectra measurements of surfaces using coherence scanning interferometry. In *Optical Micro and Nanometrology*. International Society for Optics and Photonics, Bellingham.

Claveau, R., Montgomery, P., Flury, M., Montaner, D. (2017). Depth-resolved local reflectance spectra measurements in full-field optical coherence tomography. *Optics Express*, 25(17), 20216–20232.

Claveau, R., Montgomery, P., Flury, M., Ferblantier, G. (2018). Local inspection of refractive index and thickness of thick transparent layers using spectral reflectance measurements in low coherence scanning interferometry. *Optical Materials*, 86, 100–1005.

Claveau, R., Montgomery, P., Flury, M. (2020). Coherence scanning interferometry allows accurate characterization of micrometric spherical particles contained in complex media. *Ultramicroscopy*, 208, 112859–112876.

Creath, K. (1988). Phase-measurement interferometry techniques. *Progress in Optics*, 26, 349–393.

Darafsheh, A., Walsh, G., Dal Negro, L., Astratov, V. (2012). Optical super-resolution by high-index liquid-immersed microspheres. *Applied Physics Letters*, 101(14), 141128.

Davidson, M., Kaufman, K., Mazor, I., Cohen, F. (1987). An application of interference microscopy to integrated circuit inspection and metrology. In *Integrated Circuit Metrology, Inspection, & Process Control*. International Society for Optics and Photonics, Bellingham.

De Chiffre, L., Lonardo, P., Trumpold, H., Lucca, D., Goch, G., Brown, C., Raja, J., Hansen, H. (2000). Quantitative characterisation of surface texture. *CIRP Annals*, 49(2), 635–652.

DigitalSurfé (2021). Paramètres surfaciques de champ [Online]. Available at: https://guide.digitalsurf.com/fr/guide-parametres-surfaciques-champ.html.

Dubois, A. (2004). Effects of phase change on reflection in phase-measuring interference microscopy. *Applied Optics*, 43(7), 1503–1507.

Dubois, A., Vabre, L., Boccara, A., Montgomery, P., Cunin, B., Reibel, Y., Draman, C. (2002). Real-time high-resolution topographic imagery using interference microscopy. *European Physical Journal – Applied Physics*, 20, 169.

Dubois, A., Grieve, K., Moneron, G., Lecaque, R., Vabre, L., Boccara, C. (2004). Ultrahigh-resolution full-field optical coherence tomography. *Applied Optics*, 43(14), 2874–2883.

Ghiglia, D. and Pritt, M. (1998). *Two-dimensional Phase Unwrapping: Theory, Algorithms and Software*. John Wiley & Sons, New York.

Giusca, C. and Leach, R. (2013). Calibration of the scales of areal surface topography measuring instruments: Part 3. Resolution. *Measurement Science and Technology*, 24(10), 105010.

de Groot, P. (2015). Principles of interference microscopy for the measurement of surface topography. *Advances in Optics and Photonics*, 7(1), 1–65.

de Groot, P. and Biegen, J. (2016). Interference microscope objectives for wide-field areal surface topography measurements. *Optical Engineering*, 55(7), 1–6.

de Groot, P. and Deck, L. (1995). Surface profiling by analysis of white-light interferograms in the spatial frequency domain. *Journal of Modern Optics*, 42(2), 389–401.

Guellil, M., Montgomery, P., Pfeiffer, P., Serio, B. (2014). Comparison of areal measurements of the same zone of etched Si and hydroxyapatite layers on etched Si using different profiling techniques. In *Proc. SPIE*. International Society for Optics and Photonics, Bellingham.

Harasaki, A., Schmit, J., Wyant, J. (2000). Improved vertical-scanning interferometry. *Applied Optics*, 39(13), 2107–2115.

Harris, P., Smith, I., Leach, R., Giusca, C., Jiang, X., Scott, P. (2012). Software measurement standards for areal surface texture parameters: Part 1. Algorithms. *Measurement Science and Technology*, 23(10), 105008.

Heintzmann, R. and Ficz, G. (2006). Breaking the resolution limit in light microscopy. *Briefing in Functional Genomics*, 5(4), 289–301.

Huang, D., Swanson, E., Lin, C., Schuman, J., Stinson, W., Chang, W., Hee, M., Flotte, T., Gregory, K., Puliafito, C., Fujimoto, J. (1991). Optical coherence tomography. *Science*, 254(5035), 1178–1181.

ISO (2012). Geometrical product specifications (GPS) – Indication of surface texture in technical product documentation. Standard, ISO 1302:2002.

ISO (2019). Geometrical product specifications (GPS) – Surface texture: Areal – Part 600: Metrological characteristics for areal topography measuring methods. Standard, ISO 25178-600.

Jain, M., Shukla, N., Manzoor, M., Nadolny, S., Mukherjee, S. (2011). Modified full-field optical coherence tomography: A novel tool for rapid histology of tissues. *Journal of Pathology Informatics*, 2(28).

Kassamakov, I., Lecler, S., Nolvi, A., Leong-Hoi, A., Montgomery, P., Haeggstrom, E. (2017). 3D super-resolution optical profiling using microsphere enhanced Mirau interferometry. *Scientific Reports*, 7(3683).

Kino, G. and Chim, S. (1990). Mirau correlation microscope. *Applied Optics*, 29(26), 3775–3783.

Larkin, L. (1996). Efficient nonlinear algorithm for envelope detection in white light interferometry. *Journal of the Optical Society of America*, 13(4), 832–843.

Latour, G., Moreau, J., Elia, M., Frigerio, J.-M. (2010). Micro-spectrometry in the visible range with full-field optical coherence tomography for single absorbing layers. *Optics Communications*, 283(23), 4810–4815.

Latychevskaia, T. (2019). Lateral and axial resolution criteria in incoherent and coherent optics and holography, near- and far-field regimes. *Applied Optics*, 58(13), 3597–3603.

Leach, R. (2011). *Optical Measurement of Surface Topography*. Springer, Berlin.

Lecler, S., Perrin, S., Leong-Hoi, A., Montgomery, P. (2019). Photonic jet lens. *Scientific Reports*, 9(4725).

Lee, B. and Strand, T. (1990). Profilometry with a coherence scanning microscope. *Applied Optics*, 29(26), 3784–3788.

Lehmann, P., Tereschenko, S., Xie, W. (2016). Fundamental aspects of resolution and precision in vertical scanning white-light interferometry. *Surface Topography: Metrology and Properties*, 4(2), 024004.

Leitgeb, R., Hitzenberger, C.K., Fercher, A.F. (2003). Performance of Fourier domain vs. time domain optical coherence tomography. *Optics Express*, 11(8), 889–894.

Leong-Hoi, A., Montgomery, P.C., Serio, B., Twardowski, P., Uhring, W. (2016). High dynamic range microscope imaging based on exposure bracketing in full field OCT. *Optics Letters*, 41(7), 1313.

Leong-Hoi, A., Hairaye, C., Perrin, S., Lecler, S., Pfeiffer, P., Montgomery, P. (2018). High resolution microsphere-assisted interference microscopy for 3D characterization of nanomaterials. *Physica Status Solidi (a)*, 215(6), 1700858.

Leroux, C.-E., Palmier, J., Boccara, C., Cappello, G., Monnier, S. (2015). Elastography of multicellular aggregates submitted to osmo-mechanical stress. *New Journal of Physics*, 17, 073035.

Leroux, C.-E., Bertillot, F., Thouvenin, O., Boccara, C. (2016). Intracellular dynamics measurements with full field optical coherence tomography suggest hindering effect of actomyosin contractility on organelle transport. *Biomedical Optics Express*, 7(11), 4501–4513.

Li, M.-C., Wan, D.-S., Lee, C.-C. (2012). Application of white-light scanning interferometer on transparent thin-film measurement. *Applied Optics*, 51(36), 8579–8586.

Lin, Q., Wang, D., Wang, Y., Rong, L., Zhao, J., Guo, S., Wang, M. (2016). Super-resolution imaging by microsphere-assisted optical microscopy. *Optical and Quantum Electronics*, 48, 557.

Liu, H., Bailleul, J., Simon, B., Debailleul, M., Colicchio, B., Haeberlé, O. (2014). Tomographic diffractive microscopy and multiview profilometry with flexible aberration correction. *Applied Optics*, 53(4), 748–755.

Malacara, D. (2007). *Optical Shop Testing*, 3rd edition. John Wiley & Sons, New York.

Marbach, S., Claveau, R., Wang, F., Schiffler, J., Montgomery, P., Flury, M. (2021). Wide-field parallel mapping of local spectral and topographic information with white light interference microscopy. *Optics Letters*, 46(4), 809–812.

Masters, B.P. (2020). *Superresolution Optical Microscopy: The Quest of Enhanced Resolution and Contrast*. Springer, Berlin.

Montgomery, P. and Fillard, J. (1992). Peak fringe scanning microscopy (PFSM): Submicron 3D measurement of semiconductor components. In *Proc. SPIE*. International Society for Optics and Photonics, Bellingham.

Montgomery, P. and Montaner, D. (1999). Deep submicron 3D surface metrology for 300 mm wafer characterization using UV coherence microscopy. *Microelectronic Engineering*, 45(2–3), 291–297.

Montgomery, P., Montaner, D., Salzenstein, F. (2012). Tomographic analysis of medium thickness transparent layers using white light scanning interferometry and XZ fringe image processing. In *Proc. SPIE*. International Society for Optics and Photonics, Bellingham.

Montgomery, P., Anstotz, F., Salzenstein, F., Montaner, D. (2016). Real time and high quality on-line 4D FF-OCT using continuous fringe scanning with a high speed camera and FPGA image processing. In *Full-Field Optical Coherence Microscopy: Technology and Applications*, Dubois, A. (ed.). Jenny Stanford Publishing, New York.

Montgomery, P., Claveau, R., Marbach, S., Flury, M. (2021). Spatially resolved optical characterization of functional materials using coherence scanning interferometry. *Physica status solidi (a)*, 2000683.

Nahas, A., Bauer, M., Roux, S., Boccara, C. (2013a). 3D static elastography at the micrometer scale using full field OCT. *Biomedical Optics Express*, 4(10), 2138–2149.

Nahas, A., Tanter, M., Nguyen, T.-M., Chassot, J.-M., Fink, M., Boccara, C. (2013b). From supersonic shear wave imaging to full-field optical coherence shear wave elastography. *Journal of Biomedical Optics*, 18(12), 121514.

Perrin, S. (2016). Development and characterization of an optical coherence tomography micro-system: Application to dermatology. PhD thesis, Université de Franche-Comté, Besançon.

Perrin, S., Leong-Hoï, A., Lecler, S., Pfeiffer, P., Kassamakov, I., Nolvi, A., Hæggström, E., Montgomery, P. (2017). Microsphere-assisted phase-shifting profilometry. *Applied Optics*, 56(25), 7249–7255.

Perrin, S., Li, H., Lecler, S., Montgomery, P. (2019). Unconventional magnification behaviour in microsphere-assisted microscopy. *Optics & Laser Technology*, 114, 40–43.

Perrin, S., Donie, Y.J., Montgomery, P., Gomard, G., Lecler, S. (2020). Compensated microsphere-assisted interference microscopy. *Physical Review Applied*, 13, 014068.

Petitgrand, S. (2006). Méthodes de microscopie interférométrique 3D statiques et dynamiques, pour la caractérisation de la technologie et du comportement des microsystèmes. PhD thesis, Université Paris XI.

Saleh, B. and Teich, M. (1991). *Fundamentals of Photonics*. John Wiley & Sons, New York.

Salzenstein, F., Montgomery, P., Boudraa, A. (2014). Local frequency and envelope estimation by Teager-Kaiser energy operators in white-light scanning interferometry. *Optics Express*, 22(15), 18325–18334.

Sandoz, P. (1997). Wavelet transform as a processing tool in white light interferometry. *Optics Letters*, 22(14), 1065–1067.

Sandoz, P. and Tribillon, G. (1993). Profilometry by zero-order interference fringe identification. *Journal of Modern Optics*, 40(9), 1691–1700.

Schmit, J., Reed, J., Novak, E., Gimzewski, J. (2008). Performance advances in interferometric optical profilers for imaging and testing. *Journal of Optics A: Pure Applied Optics*, 10(064001), 1–7.

Scholler, J., Mazlin, V., Thouvenin, O., Groux, K., Xiao, P., Sahel, J.-A., Fink, M., Boccara, C., Grieve, K. (2019). Probing dynamic processes in the eye at multiple spatial and temporal scales with multimodal full field OCT. *Biomedical Optics Express*, 10(2), 731–746.

Scholler, J., Groux, K., Goureau, O., Sahel, J.-A., Fink, M., Reichman, S., Boccara, C., Grieve, K. (2020). Dynamic full-field optical coherence tomography: 3D live-imaging of retinal organoids. *Light: Science & Applications*, 9(1), 1–9.

Schulz, G. and Elssner, K.-E. (1991). Errors in phase-measurement interferometry with high numerical apertures. *Applied Optics*, 30(31), 4500–4506.

Thouvenin, O., Apelian, C., Nahas, A., Fink, M., Boccara, C. (2017a). Full-field optical coherence tomography as a diagnosis tool: Recent progress with multimodal imaging. *Applied Sciences*, 7(3), 236.

Thouvenin, O., Boccara, C., Fink, M., Sahel, J., Pâques, M., Grieve, K. (2017b). Cell motility as contrast agent in retinal explant imaging with full-field optical coherence tomography. *Investigative Ophthalmology & Visual Science*, 58(11), 4605–4615.

Wang, Z., Guo, W., Li, L., Luk'yanchuk, B., Khan, A., Liu, Z., Chen, Z., Hong, M. (2011). Optical virtual imaging at 50 nm lateral resolution with a white-light nanoscope. *Nature Communications*, 2(218).

Wang, F., Liu, L., Yu, P., Liu, Z., Yu, H., Wang, Y., Li, W. (2016). Three-dimensional super-resolution morphology by near-field assisted white-light interferometry. *Scientific Reports*, 6, 24703.

7

Multimodal and Multispectral Endoscopic Imaging with Extended Field of View

Christian DAUL and Walter BLONDEL
CRAN, CNRS, Université de Lorraine, Vandœuvre-lès-Nancy, France

7.1. Introduction to conventional endoscopy

7.1.1. *Principle and medical applications of endoscopy*

In the medical field, endoscopy is a method for visually exploring the interior of the human body and a reference examination for the diagnosis of pathologies such as benign or malignant tumors, ulcers or inflammatory lesions. This examination uses a medical device called an endoscope. This instrument is composed of an optical tube with an external diameter of a few millimeters that makes it possible to send light to the internal tissues to illuminate them (illumination function) and to acquire, by means of a camera, images of the tissues thus illuminated (visualization function).

Endoscopy is used to visualize the interior of hollow organs and cavities of the human body that are accessible (i) by natural means, that is, non-invasively, such as the bronchial tubes (bronchoscopy), the colon (colonoscopy), the cervix (hysteroscopy), the esophagus and the stomach (gastroscopy) or the bladder (cystoscopy) and (ii) through the skin by means of microsurgical incisions such as in the abdominal cavity (coelioscopy) or the joints (arthroscopy)

Unconventional Optical Imaging for Biology,
coordinated by Corinne FOURNIER and Olivier HAEBERLÉ. © ISTE Ltd 2024.

With endoscopy, the physician has the possibility of performing clinical diagnosis (simple observation) and/or a surgical intervention (biopsy, resection, etc.) through an operating channel intended for the insertion of microsurgical tools within the endoscopic tube. The latter can be rigid or flexible, depending on whether the image acquisition channel comprises lenses or optical fibers, respectively. The flexible endoscope (or fiberscope) allows for lengths of endoscopic conduit longer than 1 m that are well adapted to the exploration of the air and digestive tracts, as well as articulated mechanisms making it possible to mechanically orient the endoscope tip inside the observed organ in the direction of its internal wall.

Finally, technological progress in terms of miniaturization has now led to the emergence of video endoscopes in which the camera (image sensor and its lens) and the light source (LED) are directly integrated into the distal tip of the endoscope (see Figure 7.1).

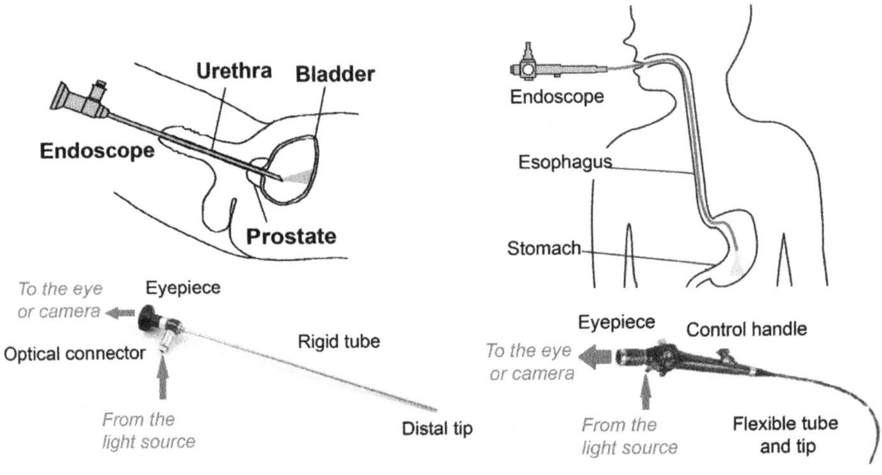

Figure 7.1. *Illustrations of endoscopic examinations using an endoscope: (a) rigid for cystoscopy; (b) flexible for gastroscopy*

7.1.2. *Relevance and limitations of conventional endoscopy*

Medical endoscopy, known as "conventional endoscopy", uses a white-light source to illuminate biological tissue. It is the major endoscopic modality for monitoring and detecting tissue anomalies. White light (WL) includes all visible wavelengths of the light spectrum from approximately 400 to 800 nm. This WL imaging modality enables clinicians to make a diagnosis based on their acquired knowledge and experience of the anatomical and morphological characteristics of biological tissues seen "under natural color illumination" (Figure 7.2). When a suspicious lesion is visually detected, a small sample of tissue can be taken (a biopsy is achieved through the operating channel of the endoscope by means of surgical microtips) and then transferred to the anatomical pathologist to formulate the final medical diagnosis by determining the exact biological status of the tissue (inflammatory, cancerous, etc.).

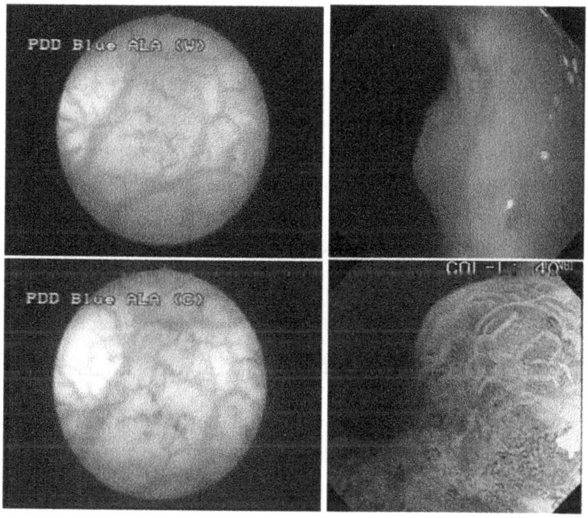

Figure 7.2. *Examples of endoscopic images of (a) the bladder and (b) the stomach, acquired in white light (top) and in different multispectral modalities (bottom) providing enhanced contrast between healthy tissues and pathological lesions: fluorescence cystoscopy with a cancerous lesion visible in pink on a blue background (Geavlete et al. 2008) and narrow band imaging gastroscopy bringing forward microsurface structures and microvascularization (Song and Ang 2014), respectively. For a color version of this figure, see www.iste.co.uk/fournier/unconventional.zip*

Despite these advantages, WL endoscopy has several limitations when it comes to discerning between healthy and pathological tissues. These limitations have motivated the development of new technical and methodological solutions for several years, namely by combining different images acquired in distinct spectral bands within the visible spectrum (sections 7.3 and 7.4).

From a medical point of view, the problems concern the invasive nature of the biopsy procedure (several pieces of tissue of a few mm^3 are taken) and the limited sensitivity of this procedure linked to the tradeoff that the clinician must achieve with the quantity of samples to be taken: this number of samples must be (i) "sufficient" to provide a reliable diagnosis but (ii) "limited" to preserve the integrity of the organ being considered. Furthermore, the difference between some healthy and pathological tissues or between some benign and malignant lesions may be difficult to detect due to the lack of visual contrast in WL observation (see Figure 7.2). For example, in cystoscopy, the rate of recurrence of bladder cancer 12 months after resection of the lesions that can be seen in conventional endoscopy may be as high as 40% (Amouroux et al. 2019).

From a technical point of view, the problems are linked to the intrinsic optical technological characteristics of endoscopes. Their short focal length eyepieces allow the internal surface of the organs to be visualized in a reduced motion space and with an intrinsically limited field of view (about a cm^2), given the distance available (a few millimeters) between the endoscope distal tip and the wall of the organ under observation. The risk of this "fragmented" observation is that a non-exhaustive visualization of the entire organ can be achieved, which potentially tends not to detect lesions in the uncovered areas.

7.1.3. *Chapter objectives and content*

The objective of this chapter is to present the technical and methodological solutions that have recently been developed or are under development to meet the medical and technical challenges of improving visual contrast between different types of tissue, optimizing surgical guidance and improving the efficiency of lesion detection. The approaches developed consist of (i) adding to the morphological or anatomical images available in WL "functional" information from complementary optical imaging modalities (multispectral and/or multimodal approaches, section 7.4) and (ii) superimposing this information on an extended mapping of the organ under examination (image registration and mosaicing, section 7.3).

Section 7.2 starts by providing a more detailed introduction to the main characteristics of the component parts of rigid and flexible medical endoscopy devices, that is, light sources, cameras and endoscopes (section 7.2.1). This introduction to endoscopes is followed by the main modeling elements of the image acquisition system. These include the pinhole model of an ideal camera (section 7.2.2) as well as the effects of radial distortion (section 7.2.3) and vignetting (section 7.2.4) that are characteristic of endoscopic optics.

7.2. The functioning of endoscopes

7.2.1. *Components of an endoscopic system*

A complete endoscopic imaging system (endoscopic column) typically includes a light source, an endoscope (rigid or flexible) and an imaging system comprising a viewing screen (typically a monitor ranging in size from 27 to 32 inches). An optical cable connects the light source and the endoscope. The imaging unit allows for the visualization and recording of image sequences acquired by a camera. It is either attached to the proximal end of the endoscope (on the eyecup, Figure 7.1) or integrated into its distal end (videoendoscopes, *chip-on-tip* technology).

7.2.1.1. *Endoscope*

A rigid endoscope consists of a stainless steel tube, about 3–15 mm in diameter and 10–50 cm long, inside which can be found (i) a bundle of optical fibers that conducts the light from the external source to the distal end of the endoscope in order to illuminate the interior of the organ cavity, (ii) a visualization channel consisting of a system of cylindrical lenses and a proximal eyepiece to which a camera is attached and (iii) if necessary (according to the model), a (hollow) operating channel making it possible to insert surgical micro-instruments such as grasping and biopsy forceps, irrigation and suction catheters or coagulation probes.

The lens located at the distal end of the vision conduit is characterized by a short focal length (less than 10 mm). This lens is fixed onto the tube by gold soldering for reasons of biological compatibility and for resistance to disinfection/sterilization procedures (detergents, autoclave). Depending on the organ, the tissue area to be observed, and the needs of the clinician, rigid endoscopes with different viewing angles with respect to the tube axis can be employed, namely direct-view (0°), forward-view (up to 60°) and side-view (up to 90°) optics (see Figure 7.3(a)). Conventionally, endoscopic optics offer a depth of field ranging from a few millimeters to a few centimeters and a field of view in the cm^2 range at a distance of about 1 cm from the tissue (aperture angles from 80° to 120°).

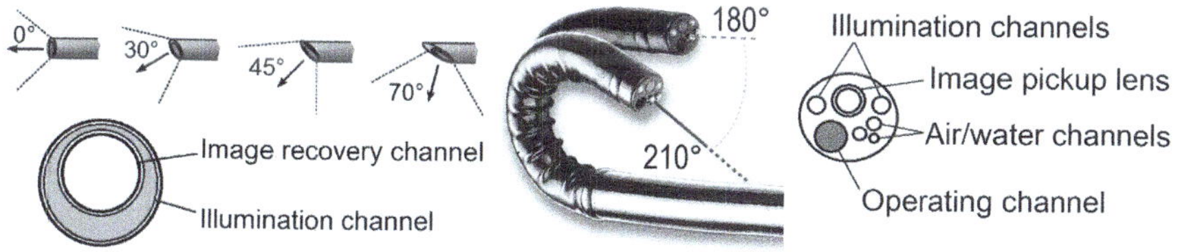

Figure 7.3. *Channels and angulations at the distal end of (a) rigid and (b) flexible endoscopes. For a color version of this figure, see www.iste.co.uk/fournier/unconventional.zip*

A flexible endoscope comprises a flexible tube with a diameter of a few millimeters and a length of 30–120 cm, within which the viewing channel consists of a bundle of several tens of thousands of optical fibers. The endoscope conduit contains an articulated mechanism that the clinician manipulates by means of a lever located on the endoscope handle. With it, the distal tip can be oriented within a range of directions in space, such as an articulation of 210° upward and 140° downward in cystoscopy (see Figure 7.3(b)).

At the end of the endoscope, the configuration of the illumination channel(s), made up of fiber optic bundles, takes into account the geometrical characteristics of each type of endoscope (rigid or flexible). Incidentally, it should be noted that these configurations produce an illumination whose spatial inhomogeneity on the tissue varies according to the position of the endoscope tip with respect to the tissue.

7.2.1.2. *Cameras*

As a result of technological progress in terms of integration of electronic and optical components, the color CCD (*charge-coupled device*) sensors that equipped medical endoscopes until the mid-2010s have now largely been replaced by CMOS (*complementary metal oxide semiconductor*) technology, which enables, at lower costs, levels of miniaturization significantly higher than those of CCD technology. For example, current endoscopes are typically equipped with high-definition (Full HD, 1,920 × 1,080 pixels) or even very high-definition cameras (UHD, 3,840 × 2,160 pixels). Both formats can be available on the same device for recording video sequences (in Full HD) and still photographs (single images in UHD), respectively. The advantage of these high-definition WL endoscopy systems is that they are capable of achieving high optical magnifications (×30) while maintaining very good image quality. In high-magnification endoscopy, an additional optical magnification (×100–150) can be obtained by means of a magnifying lens located at the distal end of the endoscope.

7.2.1.3. *Light sources*

Also due to recent technological developments and reduced costs of light sources, traditional technologies based on external xenon and halogen lamps are gradually being replaced by light-emitting diodes (LEDs), which have a service life (several tens of thousands of hours) that is 2–3 orders of magnitude longer than that of classical lamps. Some fiberscope technologies, particularly disposable ones, now include LED sources integrated into the distal end of the endoscopic tube.

The criteria for choosing an endoscope, in terms of technical characteristics (quality and performance) and costs (purchase and maintenance), depend on the clinical need, the pathology and the targeted organ. However, the camera of an endoscope can be described by using optical and physical models identical to those of consumer cameras (such as computer or cell phone cameras, for instance). These models are presented in the following section.

7.2.2. Pinhole camera model

The geometrical link between a point P_{3D} of the scene (see Figure 7.4(a)) and its projection (point P_{2D}) seen in a two-dimensional (2D) image depends on the pose (namely the position and orientation) of the camera within a three-dimensional (3D) "world" coordinate system and the optical parameter values of the camera.

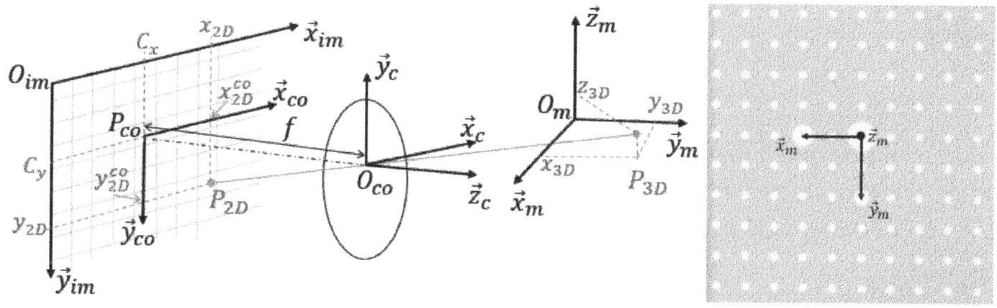

Figure 7.4. *Pinhole camera model and parameter calibration. (a) Pinhole model that can be used for any type of camera: a standard CCD or CMOS camera, an endoscope, a cell phone or a computer camera. (b) Example of a calibration plate that can be used to determine the value of extrinsic and intrinsic parameters*

The extrinsic parameters define the camera pose. In equation [7.1], the nine elements r_{ij} of a rotation matrix R and the translation vector $\vec{T} = (t_x, t_y, t_z)^T$ relate the coordinates of the point P_{3D} expressed in the world coordinate system $(O_m, \vec{x}_m, \vec{y}_m, \vec{z}_m)$ with its position within the camera coordinate system $(O_{co}, \vec{x}_c, \vec{y}_c, \vec{z}_c)$ whose origin O_{co} corresponds to the optical center of the lens:

$$\begin{pmatrix} x_c \\ y_c \\ z_c \end{pmatrix} = \begin{pmatrix} r_{11} & r_{12} & r_{13} \\ r_{21} & r_{22} & r_{23} \\ r_{31} & r_{32} & r_{33} \end{pmatrix} \begin{pmatrix} x_{3D} \\ y_{3D} \\ z_{3D} \end{pmatrix} + \begin{pmatrix} t_x \\ t_y \\ t_z \end{pmatrix} = R\,P_{3D} + \vec{T} \qquad [7.1]$$

The intrinsic parameters link the camera coordinate system $(O_{co}, \vec{x}_c, \vec{y}_c, \vec{z}_c)$ with the image coordinate system $(O_{im}, \vec{x}_{im}, \vec{y}_{im})$. The focal length f, which ranges from a few millimeters to 1 cm in the case of endoscopes, corresponds to the distance between the image plane and the lens plane that includes the position of the camera optical center. Ideally, these two planes are parallel and both perpendicular to the optical axis that runs through point P_{co} and that is carried by the axis $\vec{z}_c$. For distortion free optics, the projection of a 3D point in the coordinate system $(P_{co}, \vec{x}_{co}, \vec{y}_{co})$ depends on a single intrinsic parameter, namely the focal length f:

$$x_{co} = f\frac{x_c}{z_c} \quad \text{et} \quad y_{co} = f\frac{y_c}{z_c} \qquad [7.2]$$

The matrix sensor (CCD or CMOS), which corresponds to the image plane ideally placed in the middle of the depth of focus, comprises rectangular photosensitive elements (pixels) whose width S_x and height S_y are about 10 μm. The coordinates of the projection P_{co} of the optical center O_{co} in the image define the 2D translation vector $(C_x, C_y)^T$, which links the image coordinate system $(O_{im}, \vec{x}_{im}, \vec{y}_{im})$ with the camera coordinate system $(P_{co}, \vec{x}_{co}, \vec{y}_{co})$:

$$x_{im} = \frac{x_{co}}{S_x} + C_x \quad \text{and} \quad y_{im} = \frac{y_{co}}{S_y} + C_y \qquad [7.3]$$

It should be noted that the coordinates (x_{co}, y_{co}) and the intrinsic parameters (S_x and S_y) have a unit of length, whereas the coordinates (x_{im}, y_{im}) and the position (C_x, C_y) of the optical center are expressed in pixels.

Combining equations [7.1]–[7.3], matrix M_{cam} describes the projection in the image of a 3D point whose position is expressed in a world coordinate system:

$$M_{cam} = \begin{pmatrix} f\frac{r_{11}}{S_x} + C_x r_{31} & f\frac{r_{12}}{S_x} + C_x r_{32} & f\frac{r_{13}}{S_x} + C_x r_{33} & f\frac{t_x}{S_x} + C_x t_z \\ f\frac{r_{21}}{S_x} + C_x r_{31} & f\frac{r_{22}}{S_x} + C_x r_{32} & f\frac{r_{23}}{S_x} + C_x r_{33} & f\frac{t_y}{S_y} + C_y t_z \\ r_{31} & r_{32} & r_{33} & t_z \end{pmatrix} \qquad [7.4]$$

In equation [7.5], which expresses the link between the coordinates (x_{3D}, y_{3D}, z_{3D}) and (x_{im}, y_{im}), α is a real value whose interpretation is as follows: any 3D point located on the same line in space is projected onto the same pixel. In other words, the value of the real α depends on the position of the point on the line:

$$\begin{pmatrix} \alpha\, x_{im} \\ \alpha\, y_{im} \\ \alpha \end{pmatrix} = \begin{pmatrix} M_{cam} \end{pmatrix} \begin{pmatrix} x_{3D} \\ y_{3D} \\ z_{3D} \\ 1 \end{pmatrix} \qquad [7.5]$$

Calibration plates are conventionally utilized to determine the value of extrinsic (R and $\vec{T}$, see equation [7.1]) and intrinsic parameters (f, S_x, S_y, C_x and C_y, see equations [7.2] and [7.3]). As an example, for the plate in Figure 7.4(b), the exact position in millimeters of the disk centers is known by construction in the world coordinate system $(O_m, \vec{x}_{3D}, \vec{y}_{3D}, \vec{z}_{3D})$. One hundred disks are placed in the plane $(O_m, \vec{x}_{3D}, \vec{y}_{3D})$ and the three disks that have diameters greater than the 97 other disks define the world coordinate system. An image of the plate is acquired and the equations of the ellipses of each disk (depending on the viewpoint, the disk edge has an elliptical shape) can be determined automatically (Daul et al. 1998). Not only do these equations give the center positions, but also the value of the length of the axes of the ellipses that make it possible to identify the three disks that define the world coordinate system. This latter information facilitates the matching of the centers seen in the images (points $P_{im} = (x_{im}, y_{im})$) and their positions in the world coordinate system (points $P_{3D} = (x_{3D}, y_{3D}, z_{3D})$). The 100 pairs of points (P_{3D}, P_{im}) must each verify the three equations of relation [7.5]. To find the value of the extrinsic and intrinsic parameters, an overdetermined system of linear equations has thus simply to be solved by a least squares method.

Two observations finalize this section on camera modeling. On the one hand, the computed values of the extrinsic parameters are only valid for the pose the camera has been calibrated with, while those of the intrinsic parameters are independent of this pose (all optical parameters are fixed if f is constant). On the other hand, the intrinsic and extrinsic parameters not only make it possible to model the projection of the 3D points in the image but can also be used to determine, for each pixel, the equation of the line segment followed by the photons, which reach the corresponding photosite of the matrix sensor.

7.2.3. *Distortion modeling and correction*

The optics of the endoscopes (i.e. the distal tip of the instrument) is usually very close to the internal surface (epithelial tissues) of the explored hollow organs in order to observe a surface of a few square centimeters in high resolution. Under these conditions, the focal length f of the optics must be short to yield the minimal field of view sought. This type of optics creates geometrical barrel distortions. In Figure 7.5(a), the projection P_{co} of the optical center in an image without distortion is located at coordinates (C_x, C_y) and is also the center of symmetry of a grid with regularly spaced vertical and horizontal lines. In Figure 7.5(b), which illustrates the barrel distortion effect, the only pixel not affected by the distortion corresponds to the point P_{co}. The distance between this point and a point P_{sd} of coordinates (x_{sd}, f_{sd}) in the image without distortion is increased by the barrel effect to lead to the point P_{ad} of coordinates (x_{ad}, f_{ad}) in the image with distortions. This distance increases monotonically further away from the optical center and explains the barrel shape originating from the deformation of the grid (straight lines modified into convex curves). The distortion is mathematically modeled by using a $2n$-order polynomial, n coefficients k_i $(i \in [1, n])$ and radius r between points P_{co} and P_{ad} (see Figure 7.5 for the position of these points):

$$\begin{cases} x_{sd} = x_{ad} + (x_{ad} - C_x)(k_1 r^2 + k_2 r^4 + ... + k_n r^{2n}) \\ y_{sd} = y_{ad} + (y_{ad} - C_y)(k_1 r^2 + k_2 r^4 + ... + k_n r^{2n} \\ r = \sqrt{(x_{ad} - C_x)^2 + (y_{ad} - C_y)^2} \end{cases} \quad [7.6]$$

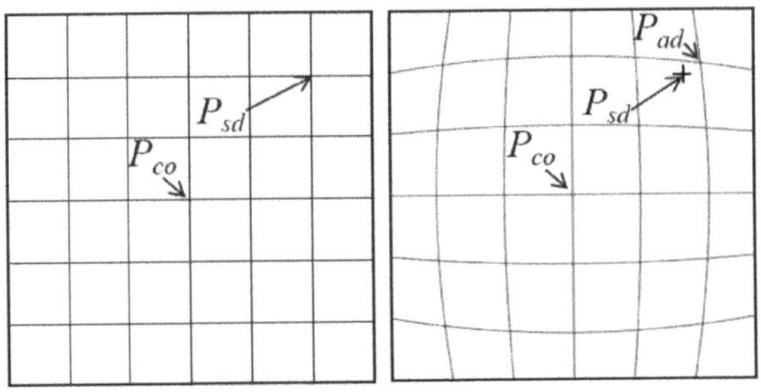

Figure 7.5. *Illustration of the barrel distortion effect. (a) Image without distortions including regularly spaced vertical and horizontal lines. (b) The barrel effect shifts the point P_{sd} from its undistorted position to the position of point P_{ad}. The distances $\overline{P_{sd}P_{ad}}$ and $r = \overline{P_{co}P_{ad}}$ increase as we get closer to the periphery of the field of view*

The parameters of the barrel distortion defined in equation [7.6] can be obtained using calibration charts constructed from geometric features with reference points that can be automatically located in the images. These reference points can be square corners (Zhang 2000) or disk centers (Daul et al. 2005), for example. In Figure 7.6(a), the reference points are given by a quasi-checkerboard pattern that has been printed on a sheet of paper, an image of which has been acquired with an endoscope (image with barrel distortion).

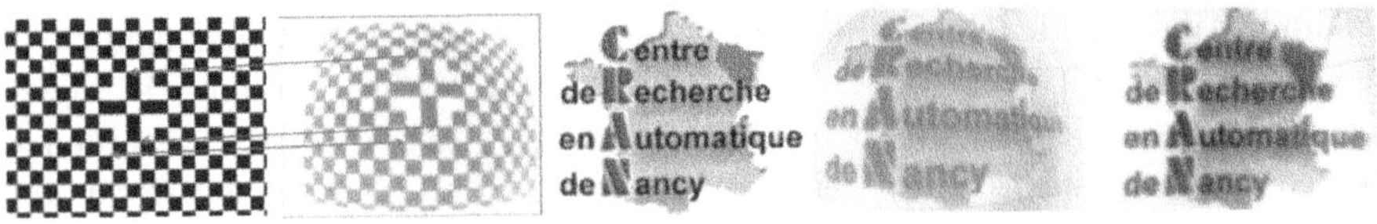

Figure 7.6. *Calibration and distortion correction. For a color version of this figure, see www.iste.co.uk/fournier/unconventional.zip*

COMMENT ON FIGURE 7.6.– *(a) Test pattern without distortion (left) and illustration of the calibration chart acquired with an endoscope, that is, with distortion (right). The red arrows highlight three of the many pairs of homologous points whose coordinates are used for determining the value of the distortion coefficients. (b) From left to right: image without distortions, previous image acquired with an endoscope and acquired image after distortion correction.*

Since the calibration chart was designed with a CAD software program, the unit of the reference point positions and the dimensions of the squares are the millimeter. However, since the values of the two resolution parameters S_x and S_y are known for the position of the endoscope in which the image of the calibration chart was acquired (section 7.2.2), it is possible to express the positions of the reference points (x_{sd}, x_{ad}) in pixels. The pixel positions of the points (x_{ad}, x_{ad}) are automatically located in the image with distortion and the rectangular features are used as a reference to facilitate the matching of the homologous points P_{sd} and P_{ad} (this matching is also facilitated by the similar points of view of the two images in Figure 7.6(a)). For each pair of points (P_{sd}, P_{ad}), it is therefore possible to write the following two equations from relation [7.6]:

$$\begin{cases} k_1 r^2 + k_2 r^4 + ... + k_n r^{2n} = \frac{x_{sd} - x_{ad}}{x_{ad} - C_x} \\ k_1 r^2 + k_2 r^4 + ... + k_n r^{2n} = \frac{y_{sd} - y_{ad}}{y_{ad} - C_y} \end{cases} \quad [7.7]$$

where the values of (x_{sd}, x_{sd}), (x_{ad}, x_{ad}), (C_x, C_y) and r are all known (C_x and C_y are calibrated and r is defined in [7.6]). In practice, the calibration charts are designed to obtain many pairs (P_{sd}, P_{ad}), and therefore we simply have to solve an overdetermined linear system ($2m > n$) formed by $2m$ equations, with m the number of homologous points and n the number of unknown coefficients k_i. Studies in the literature (Miranda-Luna et al. 2004; Zhang 2000) have shown that barrel distortions of endoscope optics are accurately modeled using fourth-order polynomials ($n = 2$). Figure 7.6(b) shows a distortion correction result using equation [7.7].

7.2.4. *Vignetting modeling and correction*

Vignetting designates the monotonic decrease of the light intensity between the optical center and any point located at the periphery of the image. For endoscopes, vignetting is a combination of two effects: one is optical and the other is numerical.

Optical vignetting is related to the fact that the illumination of a matrix sensor is most important for light rays that fall perpendicularly on the image plane and decreases when the angle θ between the photon path and the optical axis Δ increases. Figure 7.7 shows that, for a convergent lens L, the illumination in the image plane P decreases closer to the periphery of the image (θ increases). It is accepted in optics that illumination through a lens decreases following a $\cos^4(\theta)$ distribution.

Digital vignetting is superimposed on the optical vignetting. This second effect is due to the fact that the energy delivered by the photosites of the digital matrix sensors also depends on the angle of incidence of the photons. For the same amount of photons, a photosite/pixel located near the projection of the optical center of the sensor/image generates a more energetic signal than a photosite/pixel located at the periphery of the sensor/image.

A conventional approach for modeling the vignetting effect consists of modeling the illumination drop with a sixth-order polynomial (Doutre and Nasiopoulos 2009) and to use the pixel values of a calibration image I_e representing a surface of homogeneous color (such as a white surface, for example). In equation [7.8], $I_e(C_x, C_y)$ is the intensity of the pixel corresponding to the optical center, with $I_e(C_x, C_y) > I_e(x, y) \; \forall \; (C_x, C_y) \neq (x, y)$:

$$\begin{cases} v(r) = \frac{I_e(C_x, C_y)}{I_e(x,y)} & = (1 + k_1 r^2 + k_2 r^4 + k_3 r^6) \\ \text{with } r & = \sqrt{(C_x - x)^2 + (C_y - y)^2} \end{cases} \quad [7.8]$$

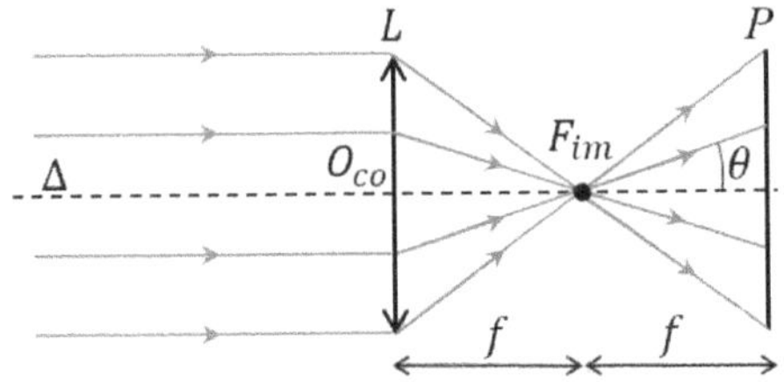

Figure 7.7. *Origin of the vignetting effect (f and O_{co} are, respectively, the focal length and the optical center). The illumination by the rays that follow the optical axis Δ ($\theta = 0$) is maximal, whereas the light energy per surface unit decreases when the value of the angle θ increases*

The coordinates C_x and C_y are known as a result of the camera calibration and the values $v(r)$ are determined using the calibration image $I_e(x, y)$ for the pixels belonging to the circles of radius r. The values of the coefficients k_i (i = 1, 2 or 3) are obtained by solving a system of overdetermined linear equations formed by the first relation of system [7.8]. A vignetting corrected image is computed using the coefficients $v(r)$ that compensate for the drop in intensities in the acquired image $I_a^c(x, y)$: $I_{cv}^c(x, y) = v(r) I_a^c(x, y)$. We should bear in mind that for a monochromatic camera c denotes the intensity image and for color cameras c represents the three color channels ($c = r$, v or b). The coefficients $v(r)$ are valid for a given value of f (the focal length is generally fixed for endoscopes).

Other solutions for vignetting correction use more complex models and/or no calibration images (these methods correct vignetting effects only with the acquired images at the expense of computation time, which is significant (Zheng et al. 2009)). The polynomial-based method can be implemented in real time and yields an efficient correction of the endoscopic images.

7.3. 3D cartography of endoscopic scenes

A panoramic image, namely with an extended field of view of the internal surface of an organ, can be obtained either by employing only 2D endoscopic images, or by utilizing data from endoscopes whose functionalities have been extended to the acquisition of 3D points. Regardless of the method being used, the registration (or matching) of homologous 2D or 3D points acquired from two endoscope viewpoints form the basis of 3D mapping (or mosaicing) methods. 2D/2D or 3D/3D registration techniques that can be implemented in the endoscopic domain are introduced in section 7.3.1. These methods are then used in section 7.3.2 to briefly present the principle of two 3D mosaicing approaches, one based on active vision, the other on passive vision (these two approaches rely on the models described in section 7.2 for cameras).

7.3.1. *Data registration from two viewpoints*

This section presents two complementary principles for finding the homologous data of two datasets. In a first family of approaches, optimization algorithms are used for simultaneously finding a geometric model that links the data and the correspondences between homologous points (matching with a geometric model). The second family consists of approaches that first search for the correspondence between homologous points and then use this knowledge to determine the geometric relationship that globally links two datasets (matching without a geometric model).

7.3.1.1. *Principle of registration with a geometric model*

Equations [7.9] describe the principle of the iterative process for determining the geometric transformation T_{geo} that superimposes the data from two viewpoints of the endoscopic camera. These equations minimize (maximize) a dissimilarity Dis (a similarity Sim) by superimposing the data $\mathcal{D}_s$ extracted from the source image I_s onto the data $\mathcal{D}_c$ from the target image I_c. The dissimilarity measure Dis or similarity measure Sim can be computed from very different types of data (for example, directly from the gray levels of the two images, or with the distances that separate homologous points, contours or surfaces observed in the two images). The vector $\vec{T}$ contains the parameters of the geometrical transformation T_{geo} and the solution $\vec{T}_{sol}$ is supposed to be found when the data $\mathcal{D}_s$ of the source image I_s (which are "displaced" by T_{geo} on the static target I_c) superimpose $\mathcal{D}_c$. With equations [7.9], it is assumed that the data are registered when Dis (or Sim) reaches a global minimum (or maximum):

$$\vec{T}_{sol} = \min_{\vec{T}} (Dis(T_{geo}(\mathcal{D}_s), \mathcal{D}_c)) \text{ and } \vec{T}_{sol} = \max_{\vec{T}} (Sim(T_{geo}(\mathcal{D}_s), \mathcal{D}_c)) \qquad [7.9]$$

The choice of optimization method depends on the nature of the data (discrete or not), on the differentiability of the measures Dis or Sim, on the proximity of the initial conditions of $\vec{T}$ to the solution $\vec{T}_{sol}$ or on the size of the parameter space (number of components of $\vec{T}$) in which a solution is sought.

For endoscopic images, the optics are close to the internal walls, which classically correspond to locally smooth surfaces without geometric discontinuities. The surfaces in the 2D images thus being quasi-planar, a homography makes it possible to accurately model the geometrical link between the coordinates (x_s, y_s) and (x_c, y_c) of the pixels of the images I_s and I_c. The transformation T_{geo} of equation [7.9] is thus a homography H_{sc} defined by an in-plane rotation (angle ϕ), by scale factors k_x and k_y along the abscissa and ordinate of the images, by shear parameters S_x and S_y along the axes $\vec{x}$ and $\vec{y}$, and by a 2D translation of components t_x and t_y. The value of the parameter α^i of each pair i of homologous pixels is entirely defined by the perspective parameters p_x and p_y whose values are related to the two out-of-image plane rotations:

$$\alpha^i \begin{pmatrix} x_c^i \\ y_c^i \\ 1 \end{pmatrix} = \begin{pmatrix} k_x \cos\phi & -S_x \sin\phi & t_x \\ S_y \sin\phi & k_y \cos\phi & t_y \\ p_x & p_y & 1 \end{pmatrix} \begin{pmatrix} x_s^i \\ y_s^i \\ 1 \end{pmatrix} = \underbrace{\begin{pmatrix} a_{11} & a_{12} & a_{13} \\ a_{21} & a_{22} & a_{23} \\ a_{31} & a_{32} & a_{33} \end{pmatrix}}_{H_{sc}} \begin{pmatrix} x_s^i \\ y_s^i \\ 1 \end{pmatrix} \quad [7.10]$$

The solution vector $\vec{T}_{sol} = (a_{11}, a_{12}, a_{13}, a_{21}, a_{22}, a_{23}, a_{31}, a_{32})^T$ includes the values of the eight linearly independent parameters a_{ij} defined by the matrix H_{sc}, which superimposes the pixels of coordinates (x_s^i, y_s^i) onto their homologous pixels in the image I_c (see equation [7.10]).

If, in addition to the images I_s and I_c, two sets $\mathcal{D}_s^{3D} = \{P_s^{3D,i}\}$ and $\mathcal{D}_c^{3D} = \{P_c^{3D,i}\}$ of 3D points are known for the two camera viewpoints, then there exists a 3D transformation that establishes the geometric link between each pair i of corresponding points $P_s^{3D,i} = (x_s^i, y_s^i, z_s^i)^T$ and $P_c^{3D,i} = (x_c^i, y_c^i, z_c^i)^T$. The transformation T_{geo} in equation [7.9] is therefore a rigid transformation T_{sc}^{3D} defined in equation [7.11] by a rotation matrix $R_{sc} = (r_{ij})_{1\leq i\leq 3, 1\leq j\leq 3}$ and a translation $\vec{T}_{sc} = (t_x, t_y, t_z)^T$. The parameters r_{ij} of the matrix R_{sc} can be defined for three successive rotations around the axes $\vec{x}$, $\vec{y}$ and $\vec{z}$ of the camera "source" position reference. However, the expression of these parameters can also be defined from the Euler angles (Daul et al. 2005). In the "x"-convention of Euler angles, the first rotation $\phi \in [0, 2\pi]$ is carried out around the $\vec{z}$ axis, the second rotation $\theta \in [0, \pi]$ is carried out around the new $\vec{x}$ axis, and the last rotation $\psi \in [0, 2\pi]$ takes place around the new $\vec{z}$ axis. Euler angles are often preferred over successive rotations around the three axes because smaller rotations often lead to the desired solution, thus resulting in a faster optimization.

$$\begin{pmatrix} x_c^i \\ y_c^i \\ z_c^i \\ 1 \end{pmatrix} = \underbrace{\begin{pmatrix} R_{sc} & \vec{T}_{sc} \\ 0 & 1 \end{pmatrix}}_{T_{sc}^{3D}} \begin{pmatrix} x_s^i \\ y_s^i \\ z_s^i \\ 1 \end{pmatrix} = \begin{pmatrix} r_{11} & r_{12} & r_{13} & t_x \\ r_{21} & r_{22} & r_{23} & t_y \\ r_{31} & r_{32} & r_{33} & t_z \\ 0 & 0 & 0 & 1 \end{pmatrix} \begin{pmatrix} x_s^i \\ y_s^i \\ z_s^i \\ 1 \end{pmatrix} \quad [7.11]$$

The solution vector $\vec{T}_{sol} = (r_{11}, r_{12}, r_{21}, r_{22}, r_{31}, r_{32}, t_x, t_y, t_y)^T$ comprises the values of nine linearly independent parameters (the values of the parameters r_{13}, r_{23} and r_{33} are determined from the values of the other six parameters r_{ij}, see Daul et al. (2005)). From this vector, the element of the matrix T_{sc}^{3D} that superimposes the corresponding 3D points can be deduced (see equation [7.11]).

7.3.1.2. *Example of 2D/2D registration using a homography*

The most direct measure of dissimilarity is based on the idea that the gray levels[1] of the homologous pixels from two images are comparable. In other words, small changes in the endoscope viewpoint result in moderate changes in the light reflected from the tissue surface and captured by the camera. The principle of registration consists therefore of moving the source image I_s on the target image I_c; this displacement is achieved by adjusting the parameters of the homography H_{sc} (see equation [7.10]) for the purpose of minimizing, by using equation [7.9], the dissimilarity measure $Dis(H_{sc}(I_s), I_c)$ defined hereafter:

$$Dis(H_{sc}(I_s), I_c) = \sum_{I_s \cap I_c} |H_{sc}(I_s(x,y)) - I_c(x,y)|^2 \quad [7.12]$$

This dissimilarity measure is zero when all homologous pixels in the common parts of the two images ($I_s \cap I_c$) are superimposed and have exactly the same gray level ($I_s(x,y) = I_c(x,y)$, $\forall\, x$ and y). The value of $Dis(H_{sc}(I_s), I_c)$ is minimized with respect to the eight independent parameters a_{ij} (see relation [7.10]) stored in the vector $\vec{T}$. At each iteration k, $\vec{T}$ is updated by an increment $\Delta\vec{T}_k$. In other words, for each $\vec{T}_k = \vec{T}_{k-1} + \Delta\vec{T}_k$, the homography H_{sc}^k moves the image I_s to the desired position on I_c. The dissimilarity measure is minimized using the first-order Taylor

1 Color images are in general converted into gray level images before their registration.

series expansion of $Dis^k(H_{sc}(I_s), I_c)$ with respect to ΔT_k and its derivative with respect to T_k:

$$\begin{cases} Dis^k(H^k_{sc}(I_s),I_c) = \sum_{I_s \cap I_c} \left(H^k_{sc}(I_s(x,y)) + \nabla I_s(x,y) J(\vec{T}_k) \Delta \vec{T}_k - I_c(x,y)\right)^2 \\ \frac{\partial Dis^k(H^k_{sc}(I_s),I_c)}{\partial \vec{T}_k} = \sum_{I_s \cap I_c} \left(\left[\nabla I_s(x,y) J(\vec{T}_k)\right]^T \right. \\ \qquad \left. -\left[H^k_{sc}(I_s(x,y)) + \nabla I_s(x,y) J(\vec{T}_k) \Delta \vec{T}_k - I_c(x,y)\right]\right) \end{cases} \quad [7.13]$$

In equation [7.13], $J(\vec{T}_k)$ is the Jacobian of the derivatives of parameters a_{ij}, whereas $\nabla I_s(x, y)$ corresponds to the gradient of the gray levels at the coordinates (x, y) of the source image. At each iteration k, the vector $\Delta \vec{T}_k$ is obtained by the Gauss–Newton nonlinear optimization method. The homographic matrix for iteration $k + 1$ is updated as follows:

$$H^{k+1}_{sc} = H^k_{sc} + \frac{\partial H^k_{sc}}{\partial \vec{T}_k} \Delta \vec{T}_k \quad [7.14]$$

The details of this method, as well as its acceleration by fast computation of initial conditions for the translation parameters a_{13} and a_{23} (see equation 7.10), are described in Hernandez-Mier et al. (2010). Another example of 2D/2D registration using a homography for endoscopic image registration (Miranda-Luna et al. 2008) relies on the maximization (see equation [7.9]) of a similarity measure based on the mutual information of gray levels (Viola and Wells 1995).

7.3.1.3. *Example of 3D/3D registration using a rigid transformation*

Let two point clouds $\mathcal{D}^{3D}_s$ and $\mathcal{D}^{3D}_c$ represent two parts P_s and P_c of the same surface and whose common subset $P_s \cap P_c$ is large enough to allow for data registration using equation [7.9]. The two sets of points $\mathcal{D}^{3D}_s = \{P^{3D}_{s,i}\}$ and $\mathcal{D}^{3D}_c = \{P^{3D}_{c,j}\}$ are each acquired or reconstructed in 3D for a given camera viewpoint, and their size ($i \in [1, I]$ and $j \in [1, J]$) can be different ($I \neq J$). A point $P^{3D}_{s,i}$ in the source data $\mathcal{D}^{3D}_s$ does not have an "exact" homologous point $P^{3D}_{c,j}$ in the target data $\mathcal{D}^{3D}_c$. In other words, equation [7.11] is not exactly verified regardless of the pair $(P^{3D}_{s,i}, P^{3D}_{c,j})$. The Hausdorff distance $H(\mathcal{D}^{3D}_s, \mathcal{D}^{3D}_c)$ is used to measure the distance between two surface parts represented by this type of 3D point clouds (Kirchberg et al. 2002):

$$H(\mathcal{D}^{3D}_s, \mathcal{D}^{3D}_c) = \max\left(Hd(\mathcal{D}^{3D}_s, \mathcal{D}^{3D}_c), Hd(\mathcal{D}^{3D}_c, \mathcal{D}^{3D}_s)\right) \quad [7.15]$$

with:

$$Hd(\mathcal{D}^{3D}_s, \mathcal{D}^{3D}_c) = \max_{P^{3D}_{s,i} \in \mathcal{D}^{3D}_s} \min_{P^{3D}_{c,j} \in \mathcal{D}^{3D}_c} \|P^{3D}_{s,i} - P^{3D}_{c,j}\| \quad [7.16]$$

The directed Hausdorff distance defined in equation [7.16] represents the largest Euclidean distance chosen among all the smallest distances from a point $P^{3D}_{s,i} \in \mathcal{D}^{3D}_{s}$ to all points $P^{3D}_{c,j} \in \mathcal{D}^{3D}_{c}$. For two identical and superposed surfaces P_s and P_c, the values of $Hd(\mathcal{D}^{3D}_{s}, \mathcal{D}^{3D}_{c})$ and $Hd(\mathcal{D}^{3D}_{c}, \mathcal{D}^{3D}_{s})$ are very close to one another and both tend to 0 (these distances are not zero if the points $P^{3D}_{s,i}$ and $P^{3D}_{c,j}$ are not homologous). In this example, the Hausdorff distance also tends to 0. When P_s and P_c are not identical but share a common subset, then the non-zero Hausdorff distance is minimal when the common subsets are actually overlapping. The Hausdorff distance increases when the surfaces P_s and P_c move apart. The value of $H(\mathcal{D}^{3D}_{s}, \mathcal{D}^{3D}_{c})$ can therefore be used as a measure of dissimilarity Dis in the minimization process of equation [7.9].

In Posada et al. (2007), the authors used two optimization methods to minimize the Hausdorff distance and thus found the parameters of the 3D rotation and translation (see relation [7.11]) that overlay the common subsets of the surfaces P_s and P_c. A descending gradient is first used to quickly approximate the solution while avoiding local minima in the parameter space. The simplex method (Nelder and Mead 1965) is then used to find an accurate solution (this last optimization is particularly well adapted for discrete data and initial conditions close to the solutions).

7.3.1.4. *Mapping principle without a geometric model*

While in the previous sections the parameters of the homographic model (global geometric link between two images) and the correspondences between homologous pixels are simultaneously determined by way of optimization (equations [7.9]), the methods presented in the following sections first search for correspondences between homologous points; they then use this information for the determination of the homography that geometrically links two images. This section first explains how it is possible to determine a homography based on a set of known correspondences between homologous points. The next two sections each present a method for determining a set of homologous points.

The homography of equation [7.10] comprises eight independent unknowns a_{ij} gathered in $\vec{T}_{sol} = (a_{11}, a_{12}, a_{13}, a_{21}, a_{22}, a_{23}, a_{31}, a_{32})^T$. Four pairs of homologous points lead to a number of equations that will suffice to determine the parameters a_{ij}. However, because the coordinates of the homologous points are never exactly known (in particular, because of the discrete nature of the images), an overdetermined system consisting of equations derived from relation [7.10] is formed for a number of pairs of homologous points greater than four. The parameters of $\vec{T}_{sol}$ are classically computed using a least squares method such as DLT (*direct linear transform*; Hartley and Zisserman (2004)).

Nevertheless, if n pairs of points ($n > 4$) are chosen among m available matches ($m \gg n$ in general), the accuracy of the computed parameters a_{ij} may be affected by erroneous matches (matching algorithms are not infallible) or by the localization of the homologous points (homologous points distributed over all regions of the images are to be preferred). The RANSAC algorithm (*Random Sample Consensus*; Fischler and Bolles (1981)) is usually associated with DLT to utilize the best matches (accurate and distributed over the images). In this iterative algorithm, n pairs of points are randomly drawn and DLT is employed to compute a vector $\vec{T}_{sol}$. The remaining pairs of homologous points (totaling $m - n$) are used to quantify the accuracy of the homography at iteration k. This operation is iterated a number of times depending on the value of m and the homography selected is the one that maximizes the number of matches above a predefined accuracy threshold.

7.3.1.5. *Example of data mapping using a sparse optical flow*

The homologous points of two consecutive images $I(x, y, t)$ and $I(x + v_x, y + v_y, t + \Delta t)$ acquired at times t and $t + \Delta t$ (for a camera, Δt is typically 40 ms) are linked by displacement vectors $\vec{v} = (v_x, v_y)^T$. The field $\mathbf{u}$ of vectors $\vec{v}$ is referred to as the optical flow. Assuming that the intensities of the homologous points of a grayscale image do not change between two consecutive acquisitions, it is necessary to find the set of vectors $\vec{v} = (v_x, v_y)^T$ of $\mathbf{u}$ that verify the following relation:

$$I(x + v_x, y + v_y, t + \Delta t) - I(x, y, t) = 0 \qquad [7.17]$$

The value of the gray levels of the image $I(x + v_x, y + v_y, t + \Delta t)$ can be rewritten as follows using a first-order Taylor expansion:

$$I(x + v_x, y + v_y, t + \Delta t) \approx I(x, y, t) + I_x v_x + I_y v_y + I_t \qquad [7.18]$$

with:

$$\begin{cases} I_x = \frac{\partial I(x,y,t)}{\partial x} \\ I_y = \frac{\partial I(x,y,t)}{\partial y} \\ I_t = \frac{\partial I(x,y,t)}{\partial t} = I(x + v_x, y + v_y, t + \Delta t) - I(x, y, t) \end{cases}$$

By combining equations [7.17] and [7.18], it is possible to write for a pair of homologous points: $I_x v_x + I_y v_y = -I_t$. However, because this equation has been written for a single pair of points, it includes two unknowns v_x and v_y, the values of the numerical spatial (I_x and I_y) and temporal (I_t) derivatives being computed from the gray levels. A solution to this ill-posed problem is to formulate the realistic assumption that in a small neighborhood of $n \times m$ pixels $p_{i,j}$ (with $i \in [1, n]$ and $j \in [1, m]$), the previous equation leads to an overdetermined system of $n \times m$ equations:

$$\left\{\begin{array}{rcl} I_x^{p_{1,1}} v_x + I_y^{p_{1,1}} v_y & = & -I_t^{p_{1,1}} \\ I_x^{p_{1,2}} v_x + I_y^{p_{1,2}} v_y & = & -I_t^{p_{1,2}} \\ \vdots & \vdots & \vdots \\ I_x^{p_{n,m}} v_x + I_y^{p_{n,m}} v_y & = & -I_t^{p_{n,m}} \end{array}\right. \quad [7.19]$$

System [7.19] can be reformulated in the following matrix manner:

$$A\vec{v} = \vec{b} \quad \text{with } A = \begin{pmatrix} I_x^{p_{1,1}} & I_y^{p_{1,1}} \\ I_x^{p_{1,2}} & I_y^{p_{1,2}} \\ \vdots & \vdots \\ I_x^{p_{n,m}} & I_y^{p_{n,m}} \end{pmatrix} \text{ and } \vec{b} = \begin{pmatrix} -I_t^{p_{1,1}} \\ -I_t^{p_{1,2}} \\ \vdots \\ -I_t^{p_{n,m}} \end{pmatrix} \quad [7.20]$$

whose least squares solution is given by

$$\vec{v} = \left(A^T A\right)^{-1} A^T \vec{b}. \quad [7.21]$$

The optical flow is said to be sparse because solution [7.21] of system [7.20] exists only at those locations in the images where the variations of the gray levels are large enough to accurately compute the derivatives I_x, I_y and I_t.

7.3.1.6. *Example of mapping using a dense optical flow*

The optical flow $\mathbf{u}$ is said to be dense when a vector $\vec{v}$ is sought between all homologous pixels of the two consecutive images $I(x, y, t)$ and $I(x + v_x, y + v_y, t + \Delta t)$. The values of the derivatives I_x, I_y and I_t can be employed at any point because, instead of solving a system like the one given by [7.20] for the sparse optical flow, the goal is to minimize an energy $E(\mathbf{u})$ globally computed over the images. In equation [7.22], the energy comprises a data term $E_d(\mathbf{u})$ and a regularization term $E_r(\mathbf{u})$:

$$E(\mathbf{u}) = \underbrace{\int_y \int_x (I_x v_x + I_y v_y + I_t)^2 \, dx\, dy}_{E_d(\mathbf{u})} + \underbrace{\lambda^2 \int_y \int_x \left(\|\nabla v_x\|^2 + \|\nabla v_y\|^2\right) dx\, dy}_{E_r(\mathbf{u})} \quad [7.22]$$

The objective of the data term $E_d(\mathbf{u})$ is to minimize the difference in gray levels between the two images. Following the principle described in the previous section, the expression $I_x v_x + I_y v_y + I_t$ is ideally zero for all pixels of coordinates (x, y) if the hypothesis of constancy of intensities is verified between two images. The regularization term $E_r(\mathbf{u})$ preserves small variations between the amplitudes and arguments of the vectors $\vec{v}$ of neighboring pixels (∇v_x and ∇v_y represent these variations). Therefore, the field $\mathbf{u}$ of vectors $\vec{v}$ progressively varies and without discontinuity from one image region to another, which must be the case for endoscopic scenes. This fact is illustrated for two cystoscopic images in Figure 7.8. The parameter λ sets the relative importance of the two energies. From the original solution by Horn and Schunck (1981) to the recent methods (Trinh and Daul 2019), which take into account the changes in illumination between two successive images of endoscopic scenes, there are many solutions for determining the optical flow $\mathbf{u}$ with equation [7.22].

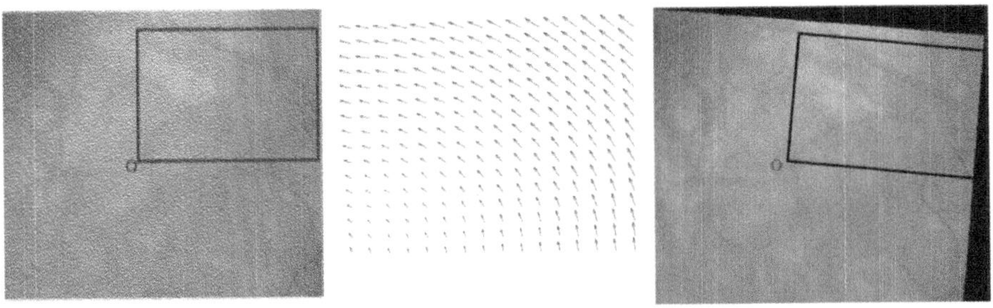

Figure 7.8. *Illustration of a dense optical flow between two consecutive images of the inner wall of a bladder seen in white light. For a color version of this figure, see www.iste.co.uk/fournier/unconventional.zip*

COMMENT ON FIGURE 7.8.– *The dense optical flow is the vector field represented in the center and which links the pixels on the right-hand side image to their homologous pixel in the image on the left side. The optical flow is that of the pixels enclosed by the black rectangles. For visibility reasons, only one vector out of 20 is represented according to the rows and columns (a displacement vector is calculated for all pixels). In this example, the vector field* u *corresponds to an image in plane rotation.*

7.3.2. *3D cartography approaches*

7.3.2.1. *The principle of stereovision*

Stereovision, whose principle is illustrated in Figure 7.9, is used for determining the position in space of a point P_{3D} using knowledge of the position of its projections $P^1_{2D} = (x^1_{2D}, y^1_{2D})^T$ and $P^2_{2D} = (x^2_{2D}, y^2_{2D})^T$ in two images acquired from different viewpoints. Assuming that both cameras are fully calibrated using the procedure described in section 7.2.2 and that any barrel distortions in the images have been compensated for with the method detailed in section 7.2.3, then the projection of the 3D point in the images can be modeled by equation [7.5] written for both images (i = 1 or 2, depending on the camera):

$$\alpha \begin{pmatrix} x_{2D}^i \\ y_{2D}^i \\ 1 \end{pmatrix} = \begin{pmatrix} M_{cam}^i \end{pmatrix} \begin{pmatrix} x_{3D}^i \\ y_{3D}^i \\ z_{3D}^i \\ 1 \end{pmatrix} \quad [7.23]$$

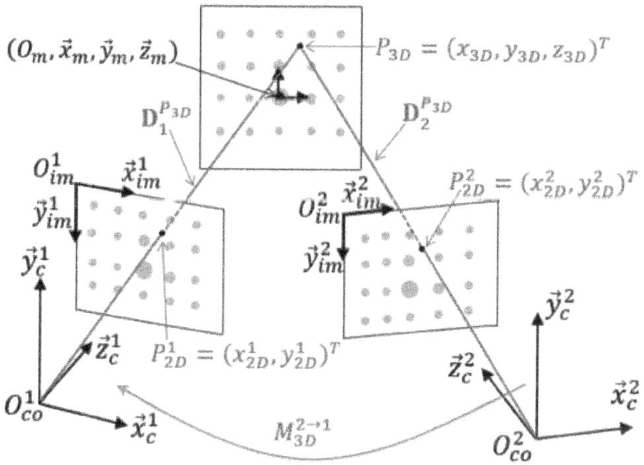

Figure 7.9. *Stereovision principle: two homologous points P_{2D}^1 and P_{2D}^2 are used to backtrack to the position of point P_{3D} in the world coordinate system $(O_m, \vec{x}_m, \vec{y}_m, \vec{z}_m)$ or in a camera reference $(O_{co}^i, \vec{x}_c^i, \vec{y}_c^i, \vec{z}_c^i)$ with i = 1 or 2*

The two matrices M_{cam}^i are entirely defined by the intrinsic and extrinsic parameters determined during the calibration procedure (see equation [7.4]). The parameters of matrices M_{cam}^i are also used to determine the equations themselves of the lines $\mathbf{D}_1^{P_{3D}}$ and $\mathbf{D}_2^{P_{3D}}$ originating from points P_{2D}^1 and P_{2D}^2 and that intersect in 3D space. These lines are however defined in their respective camera coordinate systems, namely $(O_{co}^1, \vec{x}_c^1, \vec{y}_c^1, \vec{z}_c^1)$ and $(O_{co}^2, \vec{x}_c^2, \vec{y}_c^2, \vec{z}_c^2)$. It is possible to express the position of a 3D point or the equation of the line $\mathbf{D}_2^{P_{3D}}$, both known in the coordinate system of camera 2, in that of camera 1 using the following relation (the $r^{2\to 1}$ and $t^{2\to 1}$ are rotation and translation parameters):

$$\begin{pmatrix} x_{3D}^1 \\ y_{3D}^1 \\ z_{3D}^1 \\ 1 \end{pmatrix} = \Bigg(\underbrace{\left(M_{cam}^2\right)^{-1} M_{cam}^1}_{M_{3D}^{2\to 1}} \Bigg) \begin{pmatrix} x_{3D}^2 \\ y_{3D}^2 \\ z_{3D}^2 \\ 1 \end{pmatrix} = \begin{pmatrix} r_{11}^{2\to 1} & r_{12}^{2\to 1} & r_{13}^{2\to 1} & t_x^{2\to 1} \\ r_{21}^{2\to 1} & r_{22}^{2\to 1} & r_{23}^{2\to 1} & t_y^{2\to 1} \\ r_{31}^{2\to 1} & r_{32}^{2\to 1} & r_{33}^{2\to 1} & t_z^{2\to 1} \\ 0 & 0 & 0 & 1 \end{pmatrix} \begin{pmatrix} x_{3D}^2 \\ y_{3D}^2 \\ z_{3D}^2 \\ 1 \end{pmatrix} \qquad [7.24]$$

When the equations of the lines $\mathbf{D}_1^{P_{3D}}$ and $\mathbf{D}_2^{P_{3D}}$ are expressed in the same coordinate system with $M_{3D}^{2\to 1}$ (see equation [7.24]), their intersection leads to localizing the point P_{3D} in $(O_{co}^1, \vec{x}_c^1, \vec{y}_c^1, \vec{z}_c^1)$. However, for numerical reasons, these two lines never exactly intersect. It is generally accepted that P_{3D} is located halfway along the shortest line segment between $\mathbf{D}_1^{P_{3D}}$ and $\mathbf{D}_2^{P_{3D}}$.

It should be noted that the model in Figure 7.9 not only represents the principle of 3D reconstruction with two fixed cameras whose relative position is known, but also that of a single camera whose displacement between two acquisitions is known or can be estimated.

7.3.2.2. *Example of passive vision-based 3D cartography*

Passive 3D vision only makes use of information contained in the images (as well as the camera parameters if the camera has been calibrated) to perform the construction of the scene in three dimensions. The methods that compute the structure based on the camera motion (*Structure from Motion* (SfM)) simultaneously determine the poses (position of the optical center O_{co}^i and orientation of the optical axis z_c^i at acquisition number i) of the camera along its 3D trajectory and a cloud of points P_{3D} located on the surface with the extended field of view to be calculated. Figure 7.10 illustrates the principle of SfM approaches using three images (in practice, the number of images i of a video sequence is more important, these being acquired at a rate of 25 images/s).

The dense optical flow (see section 7.3.1.6) is computed between each pair of successive (I_1, I_j) $(j = i \pm 1)$ and non-successive images $(j \neq i \pm 1)$ containing a minimal common portion of the scene (see Phan et al. (2020) for the determination of the overlapping degree of images). This optical flow gives the correspondence between many pairs of homologous points $(P_{2D}^{i,k}, P_{2D}^{j,k})$, where k is the index of the pair.

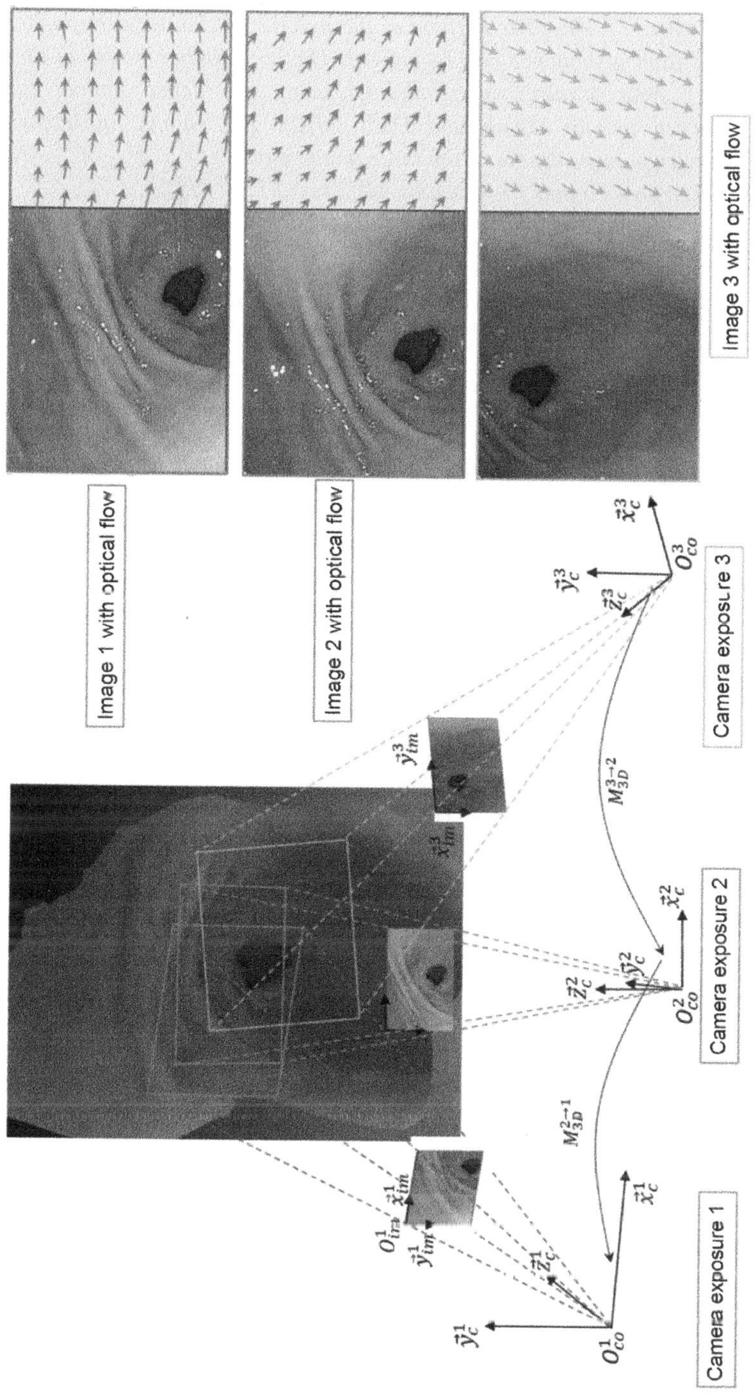

Figure 7.10. *Illustration of SfM-type approaches. For a color version of this figure, see www.iste.co.uk/fournier/unconventional.zip*

COMMENT ON FIGURE 7.10.– *The surface of the pyloric antrum (lower stomach) was reconstructed from a sequence of 173 images. The homologous points of these images with very poor texture were obtained using the dense optical flow computation between images (Trinh and Daul 2019). The change in intensity depending on the viewpoint is visible in the three image planes* $(O^i_{im}, \vec{x}^i_{im}, \vec{y}^i_{im})$. *The relationship between poses 3 and 1 is given by* $M_{3D}^{3\to1} = M_{3D}^{2\to1} M_{3D}^{3\to2}$.

As explained in the previous section, these correspondences are used to compute the position of the 3D points P_{3D} and the 3D displacement matrix $M_{3D}^{j\to i}$ of the camera. The cloud of 3D points located on the surface of the extended field of view to be constructed is determined through the following steps:

1) *Initialization*: two images I_1 and I_2 with numerous correspondences are chosen in the sequence of images, then the P_{3D} and the matrix $M_{3D}^{2\to1}$ which gives the 3D point displacements between the two camera poses are determined. The positions of these 3D points are expressed in the reference coordinate system of the first pose. In the next steps of the treatment, all point coordinates will be given in $(O^1_{co}, \vec{x}^1_c, \vec{y}^1_c, \vec{z}^1_c)$.

2) *Iterative addition of poses to the point cloud*: the image I_j which is chosen afterwards is the one that has the highest number of homologous points with all the images already used to build the point cloud. The reconstructed points P_{3D} are the shared (and homologous) points of I_j and those of all the images I_i already utilized. We should bear in mind that at this processing stage, most of the time more than two homologous points can be found (i.e. more than two images) for each point of the 3D scene. The accuracy of the triangulation described in the previous section increases with the number of homologous points. The reconstructed points are all placed in the coordinate system $(O^1_{co}, \vec{x}^1_c, \vec{y}^1_c, \vec{z}^1_c)$ using matrices $M_{3D}^{j\to i}$. Step 2 is repeated m times (if $m = 10$ the 3D points of 10 images are added to the cloud).

3) *Global adjustment*: to minimize the errors, an optimization method is employed to simultaneously adjust the position of all the 3D points and the parameters of the matrices $M_{3D}^{j\to i}$ computed at this processing stage. To this end, the dissimilarity measure that is minimized is computed from the distances between the 3D points reprojected in the images and the 2D points utilized to obtain the P_{3D}. These distances must be simultaneously as small as possible. Steps 2 and 3 are repeated as long as all the sequence images (or a selection of images) are not used.

This presentation of the principle of SfM approaches is very simplified. More details can be found in Schönberger and Frahm (2016) and Phan (2020). At this processing stage, a cloud of points P_{3D} scattered over the surface to be built is available. These points are then used to mesh the surface with triangular facets (Kazhdan et al. 2006). This mesh yields a gap-free surface onto which the texture and colors of the images are projected (Waechter et al. 2014). As illustrated in Figure 7.10, this projection of the textures can be achieved by way of knowing the camera poses along its 3D trajectory. The internal surface of the stomach shown in this same figure was obtained with the principle described here and presented in detail in Phan (2020).

7.3.2.3. *Example of active vision-based 3D cartography*

Active vision systems are based on the principle of the stereovision device, as shown in Figure 7.9, for which one of the cameras is replaced by a light projector. Thus, as illustrated in Figure 7.11, the projection perspective matrix M_{cam} that links the world coordinate system (O_m, $\vec{x}_m$, $\vec{y}_m$, $\vec{z}_m$) with the camera coordinate system (O_{co}, $\vec{x}_c$, $\vec{y}_c$, $\vec{z}_c$) is determined with a calibration plate following the procedure introduced in section 7.2.2.

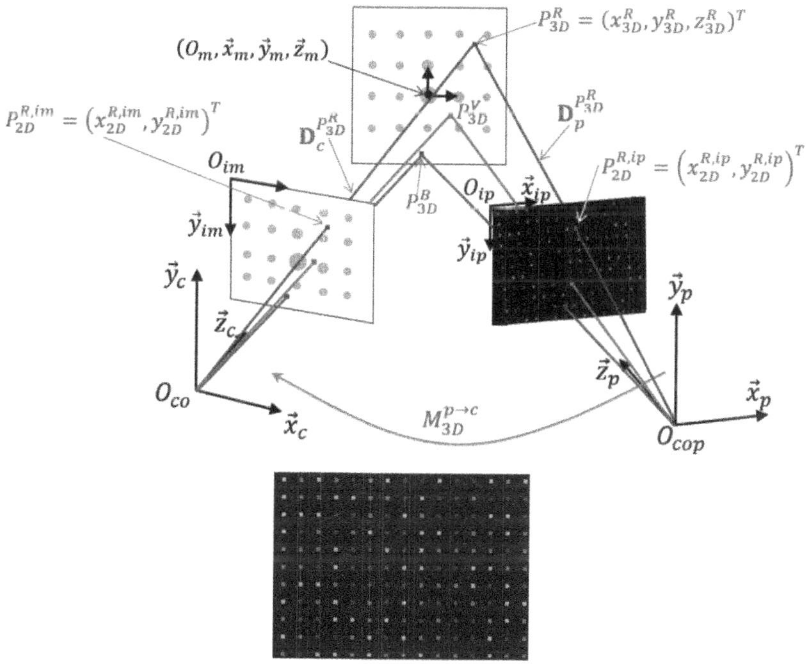

Figure 7.11. *Illustration of the active vision principle. For a color version of this figure, see www.iste.co.uk/fournier/unconventional.zip*

COMMENT ON FIGURE 7.11.– *(a) The position $P_{2D}^{k,ip}$ of the red ($k = R$), green ($k = V$) and blue squares ($k = B$) in the coordinate system (O_{ip}, $\vec{x}_{ip}$,) of the image plane is known by construction and their position P_{3D}^{k} on the calibration plate can be calculated based on the known location of the disk centers. (b) The projected image is undistorted. A barrel distortion calibration (see section 7.2.3) must therefore be performed only for the endoscope camera.*

A light projector can also be modeled by the perspective projection matrix defined by equation [7.4]. Nevertheless, in the case of a projector, this matrix reflects the operation of an "inverted camera". Indeed, for a camera, the photons falling on an image point P_{2D}^{im} (transition from 3D to 2D) follow a rectilinear trajectory defined by a line going through P_{3D} and the optical center O_{co} of the camera. For a light projector, the photons emanate from an image point P_{2D}^{ip} and propagate in 3D space (transition from 2D to 3D) along a straight line going through P_{3D} and the optical center O_{cop} of the projector. Figure 7.11(a) shows that the photons emitted by the projector at point P_{2D}^{ip} are reflected by a point P_{3D} and are absorbed by a photosite of the matrix sensor covering the point P_{2D}^{im}. The intersection of two lines $\mathbf{D}_p^{P_{3D}}$ and $\mathbf{D}_c^{P_{3D}}$ thus helps to triangulate the coordinates of a point P_{3D}.

The digital image shown in Figure 7.11(b) has been generated by a drawing software program and is placed in the image plane $(O_{ip}, \vec{x}_{ip}, \vec{y}_{ip})$. This image is projected by a pico-projector in 3D space. A line $\mathbf{D}_p^{P_{3D}}$ is computed using the intrinsic and extrinsic parameters of the perspective matrix M_{proj} of the projector that is calibrated using equation [7.5]. The latter is rewritten as follows with the notations shown in Figure 7.11(a):

$$\alpha \begin{pmatrix} x_{2D}^{k,ip} \\ y_{2D}^{k,ip} \\ 1 \end{pmatrix} = \begin{pmatrix} M_{proj} \end{pmatrix} \begin{pmatrix} x_{3D}^{k} \\ y_{3D}^{k} \\ z_{3D}^{k} \\ 1 \end{pmatrix} \quad [7.25]$$

where k refers to a red (R), green (V) or blue (B) square. The differently colored squares facilitate the establishment of the corresponding point pairs $(P_{2D}^{k,ip}, P_{3D}^{k})$ to allow for the computation of the parameters of the matrix M_{proj} by solving an overdetermined system, similar to what is done for a camera. As for a two-camera system, the equations of the lines $\mathbf{D}_p^{P_{3D}^k}$ of the projector can be expressed in the camera coordinate system using the matrix $M_{3D}^{p\to c} = (M_{proj})^{-1} M_{cam}$.

This active vision principle has been used particularly in laparoscopy for constructing internal surfaces of the abdominal cavity in the context of minimally invasive surgery (Maurice et al. 2012). The projected light image was delivered to the interior of the cavity via the operator channel of the endoscope, the coordinate systems $(O_{co}, \vec{x}_c, \vec{y}_c, \vec{z}_c)$ and $(O_{cop}, \vec{x}_p, \vec{y}_p, \vec{z}_p)$ in Figure 7.11(a) being fixed relative to one another for each acquisition. The field of view can be extended by using 3D/3D registration algorithms (see section 7.3.1) that superimpose the common area of the surface pieces represented by point clouds P_{3D}.

Figure 7.12 shows a prototype of an active vision-based 3D cystoscope. A laser beam is directed onto a diffractive lens that projects eight light rays located on a cone in 3D space. The objective is to reconstruct a few 3D points per acquisition using images that include eight laser dots, small enough to preserve the textures of the bladder. The schematic diagram shown in Figure 7.12(a) models the operation of the prototype shown in Figure 7.12(b) placed in front of a wave-shaped phantom lined with bladder images. The active vision system was calibrated using the method described in Ben-Hamadou et al. (2013) and the 3D map is constructed using the mosaicing algorithm described in Ben-Hamadou et al. (2016). Figure 7.12(c) shows the wave-like trajectory of the eight laser dots reconstructed along the image sequence, the progressive meshing of the surface and the projection of the image textures onto the reconstructed meshes. The result obtained with this prototype shows that it is possible to recover realistic surface shapes.

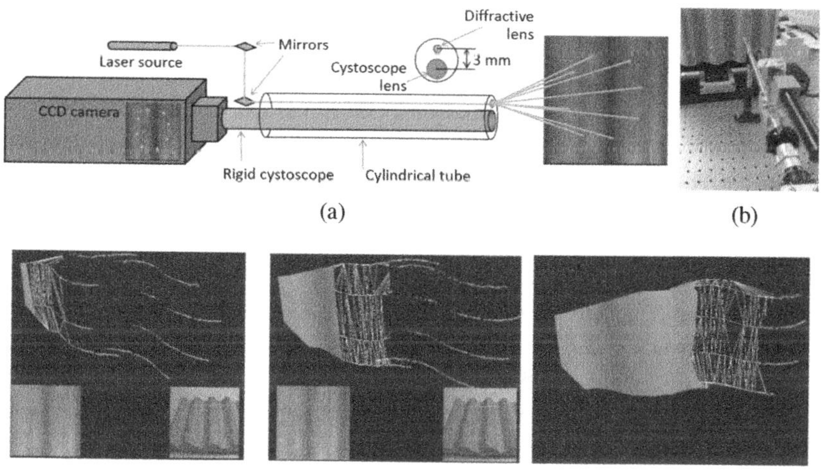

(c)

Figure 7.12. *Prototype of a 3D vision-based endoscope. (a) Principle underlying the use of active vision adapted to a rigid cystoscope manufactured by Karl Storz SE. (b) Prototype placed in front of a wave-shaped phantom which is displaced by a translation parallel to the image plane. (c) Progressive construction of the textured 3D surface. For a color version of this figure, see www.iste.co.uk/fournier/unconventional.zip*

7.4. Multimodal and multispectral endoscopic imaging systems

7.4.1. *Introduction*

Early detection of inflammatory, precancerous or early cancerous tissue lesions within hollow organs is a major medical and economic challenge that increases the chances of cure and survival, and enhances the effectiveness of treatments and results in reducing the risks of complications or sequelae. However, the sensitivity of conventional endoscopy remains limited for accurate identification of these different types of tissues, namely due to the lack of visual contrast between them on standard color images acquired in WL.

In order to improve the efficiency of this detection, new optical endoscopic imaging techniques have been developed or are under development. These techniques make use of spectral photophysical characteristics specific to biological tissues to produce images with improved and optimized contrasts between healthy and pathological tissues. The general principle of these innovative methods is based on the fact that the main optical properties of tissues such as absorption, scattering, or fluorescence vary according to the tissue condition. The resulting endoscopic imaging systems are said to be (i) multimodal because most of the time they combine the conventional WL imaging modality and a complementary modality and/or (ii) multispectral when they provide information obtained from distinct spectral bands. These systems can be classified into two broad categories: those that use a chemical marker as an additional contrast agent (section 7.4.2) and those known as label-free (Amouroux et al. 2019; Song and Ang 2014, 2017) that are based on purely optical, optoelectronic or digital contrast enhancement methods (section 7.4.3). In oncology, for example, these systems are used for detecting tumor lesions at a stage when they cannot be yet detected by WL endoscopy in order to drive biopsies and thus increase diagnostic sensitivity.

The following sections present some of the most commonly employed systems in clinical practice, as well as a few examples of systems under development that illustrate these different principles.

7.4.2. *Chemical labeling imaging systems*

7.4.2.1. *Chromoendoscopy*

Chromoendoscopy is an intravital labeling imaging technique that uses a conventional endoscope with WL illumination combined with a chromatic marker (dye) applied by the clinician to the inner wall of the organ to highlight architectural irregularities in the mucosa (the layer of tissue that covers the inner wall of hollow organs). For example, indigo carmine is a surface dye that is not absorbed by mucosal cells but instead accumulates in the crevices formed by certain lesions. This dye thus allows for better visualization of relief abnormalities, surface irregularities and the contours of these lesions (see Figure 7.13). Among the dyes that have marketing authorization (MA) and can therefore be utilized in human clinical practice, methylene blue and Lugol are eventually absorbed by the cells of the epithelium (on the surface of the mucous membrane), such that they enable better definition of the relief of the mucous membrane and improved identification of any abnormal areas.

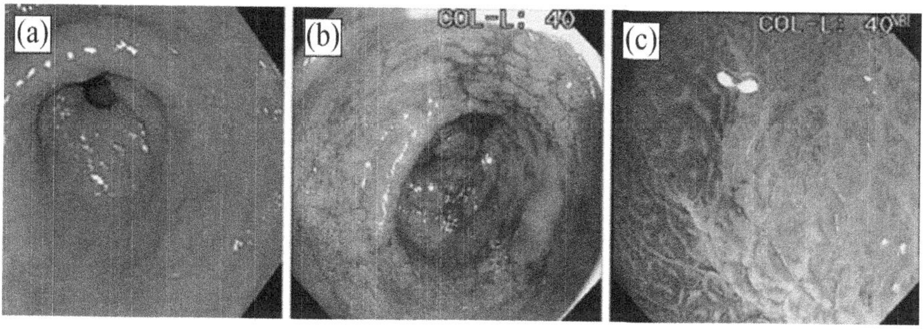

Figure 7.13. *Endoscopic images of a superficial gastric adenoma (stomach cancer) acquired (a) in white light (visible tissue elevations), (b) in chromo endoscopy with indigo carmine for enhancing the margins of the adenoma and (c) in narrow-band imaging (NBI) for visualizing regular microsurface and microvascularization structures (source: Song and Ang (2014)). For a color version of this figure, see www.iste.co.uk/fournier/unconventional.zip*

7.4.2.2. *Fluorescence endoscopy*

Endoscopic fluorescence imaging consists of visualizing the radiation emitted by a fluorescent marker (exogenous fluorophore) previously injected or applied to the biological tissue to be inspected. A fluorophore is a molecule characterized by an absorption spectrum $S_{abs}(\lambda)$ (with $\lambda \in [\lambda_{abs}^{min}, \lambda_{abs}^{max}]$) and an emission spectrum of fluorescence $S_{em}(\lambda)$ with $\lambda \in [\lambda_{em}^{min}, \lambda_{em}^{max}]$), the latter always being shifted to longer wavelengths than the former. Among the organic fluorophores with MA, and therefore usable in the clinic, we can mention in particular sodium fluorescein (with peaks for $S_{abs}(\lambda)$ and $S_{em}(\lambda)$ around [465–490] and [520–530] nm, respectively), and indocyanine green (ICG) whose absorption/emission peaks fall within the [760–800]/[790–830] nm spectral bands. These near-infrared peaks are the most suitable for deep tissue structure visualization. The high affinity of ICG for proteins contained in blood plasma leads to efficient labeling of the vascular network. Yet, the creation of new blood vessels (neovascularization) is one of the development characteristics of neoplastic lesions, which can thus be detected and visualized, even small ones, by ICG imaging.

In the context of bladder cancer detection, a particular technique for fluorescence cystoscopic imaging consists of administering to the patient, not an exogenous fluorophore, but a non-fluorescent compound, namely hexyl aminulevulinate (HAL), which promotes the selective production of an endogenous fluorophore, protoporphyrin IX (PpIX), which can then be employed as a fluorescent marker. In fact, it has been shown that the increased capacity of PpIX synthesis by tumors (compared to that of normal cells) is linked to increased enzyme activity involved in the synthesis of heme[2]. This accumulation of PpIX in neoplastic and dysplastic tissues after HAL injection is used to increase the contrast between normal and tumor tissues in endoscopic images. PpIX is a fluorescent molecule that emits a red color (spectral emission peak at 635 nm) when excited in the blue region (absorption peak at 400 nm). In addition, HAL fluorescence cystoscopy systems include a WL source and a source in the violet/blue range (380–440 nm) and are able to sequentially acquire color and fluorescence images, revealing normal and tumor tissue areas in blue/green and pink/red, respectively (see Figure 7.14).

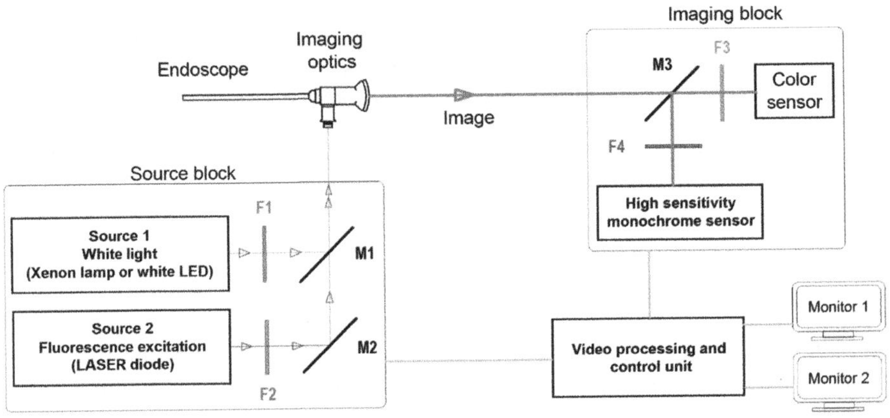

Figure 7.14. *Illustration of the principle of bimodal endoscopy systems with white light (source 1) and fluorescence with UV or NIR excitation (source 2) such that λ_{exc} = 405 or 650 nm. For a color version of this figure, see www.iste.co.uk/fournier/unconventional.zip*

COMMENT ON FIGURE 7.14.– *F1 = 405–650 nm band-pass filter; F2 = dichroic band-pass filter (narrow) centered on 405 or 650 nm; M1 = semi-transparent mirror; M2 = reflecting mirror; M3 = image splitter and coupler; F3 = 650 nm notch filter; F4 = high-pass filter 605 or 690 nm (source: Amouroux et al. 2019; Jacobson et al. 2012).*

Recent research work has led to the development and clinical validation of bimodal cystoscopic imaging systems that allow the simultaneous acquisition and visualization

2 A constituent substance of hemoglobin, which serves to transport blood gases.

of both video streams in WL and fluorescence by HAL (Amouroux et al. 2019). It is worth noting that this bimodality has made it possible to achieve for the first time the superposition of 2D panoramic images of bladders in WL and fluorescence (see Figure 7.15). A dense optical flow method was used, which provided the homologous points necessary for the calculation of the homographies, thus giving the geometrical link between the images (see section 7.3.1.1).

(a)

(b)

(c)

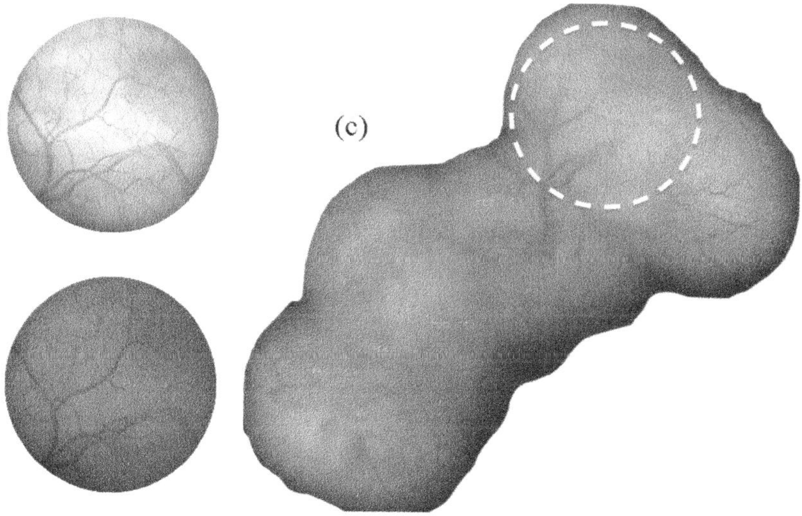

Figure 7.15. *Pictures of the inner wall of a bladder extracted from cystoscopic video sequences acquired in (a) white light (WL) and (b) HAL-induced fluorescence, corresponding to the white dotted circle located on the panoramic image (c) constructed from mosaicing 150 images; redder tissue areas (PpIX fluorescence emission) correspond to potentially cancerous lesions (source: Amouroux et al. 2019). For a color version of this figure, see www.iste.co.uk/fournier/unconventional.zip*

7.4.3. *Exogenous markerless imaging systems*

7.4.3.1. *Narrow-band Imaging*

Narrow-band imaging (NBI) is an endoscopic imaging technique that implements narrow bandpass filters in the blue ([400–430] nm) and green ranges ([520–550] nm) at the illumination source (WL). Depending on the spectral band of the illumination, the depths of penetration of the photons into the tissue (between 0.15 and 0.30 mm on average in NBI) will be different. The penetration is limited to the most superficial layers in the blue, extended to the less superficial layers in the green and the deepest in the red. Since blue and green light are more strongly absorbed by hemoglobin (with a peak absorption between 400 and 420 nm), the combination of images acquired with three wavelengths enables the construction of a new composite image clearly highlighting the subsurface vascularization of the biological tissue (darker vessels). However, the normal structure of the vascular network is altered during tumor transformation, characterized by angiogenesis and vascular hyperproliferation (production of new vessels that feed tumor growth). Therefore, with NBI endoscopy, visualization of better contrasted capillary (smaller vessels) images leads to improved detection of localized tumor lesions that may be associated with localized tumor neovascular development (see Figure 7.16).

7.4.3.2. *Autofluorescence imaging*

Autofluorescence (AF) imaging enables the visualization of radiation emitted by endogenous fluorophores naturally existing in biological tissues and carrying structural and metabolic information of major diagnostic interest; this includes those related to structural proteins of the extracellular matrix (collagen, elastin) and intracellular molecules (flavin adenine dinucleotide (FAD), porphyrins, reduced nicotinamide adenine dinucleotide (NADH)). When these fluorophores are illuminated by a light source of appropriate wavelength, typically within the [350–450] nm spectral band, part of the energy of the incident photons they absorb is converted into radiative transitions with emission of lower-energy photons, that is, with a wavelength (emission) greater than that of excitation, typically in the [400–700] nm spectral band.

AF endoscopy makes use of the differences in AF emission existing between healthy and pathological tissues such as (i) a decrease in collagen fluorescence (reduced fluorescence in the green) associated with some dysplastic tissues characterized by collagen loss or (ii) an increase in porphyrin fluorescence related to their higher level in some cancerous tissues. Based on the general principle of the scheme in Figure 7.14, AF endoscopy consists of illuminating the tissues with narrow-band light in the violet-blue (filtered WL source or LED) and acquiring the AF images on a monochrome sensor equipped with a green-red emission filter. It should be noted that the very low AF intensity level emitted by biological tissues sets several technical constraints in terms of source (irradiance, spectral width) and image acquisition (sensor sensitivity, exposure time) that limit the video flow to a few frames per second. The WL and AF images, acquired alternately, are then re-registered and combined to form a composite image leading to visualizing the morphological and functional information in pseudo-color.

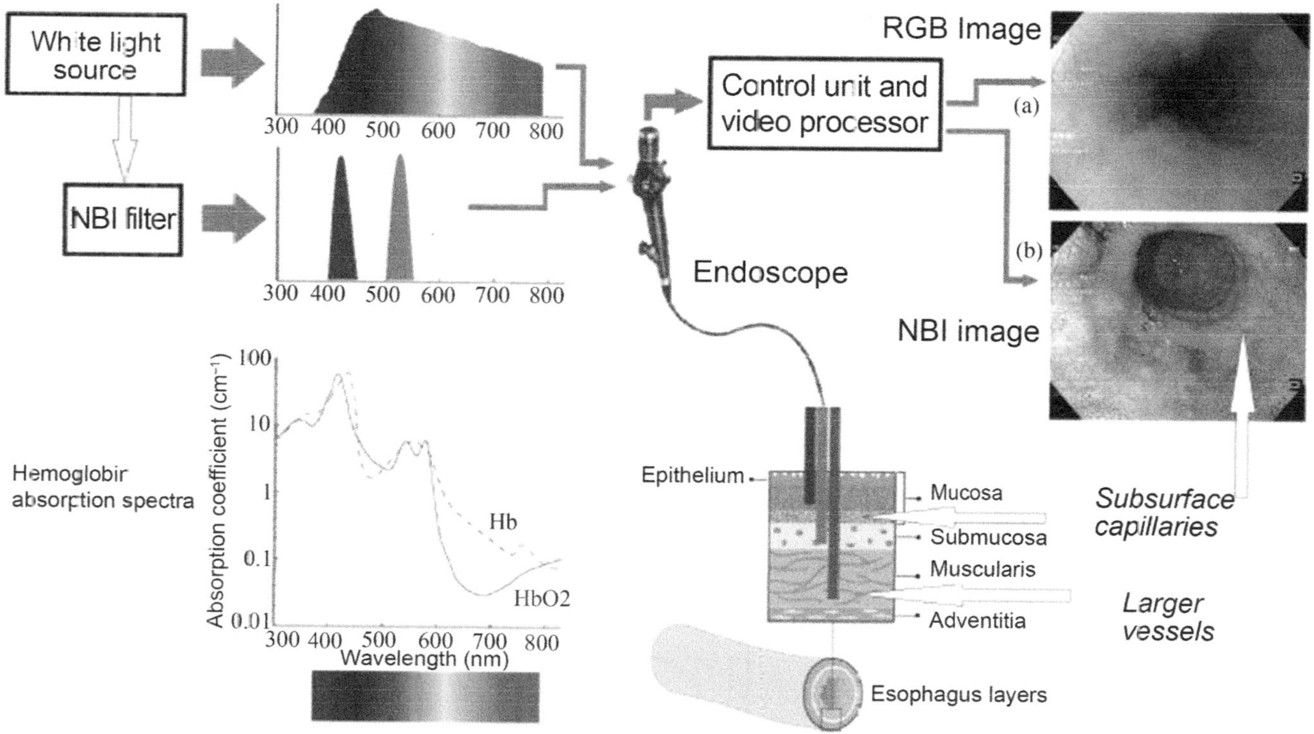

Figure 7.16. *Illustration of the principle of endoscopic narrow-band imaging (NBI) and examples of images showing a cancerous lesion of the esophagus (a) in white light and (b) NBI (images taken from Barbeiro et al. 2019). For a color version of this figure, see www.iste.co.uk/fournier/unconventional.zip*

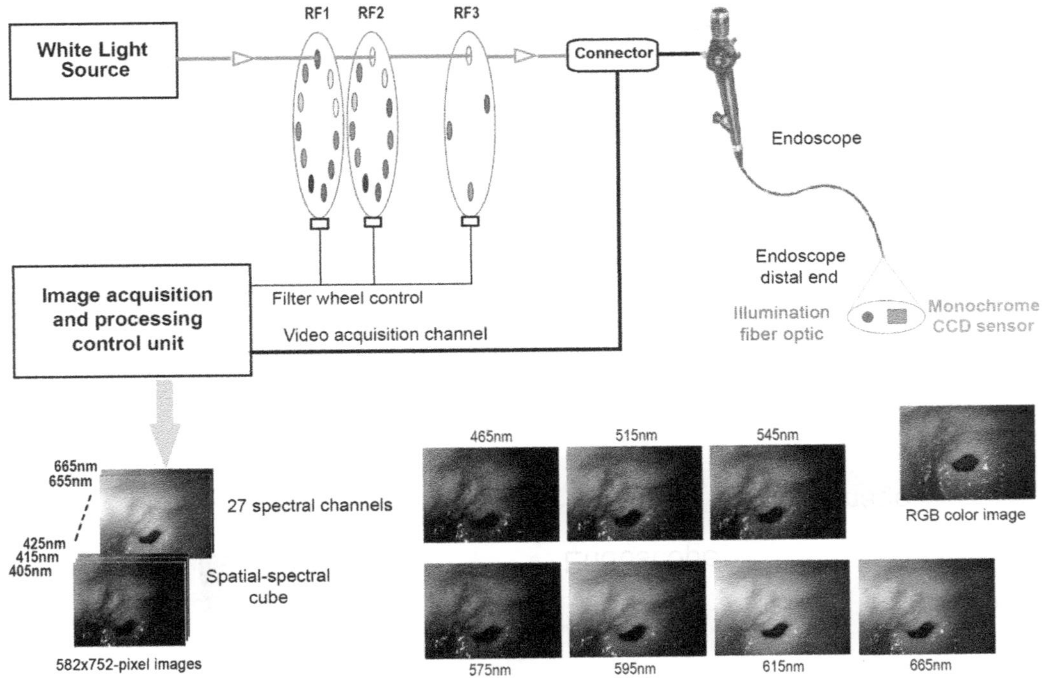

Figure 7.17. *Illustration of the principle of a 27-channel hyperspectral endoscopic imaging system of 405–665 nm. RF1 and RF2 = hyperspectral filter wheels, RF3 = RGB filter wheel. Example of pictures of a stomach ulcer acquired in RGB color with seven wavelengths in hyperspectral modality (source: Han et al. 2016; Gu et al. 2016). For a color version of this figure, see www.iste.co.uk/fournier/unconventional.zip*

Among the multimodality endoscopic imaging methods developed to further improve diagnostic specificity, AF endoscopy can be combined with conventional endoscopy and virtual chromoendoscopy (NBI) in a "tri-modal" approach that provides additional contrast by making use of the increased AF in the red of certain lesions.

7.4.3.3. *Multi- or hyperspectral imaging*

The principle of multi- or hyperspectral endoscopic imaging consists of acquiring and analyzing a set of images formed in different spectral bands or at different wavelengths. The developed systems are characterized by the size of the spatiospectral cube thus acquired (image size × number of wavelength bands) and by the construction technique for this data cube (Krebs et al. 2020). For example, a hyperspectral flexible gastroscopy system (*hyperspectral imaging* (HSI)) has been developed for the purposes of improving diagnostic efficiency for different types of stomach pathologies (Gu et al. 2016, Han et al. 2016). This device integrates 27 narrow bandpass interference filters mounted on two motorized filter wheels. The center wavelengths of these filters, as well as their 10 nm half-width, result in a spectral sampling of 405 and 665 nm in 10 nm steps. When the conventional WL mode is activated, a color image is acquired through the RGB filter wheel (Figure 7.17). When the HSI mode is activated, the 27 "monochromatic" light beams are sequentially produced in 4.2 s. A monochromatic 582 × 752-pixel CCD sensor is used to acquire the reflected images of the mucosa in spectral resolution.

The development of a spectral band selection algorithm, based on a statistical measure of information dependence, has facilitated the analysis of hyperspectral images of gastric ulcers and the identification of a combination of three discriminating wavelengths (495, 545 and 645 nm). By constructing a new enhanced composite image using these three selected bands, Han et al. (2016) showed that this new method provided superior contrast to WL images, thus improving the detection efficiency of the lesions being considered.

7.5. Conclusion

Endoscopy is the reference clinical exploration modality for observing and analyzing the internal wall of hollow organs and for performing localized surgical actions, diagnostic (biopsies) and therapeutic (resection of pathological tissues) purposes.

The development and clinical transfer of new tools and methods for multimodality endoscopic imaging, with chemical or virtual labeling, is a major technical, medical and economic challenge. By providing clinicians with optimized visual contrast inside hollow organs between healthy and pathological tissues, these innovative solutions significantly increase the sensitivity and specificity of perioperative diagnosis and the overall efficiency of biopsy procedures.

Comprehensive observation of the inner wall of hollow organs is also a critical issue for clinicians who must ensure that they have successfully visualized the entire surface without missing a potentially lesioned area. With the development of image mosaicing methods, the construction of multi-modality panoramic images provides high-resolution, wide field of view morpho-functional mappings that enable visualization of the spatial distribution of lesions, thus contrasted over large regions of interest.

7.6. References

Amouroux, M., Salleron, J., Huin-Schohn, C., Ali, S., Berthaud, S., Rizo, P., Schneider, S., Vever-Bizet, C., Bourg-Heckly, G., Guillemin, F. et al. (2019). Clinical evaluation of a device providing simultaneous white-light and fluorescence video streams as well as panoramic imaging during fluorescence assisted-transurethral resection of bladder cancer. *Journal of the Optical Society of America A*, 36(11), C62–C68 [Online]. Available at: https://doi.org/10.1364/JOSAA.36.000C62.

Barbeiro, S., Libânio, D., Castro, R., Dinis-Ribeiro, M., Pimentel-Nunes, P. (2019). Narrow-band imaging: Clinical application in gastrointestinal endoscopy. *GE Portugese Journal of Gastroenterology*, 26, 40–53.

Ben-Hamadou, A., Soussen, C., Daul, C., Blondel, W., Wolf, D. (2013). Flexible calibration of structured-light systems projecting point patterns. *Computer Vision and Image Understanding*, 117(10), 1468–1481.

Ben-Hamadou, A., Daul, C., Soussen, C. (2016). Construction of extended 3D field of views of the internal bladder wall surface: A proof of concept. *3D Research*, 7(11), 1–23.

Daul, C., Graebling, P., Hirsch, E. (1998). From the Hough transform to a new approach for the detection and approximation of elliptical arcs. *Computer Vision and Image Understanding*, 72(3), 215–236.

Daul, C., Graebling, P., Tiedeu, A., Wolf, D. (2005). 3-D reconstruction of microcalcification clusters using stereo imaging: Algorithm and mammographic unit calibration. *IEEE Transactions on Biomedical Engineering*, 52(12), 2058–2073.

Doutre, C. and Nasiopoulos, P. (2009). Fast vignetting correction and color matching for panoramic image stitching. *Proceedings of the 16th IEEE International Conference on Image Processing (ICIP)*, Cairo, 709–712.

Fischler, M. and Bolles, R. (1981). Random sample consensus: A paradigm for model fitting with applications to image analysis and automated cartography. *Communications of the ACM*, 24(6), 381–395.

Geavlete, B., Mulţescu, R., Georgescu, D., Geavlete, P. (2008). Hexvix blue light fluorescence cystoscopy – A promising approach in superficial bladder tumors diagnosis. *Journal of Medicine and Life*, 1(3), 355–362.

Gu, X., Han, Z., Yao, L., Zhong, Y., Shi, Q., Fu, Y., Liu, C., Wang, X., Xie, T. (2016). Image enhancement based on in vivo hyperspectral gastroscopic images: A case study. *Journal of Biomedical Optics*, 21(10), 101412.

Han, Z., Zhang, A., Wang, X., Sun, Z., Wang, M.D., Xie, T. (2016). In vivo use of hyperspectral imaging to develop a noncontact endoscopic diagnosis support system for malignant colorectal tumors. *Journal of Biomedical Optics*, 21(1), 16001 [Online]. Available at: https://doi.org/10.1117/1.JBO.21.1.016001.

Hartley, R. and Zisserman, A. (2004). *Multiple View Geometry in Computer Vision*, 2nd edition. Cambridge University Press, Cambridge.

Hernandez-Mier, Y., Blondel, W., Daul, C., Wolf, D., Guillemin, F. (2010). Fast construction of panoramic images for cystoscopic exploration. *Computerized Medical Imaging and Graphics*, 34(7), 579–592.

Horn, B.K. and Schunck, B.G. (1981). Determining optical flow. *Artificial Intelligence*, 17(1), 185–203.

Jacobson, M., de Vere White, R., Demos, S. (2012). In vivo testing of a prototype system providing simultaneous white light and near infrared autofluorescence image acquisition for detection of bladder cancer. *Journal of Biomedical Optics*, 17(3), 036011.

Kazhdan, M., Bolitho, M., Hoppe, H. (2006). Poisson surface reconstruction. In *Symposium on Geometry Processing*, Sheffer, A. and Polthier, K. (eds). The Eurographics Association, Cagliari, Sardinia.

Kirchberg, K., Jesorsky, O., Frischholz, R. (2002). Alignment by maximization of mutual information. *Proceedings of the ECCV Workshop on Biometric Authentication*, LNCS-2359, IEEE, Cambridge, MA.

Krebs, A., Benezeth, Y., Bazin, T., Marzani, F., Lamarque, D. (2020). Pre-cancerous stomach lesion detections with multispectral-augmented endoscopic prototype. *Applied Sciences*, 2020(10), 795.

Maurice, X., Albitar, C., Doignon, C., de Mathelin, M. (2012). A structured light-based laparoscope with real-time organs' surface reconstruction for minimally invasive surgery. *Proceedings of the Annual International Conference of the IEEE Engineering in Medicine and Biology Society*, IEEE, San Diego, CA.

Miranda-Luna, R., Blondel, W., Daul, C., Hernandez-Mier, Y., Posada, R., Wolf, D. (2004). A simplified method of endoscopic image distortion correction based on grey level registration. *Proceedings of the 2004 International Conference on Image Processing*, IEEE, Singapore.

Miranda-Luna, R., Daul, C., Blondel, W.C.P.M., Hernandez-Mier, Y., Wolf, D., Guillemin, F. (2008). Mosaicing of bladder endoscopic image sequences: Distortion calibration and registration algorithm. *IEEE Transactions on Biomedical Engineering*, 55(2), 541–553.

Nelder, J.A. and Mead, R. (1965). A simplex method for function minimization. *The Computer Journal*, 7(4), 308–313.

Phan, T.B. (2020). On the 3D hollow organ cartography using 2D endoscopic images. PhD thesis, Université de Lorraine.

Phan, T.-B., Trinh, D.-H., Wolf, D., Daul, C. (2020). Optical flow-based structure-from-motion for the reconstruction of epithelial surfaces. *Pattern Recognition*, 105, 107391.

Posada, R., Daul, C., Wolf, D., Aletti, P. (2007). Towards a noninvasive intracranial tumor irradiation using 3D optical imaging and multimodal data registration. *International Journal of Biomedical Imaging*, 2007(062030), 1–14.

Schönberger, J.L. and Frahm, J.-M. (2016). Structure-from-motion revisited. *Proceedings of the Conference on Computer Vision and Pattern Recognition (CVPR)*, Las Vegas, NV.

Song, M. and Ang, T.L. (2014). Early detection of early gastric cancer using image-enhanced endoscopy: Current trends. *Gastrointestinal Intervention*, 3, 1–7.

Song, M. and Ang, T.L. (2017). A guide to multimodal endoscopy imaging for gastrointestinal malignancy – An early indicator. *Nature Reviews: Gastroenterology & Hepatology*, 14(7), 421–434.

Trinh, D.-H. and Daul, C. (2019). On illumination-invariant variational optical flow for weakly textured scenes. *Computer Vision and Image Understanding*, 179, 1–18.

Viola, P. and Wells, W. (1995). Alignment by maximization of mutual information. *Proceedings of IEEE International Conference on Computer Vision*, IEEE, Cambridge, MA.

Waechter, M., Moehrle, N., Goesele, M. (2014). Let there be color! Large-scale texturing of 3D reconstructions. *Proceedings of the European Conference on Computer Vision (ECCV)*, Zurich.

Zhang, Z. (2000). A flexible new technique for camera calibration. *IEEE Transactions on Pattern Analysis and Machine Intelligence*, 22(11), 1330–1334.

Zheng, Y., Lin, S., Kambhamettu, C., Yu, J., Kang, S.B. (2009). Single-image vignetting correction. *IEEE Transactions on Pattern Analysis and Machine Intelligence*, 31(12), 2243–2256.

8

An Introduction to Single-Pixel Imaging

Nicolas DUCROS[1,2]
[1] *CREATIS, INSA Lyon, France*
[2] *Institut Universitaire de France (IUF), Paris, France*

8.1. Introduction

This chapter focuses on a family of computational methods for acquiring images of a scene with a single-point detector. More precisely, single-pixel imaging consists of measuring, by means of a physical device, the intensity of the scene as seen through a light pattern. By repeating this operation for different well-chosen patterns, it is possible to recover the initial image using a digital processing step called image reconstruction.

At a time when 2D sensors capable of directly measuring an image have invaded our daily lives, due to their moderate cost (a few tens of dollars per unit) and their small size (about a square centimeter), the relevance of single-sensor imaging remains twofold. First, while the availability of 2D sensors has dramatically increased in the visible wavelength range, the same cannot be said for the full range of the electromagnetic spectrum. Matrix sensors remain expensive, in particular in the infrared range (Figure 8.1) where they are moreover affected by significant measurement noise that the methods described in this chapter are capable of reducing. Second, the principle of single-pixel acquisition makes it possible to easily access a third dimension, in addition to the two traditional spatial dimensions. This

Unconventional Optical Imaging for Biology,
coordinated by Corinne FOURNIER and Olivier HAEBERLÉ. © ISTE Ltd 2024.

approach is thus naturally adapted to hyperspectral imaging that acquires the wavelength of incident photons or to time-of-flight imaging. Single-pixel computational imaging has a wide range of applications, namely, infrared imaging (Radwell et al. 2014), terahertz imaging (Chan et al. 2008), fluorescence microscopy (Studer et al. 2012), multispectral imaging (Rousset et al. 2018) or fluorescence lifetime imaging (Pian et al. 2017).

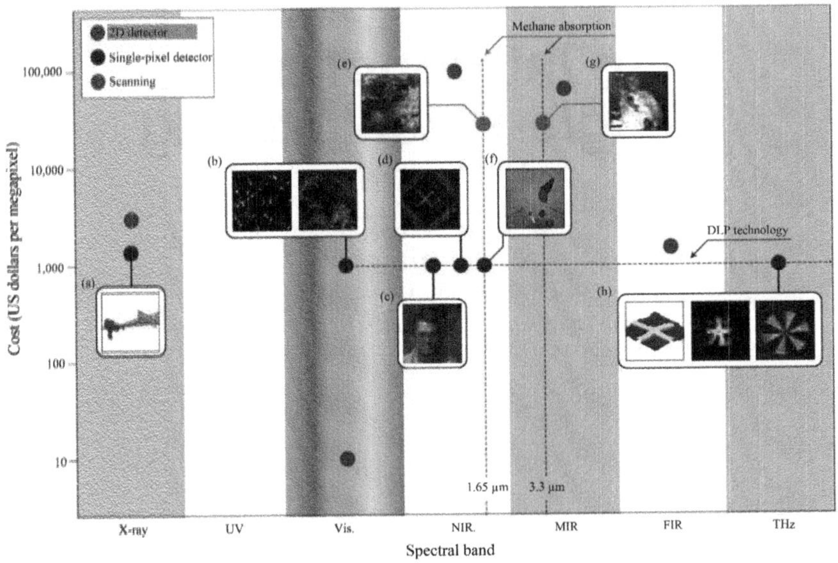

Figure 8.1. *Imaging methods available according to the wavelengths considered (source: Edgar et al. 2019). For a color version of this figure, see www.iste.co.uk/fournier/unconventional.zip*

COMMENTS ON FIGURE 8.1.– *While imaging systems based on array sensors (2D detectors) are available at low cost in the visible range (Vis), single-pixel systems are relevant alternatives in the near- (NIR), mid- (MIR) or far- (FIR) infrared.*

Single-pixel imaging is associated with the seminal paper by Duarte et al. (2008), in which it was first introduced. However, one interesting fact is that the concept of Hadamard spectroscopy, developed four decades earlier (Nelson and Fredman 1970), is based on an identical acquisition principle. Hadamard spectroscopy can thus be considered a precursor movement to *single-pixel imaging*, thus providing a complementary theoretical insight to this approach which seems to have been developed later, though independently. Computational single-pixel imaging has recently undergone a new development phase, driven by the studies of Higham et al. (2018), who introduced the use of *deep learning* methods for reconstruction.

We have chosen to structure this chapter according to these three main chronological phases, which will be the subject of three independent sections: Hadamard spectroscopy, single-pixel imaging and deep learning. We will illustrate the different methods proposed through numerous examples for which we will provide the computer code for simulation with experimental data and image reconstruction. This code is based on the Python package SPyRit (Openspyrit/Spyrit 2021), specifically dedicated to single-pixel imaging.

8.1.1. *Mathematical formulation*

Let $\boldsymbol{x} \in \mathbb{R}^N$ be the signal to be acquired, generally the image of a scene. The basic principle of computational imaging consists of measuring, by means of a physical device, not $\boldsymbol{x}$ directly but a transformed version $\boldsymbol{y} = \boldsymbol{A}\boldsymbol{x}$, from which algorithms will be able to recover $\boldsymbol{x}$. The matrix $\boldsymbol{A} \in \mathbb{R}^{M \times N}$, $M \leq N$, models the acquisition process; its rows contain multiplexing patterns which will be sequentially acquired. In situations where matrix $\boldsymbol{A}$ is invertible, the image $\boldsymbol{x}$ can be recovered by computing $\boldsymbol{A}^{-1}\boldsymbol{y}$.

To illustrate this principle, consider a simple example where an image comprising $N = 2$ pixels is to be acquired from $M = N = 2$ independent measurements. We have an experimental system that makes it possible to measure linear combinations of these two pixels. The first measurement y_1 acquires $-x_1 + x_2$, while the second y_2 acquires $x_1 - 0.5, x_2$. In this case, $\boldsymbol{A} = \begin{bmatrix} -1 & 1 \\ 1 & -0.5 \end{bmatrix}$. Since $\boldsymbol{A}^{-1} = \begin{bmatrix} 1 & 2 \\ 2 & 2 \end{bmatrix}$, the original image can be simply reconstructed from y_1 and y_2 by computing $x_1 = y_1 + 2\,y_2$ and $x_2 = 2\,y_1 + 2\,y_2$.

8.1.2. *Experimental implementation*

The previously exposed principle needs to be able to modulate the image according to different light patterns that correspond to the lines of matrix $\boldsymbol{A}$. An example of experimental implementation is represented in Figure 8.2. Early demonstrations relied on perforated masks through which light was allowed to travel or was blocked; the implementation has however been greatly simplified with the advent of spatial light modulators, whose modulation pattern can be controlled through computer software. Various modulator technologies are available. These include *digital micromirror devices* (DMDs), which are arrays made up of several million micromirrors, whose size is typically 10×10 μm^2; furthermore, these can be tilted in two different orientations at frequencies exceeding 20 kHz. This speed, coupled with a moderate cost of a few hundred euros, makes DMDs the technology mainly found in most recent implementations (Figure 8.2).

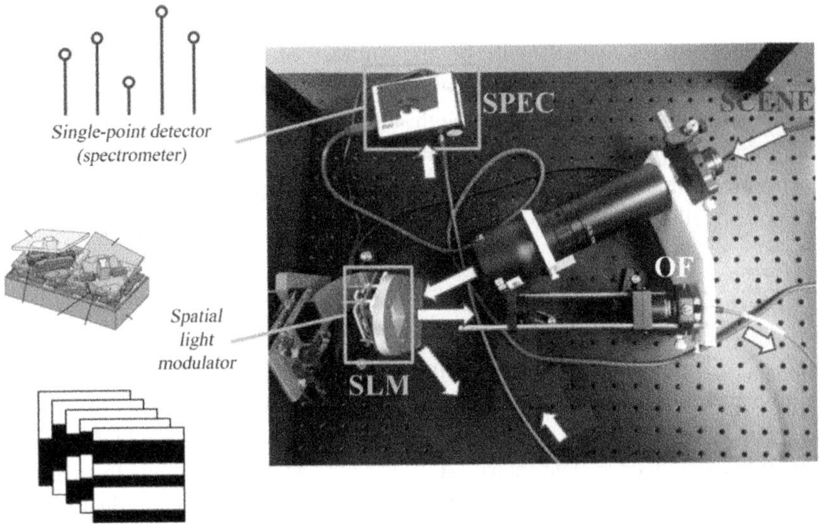

Figure 8.2. *Acquisition principle of single-pixel imaging. For a color version of this figure, see www.iste.co.uk/fournier/unconventional.zip*

COMMENTS ON FIGURE 8.2.– *The image obtained from the scene (SCENE) is projected onto a spatial light modulator (SLM) which sends, according to a given pattern, only part of the image to a single-pixel detector, here an optical fiber (OF) directing the light toward a compact spectrometer (SPEC). A complete acquisition consists of displaying different patterns on the spatial light modulator. These patterns correspond to the rows of the matrix* $\mathbf{A}$ *of equation [8.3], whereas the different values measured by the single-pixel detector form the vector* $\boldsymbol{y}$ *of this same equation. Knowing* $\mathbf{A}$ *and having measured* $\boldsymbol{y}$*, the objective is to recover the image of the scene* $\boldsymbol{x}$ *which remains unknown.*

8.2. Hadamard transform optics: the origins (1970–1980)

Hadamard transform optics is based on the noisy acquisition model:

$$y_m = a_{m,1}\, x_1 + \ldots + a_{m,N}\, x_N + \epsilon_m \qquad [8.1]$$

$$= \boldsymbol{a}_m^\top \boldsymbol{x} + \epsilon_m \qquad [8.2]$$

where y_m represents the mth measurement, $\boldsymbol{a}_m^\top = [a_{m,1} \ldots a_{m,N}]$ the mth pattern and ϵ_m is an additive noise source. Unlike the conventional scanning approach where each scene pixel x_n is successively acquired – which corresponds to the scenario where $y_m = x_m$, $1 \leq m \leq N$ – the Hadamard transform optics measures a mixture of all the pixels in the scene, and the proportions of such a mixture vary from one measurement to another. Considering M measurements, we have the following matrix notation:

$$\boldsymbol{y} = \boldsymbol{A}\boldsymbol{x} + \boldsymbol{\epsilon} \quad [8.3]$$

where $\boldsymbol{A} = [\boldsymbol{a}_1^\top, \ldots, \boldsymbol{a}_M^\top]^\top \in \mathbb{R}^{M \times N}$ is the matrix containing the M patterns and $\boldsymbol{\epsilon} \in \mathbb{R}^N$ represents the noise.

Hadamard transform optics has considered scenarios where $M = N$ in which the number of measurements is equal to the number of pixels in the image of the scene. Under the assumption that the errors are independent of each other and independent of the image, the image can be estimated in the least squares sense by:

$$\hat{\boldsymbol{x}} = \boldsymbol{A}^\dagger \boldsymbol{y} = \boldsymbol{x} + \boldsymbol{\eta}, \quad \text{with } \boldsymbol{\eta} = \boldsymbol{A}^\dagger \boldsymbol{\epsilon} \quad [8.4]$$

where $\boldsymbol{A}^\dagger$ is the pseudo-inverse of $\boldsymbol{A}$, which coincides with $\boldsymbol{A}^{-1}$ when $\boldsymbol{A}$ is invertible, and $\boldsymbol{\eta}$ represents the reconstruction error.

Assuming that the measurement errors have zero means, that is $\mathbb{E}(\boldsymbol{\epsilon}) = \boldsymbol{0}$, the reconstruction errors also have zero means. Moreover, assuming that $\boldsymbol{A}$ is invertible, we have $\mathbb{E}(\hat{\boldsymbol{x}}) = \boldsymbol{A}^{-1}\boldsymbol{y} = \boldsymbol{x}$ and it is then said that $\hat{\boldsymbol{x}}$ is an unbiased estimator of $\boldsymbol{x}$. On the other hand, the variance of the reconstruction error depends on the choice of patterns $\boldsymbol{A}$. Assuming that the measurement error has known variance σ^2, it can be shown that:

$$\mathsf{Cov}(\hat{\boldsymbol{x}}) = \sigma^2 \boldsymbol{A}^\dagger (\boldsymbol{A}^\dagger)^\top \quad [8.5]$$

where $\boldsymbol{A}^\top$ is the transposed matrix $\boldsymbol{A}$.

REMARK.–

$$\mathsf{Cov}(\hat{\boldsymbol{x}}) = \mathsf{Cov}(\boldsymbol{\eta}) = \mathsf{Cov}\left(\boldsymbol{A}^\dagger \boldsymbol{\epsilon}\right) \quad [8.6]$$

$$= \boldsymbol{A}^\dagger \, \mathsf{Cov}(\boldsymbol{\epsilon}) \, (\boldsymbol{A}^\dagger)^\top \quad [8.7]$$

Since the measurement errors $\boldsymbol{\epsilon}$ are independent and have known variance σ^2, we have $\mathsf{Cov}(\boldsymbol{\epsilon}) = \sigma^2 \boldsymbol{I}_N$, where $\boldsymbol{I}_N \in \mathbb{R}^{N \times N}$ is the identity matrix. Consequently:

$$\mathsf{Cov}(\hat{\boldsymbol{x}}) = \sigma^2 \boldsymbol{A}^\dagger (\boldsymbol{A}^\dagger)^\top \quad [8.8]$$

Many studies have been dedicated to determining "good" matrices $\boldsymbol{A}$ by seeking to reduce the reconstruction error $\boldsymbol{\eta}$. One of the main results, demonstrated by Hadamard, recommends, when it exists, the Nth-order Hadamard matrix, which is denoted by $\boldsymbol{H}_N$. This is a binary orthogonal matrix such that $\boldsymbol{H}_N \boldsymbol{H}_N^\top = N\boldsymbol{I}_N$. Figure 8.3 represents different Hadamard matrices in 1D and 2D.

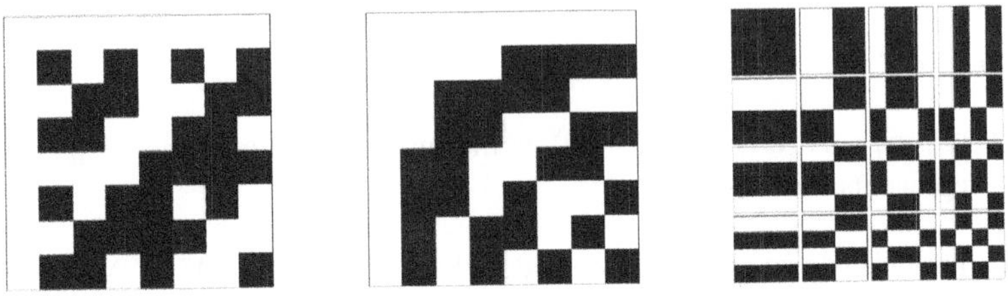

(a) (b) (c)

Figure 8.3. *1D and 2D Hadamard patterns*

COMMENTS ON FIGURE 8.3.– *(a, b) Hadamard matrix for $N = 8$. Each row of these matrices corresponds to a 1D modulation profile; the matrix rows are naturally ordered in (a), following Walsh ordering in (b). A permutation can be used to switch from one matrix to the other. (c) 2D Hadamard patterns for $N = 4 \times 4$. The 16 2D Hadamard patterns are represented from top to bottom and from left to right in Walsh order.*

The reconstruction error can be characterized when performing acquisition with the Hadamard matrix by substituting $\boldsymbol{A}^\dagger = \boldsymbol{H}^{-1} = \frac{1}{N}\boldsymbol{H}^\top$ in equation [8.5]. It is then obtained that:

$$\mathrm{Cov}\,(\eta) = \frac{\sigma^2}{N}\boldsymbol{I}_N, \quad 1 \leq n \leq N \qquad [8.9]$$

It can be observed that the errors are independent (the non-diagonal coefficients of $\mathrm{Cov}\,(\eta)$ being zero) and that each pixel will be reconstructed with the same level of noise of variance $\frac{\sigma^2}{N}$. It has been shown that the reconstruction error obtained in this way is the smallest possible and, from this point of view, Hadamard matrices are an optimal choice.

It is interesting to compare the Hadamard approach to the intuitive scanning approach where each pixel is sequentially acquired, independently of the others. In this case, we substitute $\boldsymbol{A} = \boldsymbol{I}_N$ in equation [8.5] and obtain a variance $\mathrm{Cov}\,(\epsilon) = \sigma^2\boldsymbol{I}_N$. The Hadamard approach thus achieves a noise standard deviation reduction factor of $\sqrt{N}$. This noise reduction property is illustrated in Figure 8.4, where the same reconstruction quality can be visually found for the scanning approach with $\sigma = 0.25$ and for the Hadamard approach with $\sigma = 16$, that is, an improvement of a factor of $16/0.25 = 64$, which indeed corresponds to the square root of the number of pixels considered.

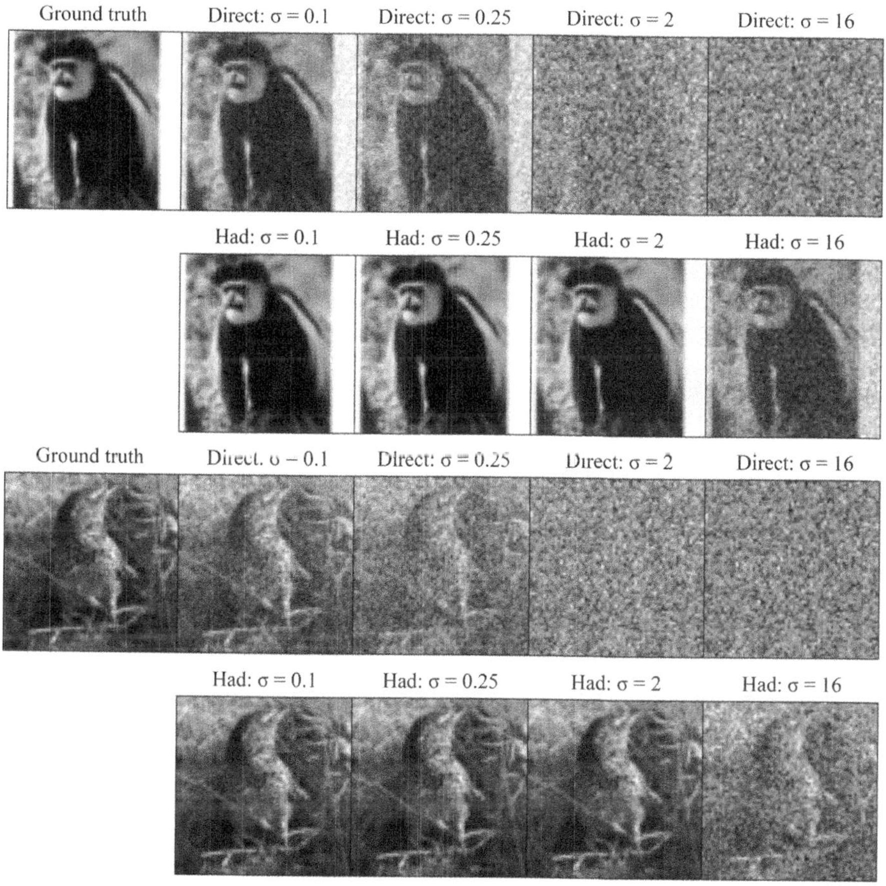

Figure 8.4. *Illustration of the improved Hadamard (Had) approach compared to scan-based acquisition (Direct) for different noise levels σ. The measurements were simulated for $N = 64 \times 64 = 4096$ 2D Hadamard patterns*

Additional constraints on the patterns, based on practical considerations, have also been the focus of particular attention. These include namely the positivity of the patterns as well as their cyclic character[1], which is necessary in order for them to be experimentally achieved by simple translation of a physical mask (Nelson and Fredman 1970; Sloane and Harwit 1976). This last condition was particularly critical before the advent of computer controllable spatial modulators.

8.3. Compressed sensing: the revival (2006–2016)

8.3.1. *Undersampled acquisition*

In order to reduce the acquisition time, it may be desirable to limit the number of measurements. The reconstruction problem is then tantamount to inverting a linear system $\boldsymbol{y} = \boldsymbol{A}\boldsymbol{x}$ for which the number of measurements is less than the number of unknowns, that is, for $\boldsymbol{A} \in \mathbb{R}^{M \times N}$ such that $M \leq N$. This is then referred to as compressed acquisition.

In the absence of noise, there exists a set of solutions satisfying $\boldsymbol{m} = \boldsymbol{A}\boldsymbol{x}$. One of the classical choices consists of retaining the minimal norm solution obtained by the constrained minimization:

$$\min_{\boldsymbol{x}} \|\boldsymbol{x}\|_2^2 \quad \text{such that} \quad \boldsymbol{y} = \boldsymbol{A}\boldsymbol{x} \qquad [8.10]$$

where $\|.\|_2$ represents the ℓ_2-norm. When the rows of $\boldsymbol{A}$ are independent, that is, when $\boldsymbol{A}$ is a full rank matrix, equation [8.10] admits the following analytical solution:

$$\boldsymbol{x} = \boldsymbol{A}^\top(\boldsymbol{A}\boldsymbol{A}^\top)^{-1}\boldsymbol{y} \qquad [8.11]$$

in which $\boldsymbol{A}^\dagger = \boldsymbol{A}^\top(\boldsymbol{A}\boldsymbol{A}^\top)^{-1}$ will denote hereafter the pseudo-inverse matrix of $\boldsymbol{A}$. When the rows of $\boldsymbol{A}$ are orthogonal, i.e., if $\boldsymbol{A}\boldsymbol{A}^\top = \boldsymbol{I}_M$, we simply have $\boldsymbol{A}^\dagger = \boldsymbol{A}^\top$.

However, the pseudo-inverse solution obtained at equation [8.11] is biased since, in general, $\boldsymbol{A}^\dagger\boldsymbol{y} = \boldsymbol{A}^\dagger\boldsymbol{A}\boldsymbol{x}^{\text{true}} \neq \boldsymbol{x}^{\text{true}}$. It is also said that the reconstruction is not perfect. When the rows of $\boldsymbol{A}$ are independent, a perfect reconstruction would imply the condition $\boldsymbol{A}^\top\boldsymbol{A} = \boldsymbol{I}_N$, which cannot be verified if $M < N$.

8.3.2. Compressed sensing *general principle*

The *compressed sensing* theory establishes a theoretical framework for the perfect reconstruction of signals from a small number of measurements. This theory has

1 The patterns can then be obtained by translating the same mask.

had a considerable impact in the field of computational imaging, during the decade following its introduction (Donoho 2006).

This theory is based on the notion of sparse representation, that is, on the existence of a sparsifying operator $\boldsymbol{\Psi}$ (typically linked to wavelet or Fourier transform) such that any image $\boldsymbol{x}$ can be represented as $\boldsymbol{x} = \boldsymbol{\Psi}\boldsymbol{\alpha}$, where $\boldsymbol{\alpha}$ is a vector containing only a few non-zero components (Candes and Wakin 2008). The reconstruction of an image $\boldsymbol{x}$ from measurements $\boldsymbol{y} = \boldsymbol{A}\boldsymbol{x}$ can then be performed by minimizing the number of non-zero components of the vector $\boldsymbol{\alpha}$ under the constraint $\boldsymbol{y} = \boldsymbol{A}\boldsymbol{x} = \boldsymbol{A}\boldsymbol{\Psi}\boldsymbol{\alpha}$.

This problem is an NP-hard combinatorial optimization problem, the solution to which is notoriously long and complex. Nevertheless, the compressed sensing theory shows that, under additional assumptions on the direct model $\boldsymbol{A}$ (and in particular its incoherence with the sparsifying operator), the minimization problem:

$$\min_{\boldsymbol{\alpha}} \|\boldsymbol{\alpha}\|_1 \quad \text{such that} \quad \boldsymbol{y} = \boldsymbol{A}\boldsymbol{\Psi}\boldsymbol{\alpha} \qquad [8.12]$$

where $\|.\|_1$ represents the ℓ_1-norm, which results in recovering the vector $\boldsymbol{\alpha}$ that corresponds to the image $\boldsymbol{x}$. This result is important because the ℓ_1 minimization problem defined in equation [8.12] is significantly simpler to solve than the original combinatorial problem.

In the presence of noise, the constraint $\boldsymbol{y} = \boldsymbol{A}\boldsymbol{x}$ is no longer verified and the following unconstrained formulation should instead be adopted:

$$\min_{\boldsymbol{x}} \|\boldsymbol{y} - \boldsymbol{A}\boldsymbol{x}\|_2^2 + \lambda\|\boldsymbol{\Phi}\boldsymbol{x}\|_1 \qquad [8.13]$$

where λ is a regularization parameter and $\boldsymbol{\Phi}$ a sparse operator (which can be seen as $\boldsymbol{\Psi}^{-1}$ when defined). Given that the ℓ_1-norm is not differentiable at 0, it is usual to use proximal methods to solve [8.13], among which Bregman methods or the alternating direction algorithm can be mentioned.

Despite the solidity of its theoretical foundations, the compressive sensing theory is inhibited by practical limitations (Adcock et al. 2017). Proximal optimization methods are iterative by nature, which leads to computation times that can prove prohibitive, even for low-dimensional problems. Moreover, as the sparsity operator $\boldsymbol{\Phi}$ is not known a priori, it is common practice to choose the discrete gradient. It is then assumed that the image jumps are localized (such as an image with low total variation), which leads to typical staircase artifacts. More advanced methods based on minimization of the isotropic total variation, the higher order total variation or the solution rank can be used to overcome this problem at the cost of significantly longer computation times. Moreover, most of these algorithms depend strongly on the setting of one or more hyperparameters (regularization parameter, descent step, number of iterations, etc.), whose optimal values depend, among other things, on the image being acquired and the level of measurement noise.

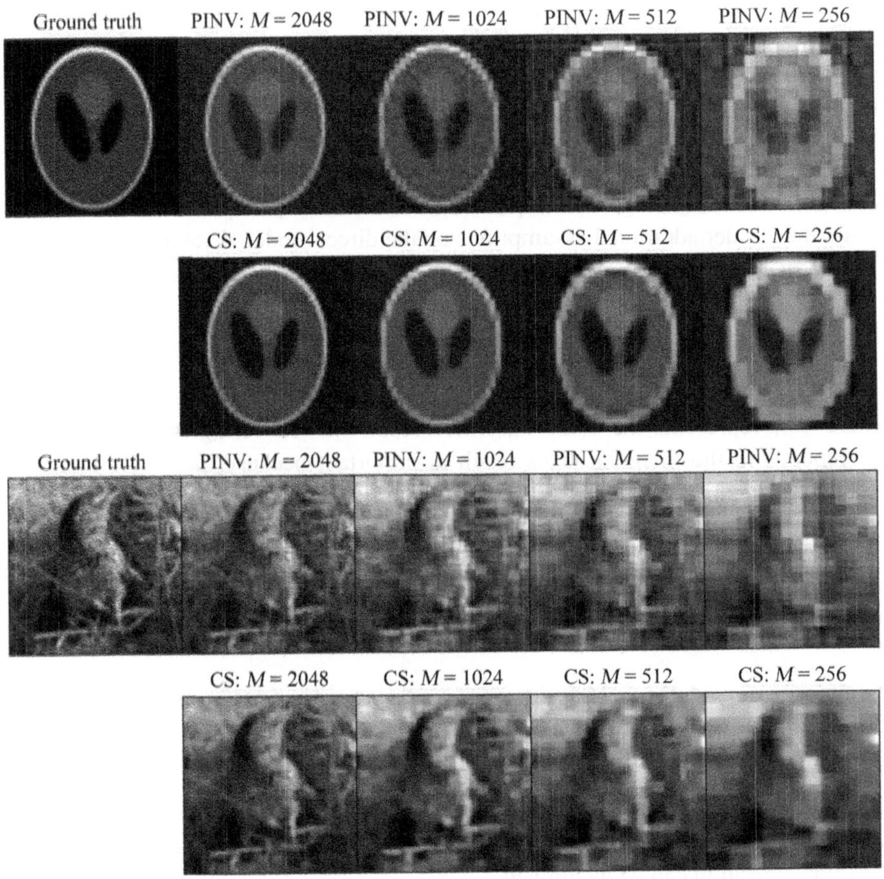

Figure 8.5. *Reconstruction from undersampled acquisitions*

COMMENTS ON FIGURE 8.5.– *PINV: least squares-based solution given by equation [8.11]. CS: compressed sensing solution obtained by minimizing* [8.13] *with* $\boldsymbol{\Phi} = [\nabla_x^\top, \nabla_y^\top]^\top$, *corresponding to the total variation* $\|\boldsymbol{\Phi} f\|_1 = \|\nabla_x f\|_1 + \|\nabla_y f\|_1$. *The different columns consider different sampling rates* $\frac{M}{N}$. *With* $N = 4096$, *the sampling rate decreases from left to right (*$\frac{1}{2}$, $\frac{1}{4}$, $\frac{1}{8}$ *and finally* $\frac{1}{16}$*).*

8.3.3. *Choice of acquisition patterns*

Usually, acquisition patterns $\boldsymbol{A}$ are chosen from a basis of patterns $\boldsymbol{H}$, which can be modeled by:

$$\boldsymbol{A} = \boldsymbol{S}_M \boldsymbol{H} \tag{8.14}$$

where $\boldsymbol{S}_M \in \{0,1\}^{M \times N}$ is an undersampling matrix that selects some of the rows of the full basis $\boldsymbol{H} \in \mathbb{R}^{N \times N}$. For example, the undersampling matrix for retaining, respectively, the second, first and sixth pattern of an $\mathbb{R}^{8 \times 8}$ basis is given by:

$$\boldsymbol{S}_3 = \begin{pmatrix} 0\,1\,0\,0\,0\,0\,0\,0 \\ 1\,0\,0\,0\,0\,0\,0\,0 \\ 0\,0\,0\,0\,0\,1\,0\,0 \end{pmatrix} \tag{8.15}$$

The choice of the matrix $\boldsymbol{A}$ then amounts to choosing a full basis $\boldsymbol{H}$ and an undersampling matrix $\boldsymbol{S}_M$. As explained in the previous section, the Hadamard basis is a natural choice due to its noise reduction properties but Fourier, discrete cosine or wavelet bases are common alternatives. A solution to the problem of choosing the undersampling matrix can be found in the compressed sensing theory, which requires the use of random matrices (Candes and Wakin 2008). A second interesting theoretical result shows that the reconstruction error obtained by a linear reconstruction method is minimized by the choice of patterns that maximize the measurement energy (Baldassarre et al. 2016). The undersampling matrix is then obtained by solving:

$$\max_{\boldsymbol{S}_M} \sum_s \|\boldsymbol{S}_M \boldsymbol{H} \boldsymbol{x}_s\|_2^2 \tag{8.16}$$

where the $\boldsymbol{x}_s$, $1 \leq s \leq S$, represent the S images constituting a database. By chance, the problem posed by equation [8.16] can be solved very simply. First, we simply have to compute the image $\sum_s (\boldsymbol{H}\boldsymbol{x}_s)^2$, where the square is applied in a pixel-wise manner, then the M largest components of this energy image are retained.

Distinct empirical choices with often honorable performance are common practice. A large number of studies have compared the results obtained by choosing different bases and undersampling methods (Higham et al. 2018; Ochoa et al. 2018; Vaz et al. 2020).

In Figure 8.6, we compare three classical approaches to undersampling the Walsh–Hadamard basis. The first strategy consists of random sampling, the second the said “natural” sampling for which the lowest frequency patterns are preserved, the third is based on maximizing measurement energy as described by equation [8.16].

Random sampling leads visually to the lowest quality images for which it is difficult to distinguish the main object in the scene. The PSNR is fairly small, typically 15–20 dB lower than with the other two approaches. The latter two approaches are also significantly better visually, with the reconstruction of fine details such as the masts of the boat in the first image. In line with theory, the energy-based approach is on average the best of both, with a higher PSNR of about 2–3 dB.

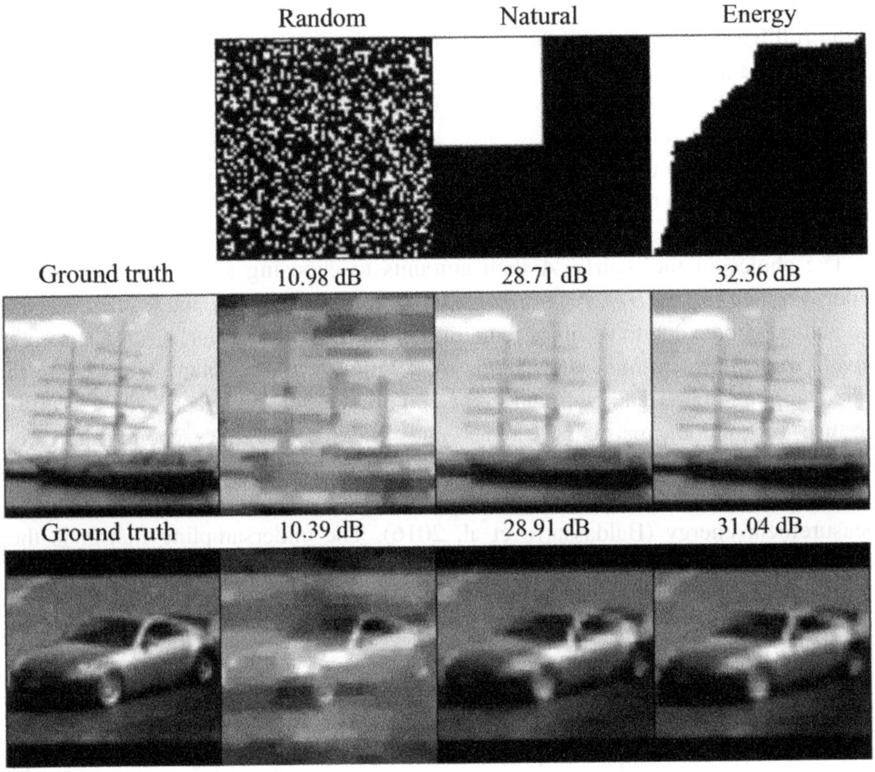

Figure 8.6. *Subsampling of acquisition patterns for different methods*

COMMENTS ON FIGURE 8.6.– *The first line represents a mask that describes the measurements retained by the sampling procedure (random: random sampling; natural: low frequency; energy: solution to [8.16]). The basis* $\boldsymbol{H}$ *chosen is the Walsh–Hadamard basis for* $N = 64 \times 64$ *and we have set* $M = \frac{1}{4}N$*. The reconstructions are obtained by solving [8.13].*

8.4. Deep learning reconstruction

8.4.1. *General principle*

Deep learning reconstruction methods attempt to reconstruct an image directly from the measurements, using a nonlinear function that depends on parameters whose values must be reasonably chosen (Barbastathis et al. 2019). More specifically, by denoting the measurements $\boldsymbol{y} \in \mathbb{R}^M$, we obtain the image $\boldsymbol{x} \in \mathbb{R}^N$ by application of the function $\mathcal{G}_{\boldsymbol{\omega}} : \mathbb{R}^M \to \mathbb{R}^N$, namely:

$$\boldsymbol{x} = \mathcal{G}_{\boldsymbol{\omega}}(\boldsymbol{y}) \quad [8.17]$$

where $\boldsymbol{\omega}$ represents the parameters of the function $\mathcal{G}$.

In the field of deep learning, the function $\mathcal{G}_{\boldsymbol{\omega}}$ is conventionally called a model and corresponds to a neural network. One of the strong points of this type of approach is that model evaluation is generally fast (less than a second, typically), which leads to a significant reduction in reconstruction time compared to the methods resulting from the compressed sensing theory.

8.4.2. *Model architecture*

The most common models in deep learning are probably feedforward neural networks. These are made of cascaded layers of neurons, which can be modeled by:

$$\mathcal{G}_{\boldsymbol{\omega}} = \mathcal{G}^L_{\boldsymbol{\omega}^L} \circ \ldots \circ \mathcal{G}^1_{\boldsymbol{\omega}^1} \quad [8.18]$$

where $\mathcal{G}^\ell_{\boldsymbol{\omega}^\ell}$, $1 \leq \ell \leq L$, represents the ℓth layer of the network and $\circ$ the composition of functions. The output of a layer is obtained by linear combination of its inputs, followed by a nonlinear transformation. By denoting the input vector of a layer by $\boldsymbol{y} \in \mathbb{R}^{M_{\text{in}}}$, its output $\boldsymbol{x} \in \mathbb{R}^{M_{\text{out}}}$ is given by:

$$\mathcal{G}_{\boldsymbol{\omega}}(\boldsymbol{y}) = g(\boldsymbol{W}\boldsymbol{y} + \boldsymbol{b}) \quad [8.19]$$

where $\boldsymbol{W} \in \mathbb{R}^{M_{\text{out}} \times M_{\text{in}}}$ and $\boldsymbol{b} \in \mathbb{R}^{M_{\text{out}}}$ are, respectively, the weights and the biases of the layer, while g is a nonlinear function, classically called the activation function. The values of the network parameters $\boldsymbol{\omega} = (\boldsymbol{W}, \boldsymbol{b})$ are determined during the training phase. On the other hand, the number of layers, the number of inputs and outputs of each layer, the structure of the weight matrices and the nature of the activation functions form the network architecture, which is usually defined, once and for all, before training.

There are different types of neural layers that satisfy equation [8.19] but differ in the structure of the connections that link inputs to outputs. Figure 8.7 describes the conventional structures of fully connected layers and convolution layers as well as the ReLU function. The latter is a typical activation function that thresholds negative values to zero. For fully connected neural layers, the weight matrices $\boldsymbol{W}$ are full and thus require $M_{\text{out}} \times M_{\text{in}}$ parameters. On the other hand, convolution layers consider structured weight matrices, which considerably reduces the number of parameters involved, typically a few 3×3 filters regardless of the size of the input image.

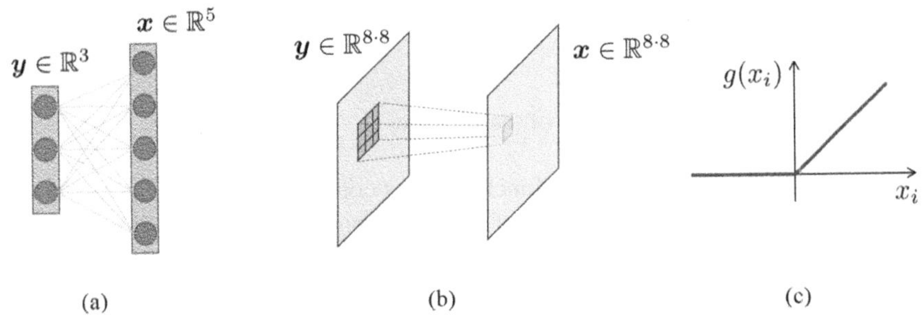

Figure 8.7. *The layers comprised in a neural network where $\boldsymbol{y}$ represents the input signal and $\boldsymbol{x}$ the output signal. For a color version of this figure, see www.iste.co.uk/fournier/unconventional.zip*

COMMENTS ON FIGURE 8.7.– *(a) Fully connected layer in which all outputs (i.e. all components of $\boldsymbol{x}$) are connected to all inputs (i.e. all components of $\boldsymbol{y}$). In the illustrated example, 5×3 connections can be found, namely 15 weights ω_i^j, $1 \leq i \leq 3$, $1 \leq j \leq 5$, characterizing the layer. (b) Convolution layer in which the output is obtained by convolving the input by a fixed size filter, here 3×3. Independently of the input and output image size, namely 8×8 in this illustration, the number of weights characterizing the layer will thus be limited to $3 \times 3 = 9$. (c) Nonlinear activation function, applied to a layer output before connecting it to the input of the next layer. The function represented here is the conventional thresholding of negative values to zero, known as the ReLU* (rectified linear unit) *function.*

As depicted in Figure 8.8, the first layer of a deep reconstruction network is typically a fully connected layer that maps the measurements $\boldsymbol{y} \in \mathbb{R}^M$ to an image $\tilde{\boldsymbol{x}} \in \mathbb{R}^N$. This first layer is typically followed by convolution layers that operate in the image domain and lead to the final solution $\hat{\boldsymbol{x}}$.

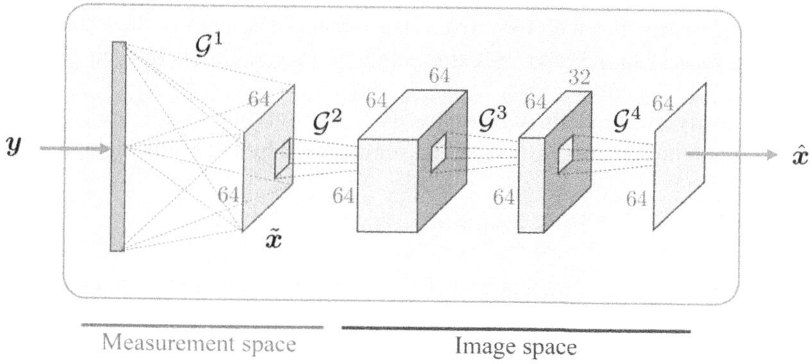

Figure 8.8. *Simple reconstruction network architecture. For a color version of this figure, see www.iste.co.uk/fournier/unconventional.zip*

COMMENTS ON FIGURE 8.8.– *This network, referred to as freeNet, is composed of four layers and inspired by Higham et al. (2018). The first layer is a fully connected layer operating in the measurement domain, followed by three convolution layers operating in the image domain. The outputs of the convolution layers are all* 64 *images but their number* n^{filt} *varies depending on the layer being considered. The value of* n^{filt} *corresponds to the number of convolution kernels used in each layer, which is 64 for the first layer, 32 for the second and 1 for the third. The size of all filter kernels of this network is* 3×3.

8.4.3. *Training*

The model parameters are obtained before reconstruction during the training phase. This phase aims at minimizing the difference between the output of the model and the images from a database. By denoting $\boldsymbol{X} = [\boldsymbol{x}_1, \ldots, \boldsymbol{x}_S]$ the image basis and $\boldsymbol{Y} = [\boldsymbol{y}_1, \ldots, \boldsymbol{y}_S]$ the corresponding measurements, such that $\boldsymbol{y}_s = \boldsymbol{A}\boldsymbol{x}_s$, the training phase minimizes a loss function $\mathcal{J}$ that reflects the similarity between the original images and the reconstructed images. Conventionally, one considers the mean square error, that is:

$$\min_{\omega} \mathcal{J}(\omega) = \min_{\omega} \frac{1}{S} \sum_{s=1}^{S} \|\mathcal{G}_{\omega}(\boldsymbol{y}_s) - \boldsymbol{x}_s\|_2^2 \qquad [8.20]$$

It should be noted that the loss function is classically computed as the sum over the training basis and, consequently, the larger the training basis, the larger the training times. However, a large number of images is generally required to obtain a network capable of reconstructing with low error images that are not part of the training basis. The training phase can therefore be extremely long (several hours or even weeks).

The majority of modern algorithms used for solving [8.20] are variants of stochastic gradient descents, which can be summarized by the following update:

$$\boldsymbol{\omega}^{(k+1)} = \boldsymbol{\omega}^{(k)} - \tau_k \nabla_\omega \mathcal{J}_{\text{batch}}^{(k)}(\boldsymbol{\omega}) \quad [8.21]$$

where ∇_ω represents the gradient and $\mathcal{J}_{\text{batch}}^{(k)}$ the partial cost function, computed by taking only a subset of the available pairs of measurements into consideration. By denoting $\mathbb{B}_k$ a subset of B randomly chosen among the S possible image indexes, we have:

$$\mathcal{J}_{\text{batch}}^{(k)}(\boldsymbol{\omega}) = \frac{1}{B} \sum_{s \in \mathbb{B}_k} \|\mathcal{G}_\omega(\boldsymbol{y}_s) - \boldsymbol{x}_s\|_2^2 \quad [8.22]$$

The parameter τ_k introduced in [8.21] is the gradient step, known as the *learning rate*, and chosen to decrease with each iteration. Many variants are capable of speeding up the convergence speed, namely through momentum techniques and descent step adaptation rules (Goodfellow et al. 2016, Chapter 8). It is important to note that gradient-based approaches are particularly widespread due to the availability of the gradient backpropagation algorithm, which enables $\nabla_\omega \mathcal{J}_{\text{batch}}^{(k)}$ to be efficiently computed.

In Figure 8.9, we represent the output of an artificial neural network at different epochs, namely at different stages of the training phase. An "epoch" is defined as a cycle of iterations at the end of which all images in the database have been included in the partial cost function of equation [8.22]. It is observed that the object is recognizable as early as the reconstructed image at the first epoch (0 epoch). The PSNR then significantly increases, reaching values around 34 dB. By the sixth epoch, the PSNR are already around 30 dB and the image is a good faithful reconstruction. The successive epochs result in reducing the artifacts present in the background of the image but also in enhancing the contrasts.

8.4.4. *Simple link with conventional methods*

The link between conventional reconstruction methods of sections 8.2 and 8.3 and the reconstructions obtained by neural networks appears clearly when freezing the parameters of certain layers instead of learning them. More specifically, the output of the first layer, denoted by $\tilde{\boldsymbol{x}} \in \mathbb{R}^N$, is written as:

$$\tilde{\boldsymbol{x}} = \boldsymbol{W}^1 \boldsymbol{y} + \boldsymbol{b}^1 \quad [8.23]$$

by removing the activation function, which amounts to choosing g^1 as the identity function. Based on this observation, it is possible to obtain, by identification with classical linear estimators, analytic expressions for the parameters $\boldsymbol{\omega}^1 = (\boldsymbol{W}^1, \boldsymbol{b}^1)$ of this layer.

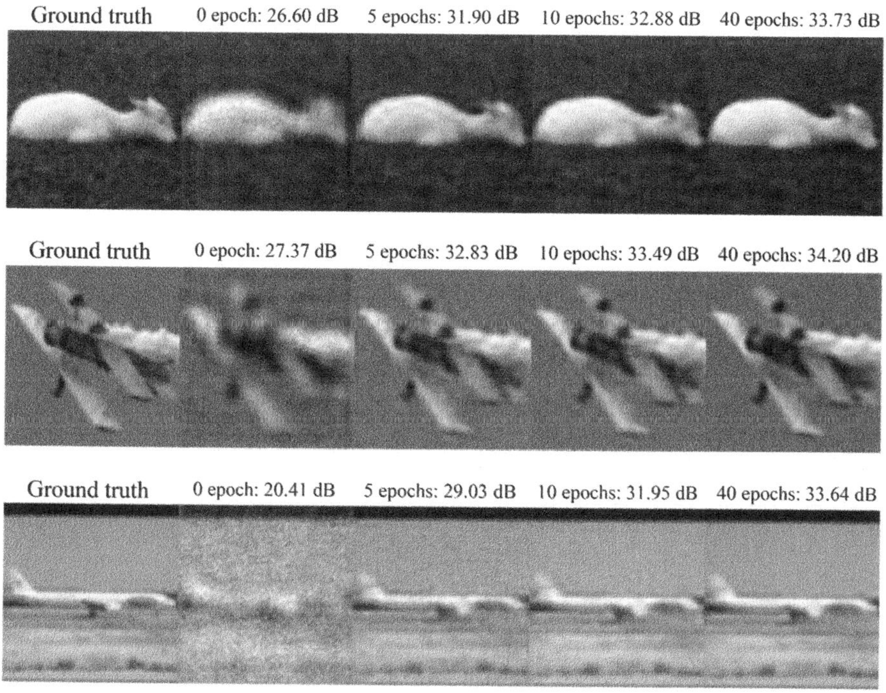

Figure 8.9. *Reconstruction network at different stages (epochs) of the training phase*

COMMENTS ON FIGURE 8.9.– *An "epoch" refers to a cycle of iterations at the end of which all the images in the database have been considered once, that is, taken into account in a minibatch, as presented in equation [8.22]. Here, the freeNet network described in Figure 8.8 is considered. We examine an example with* $N = 64 \times 64$ *and* $M = \frac{1}{4}N$ *and choose to initialize* τ_k *to* 10^{-3} *before multiplying it by 0.25 every 20 epochs. The network parameters are randomly initialized before the training starts.*

First, it is possible to identify the parameters of equation [8.23] with the pseudo-inverse solution given with equation [8.11]. When the light patterns are orthogonal, the first layer of the network generates the pseudo-inverse solution by choosing:

$$\boldsymbol{W}_{\text{pinv}}^{1} = \boldsymbol{A}^{\top} \quad \text{and} \quad \boldsymbol{b}_{\text{pinv}}^{1} = \boldsymbol{0} \tag{8.24}$$

Before going any further, we set $\tilde{\boldsymbol{y}} \in \mathbb{R}^{N}$ the full measurement vector, defined as $\tilde{\boldsymbol{y}} = \boldsymbol{H}\boldsymbol{x}$, where $\boldsymbol{H}$ is the full acquisition basis, that is, which has not been undersampled. This vector is full in that it contains both the measurements $\boldsymbol{y} \in \mathbb{R}^{M}$ acquired by the experimental system and those $\boldsymbol{y}_2 \in \mathbb{R}^{N-M}$ that were not. The full basis $\boldsymbol{H}$ can be seen as $\boldsymbol{H} = [\boldsymbol{A}, \boldsymbol{A}_2]$, where $\boldsymbol{A}_2 \in \mathbb{R}^{(N-M)\times N}$ represents the light patterns that were not acquired.

In this framework, we can note (see the observation below) that the pseudo-inverse solution $\tilde{\boldsymbol{x}} = \boldsymbol{A}^{\top}\boldsymbol{y}$ of equation [8.11] is also given by $\tilde{\boldsymbol{x}} = \boldsymbol{H}^{\top}\tilde{\boldsymbol{y}}_0$, where $\tilde{\boldsymbol{y}}_0 = [\boldsymbol{y}, \boldsymbol{0}]$ is the acquisition vector where missing data are replaced by zeros.

REMARK.–

$$\tilde{\boldsymbol{x}} = \boldsymbol{H}^{\top}\tilde{\boldsymbol{y}} = \begin{bmatrix} \boldsymbol{A} \\ \boldsymbol{A}_2 \end{bmatrix}^{\top} \tilde{\boldsymbol{y}} = \begin{bmatrix} \boldsymbol{A}^{\top} & \boldsymbol{A}_2^{\top} \end{bmatrix} \tilde{\boldsymbol{y}} \tag{8.25}$$

$$= \begin{bmatrix} \boldsymbol{A}^{\top} & \boldsymbol{A}_2^{\top} \end{bmatrix} \begin{bmatrix} \boldsymbol{y} \\ \boldsymbol{y}_2 \end{bmatrix} = \boldsymbol{A}^{\top}\boldsymbol{y} + \boldsymbol{A}_2^{\top}\boldsymbol{y}_2 \tag{8.26}$$

Therefrom, $\tilde{\boldsymbol{x}} = \boldsymbol{A}^{\top}\boldsymbol{y}$ is correctly recovered by imposing $\boldsymbol{y}_2 = \boldsymbol{0}$. ■

8.4.5. *Best linear estimator: Bayesian completion*

The previous approach can be generalized by considering filling in the missing measures with relevant non-zero values $\tilde{\boldsymbol{y}}_2$ before multiplication by the transpose of the full basis. Let:

$$\tilde{\boldsymbol{x}} = \boldsymbol{H}^{\top}\tilde{\boldsymbol{y}}, \quad \text{where} \quad \tilde{\boldsymbol{y}} = \begin{bmatrix} \boldsymbol{y} \\ \tilde{\boldsymbol{y}}_2 \end{bmatrix} \tag{8.27}$$

In a Bayesian framework, the missing measurements can be estimated from their correlation with the measurements carried out (Ducros et al. 2020), which leads to the following analytical expression:

$$\tilde{\boldsymbol{y}}_2 = \boldsymbol{\mu}_2 + \boldsymbol{\Sigma}_{21}\boldsymbol{\Sigma}_1^{-1}(\boldsymbol{y} - \boldsymbol{\mu}_1) \qquad [8.28]$$

where $\boldsymbol{\mu}_1$ and $\boldsymbol{\mu}_2$ represent the mean of the measurements, $\boldsymbol{\Sigma}_1$ and $\boldsymbol{\Sigma}_{21}$ are their covariance. More specifically, $\boldsymbol{\mu}_1 \in \mathbb{R}^M$ is the mean of the measurements carried out, $\boldsymbol{\mu}_2 \in \mathbb{R}^{N-M}$ is the mean of the missing measurements, $\boldsymbol{\Sigma}_1 \in \mathbb{R}^{M\times M}$ is the variance of the measurements carried out and $\boldsymbol{\Sigma}_{21} \in \mathbb{R}^{N-M\times M}$ is the covariance between the missing measurements and those acquired. A geometrical illustration of equation [8.28] is given in Figure 8.10, which illustrates the correlation between the second and the seventh component of the full Hadamard vector $\tilde{\boldsymbol{y}}$. In this example, if we measure $\tilde{y}_2 = 20$, we will set $\tilde{y}_7 = 9$ rather than $\tilde{y}_7 = 0$ if this component could not be measured.

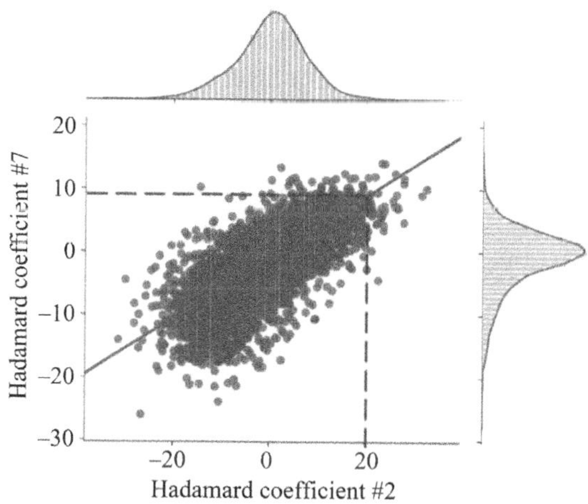

Figure 8.10. *Geometrical interpretation of the Bayesian completion. Each point represents an image of the STL-10 basis, whose position along the x-axis (respectively y-axis) depends on the value of the second (respectively, seventh) component of the full Hadamard vector $\tilde{\boldsymbol{y}}_s = \boldsymbol{H}\boldsymbol{x}_s$. The slope of the blue solid line reflects the correlation between these two components. For a color version of this figure, see www.iste.co.uk/fournier/unconventional.zip*

The different quantities involved in equation [8.28] can be estimated from a basis of images $\{\boldsymbol{x}_s\}$, $1 \leq s \leq S$, where S is the number of images contained in the basis using classical estimators of the mean:

$$\boldsymbol{\mu}_1 = \frac{1}{S}\sum_s \boldsymbol{A}\boldsymbol{x}_s \qquad [8.29]$$

$$\boldsymbol{\mu}_2 = \frac{1}{S}\sum_s \boldsymbol{A}_2\boldsymbol{x}_s \qquad [8.30]$$

and of the covariance:

$$\boldsymbol{\Sigma}_1 = \frac{1}{S-1}\sum_s (\boldsymbol{A}\boldsymbol{x}_s - \boldsymbol{\mu}_1)(\boldsymbol{A}\boldsymbol{x}_s - \boldsymbol{\mu}_1)^\top \qquad [8.31]$$

$$\boldsymbol{\Sigma}_{21} = \frac{1}{S-1}\sum_s (\boldsymbol{A}_2\boldsymbol{x}_s - \boldsymbol{\mu}_2)(\boldsymbol{A}\boldsymbol{x}_s - \boldsymbol{\mu}_1)^\top \qquad [8.32]$$

Since equations [8.27] and [8.28] are linear, a reconstruction can be obtained using Bayesian completion by means of a layer of neurons whose parameters are well chosen. By substituting [8.28] in [8.27], then by identification with [8.23], we obtain:

$$\boldsymbol{W}^1_{\text{comp}} = \boldsymbol{H}^\top \begin{bmatrix} \boldsymbol{I}_M \\ \boldsymbol{\Sigma}_{21}\boldsymbol{\Sigma}_1^{-1} \end{bmatrix} \quad \text{and} \quad \boldsymbol{b}^1_{\text{comp}} = \boldsymbol{H}^\top \begin{bmatrix} \boldsymbol{0}_M \\ \boldsymbol{\mu}_2 - \boldsymbol{\Sigma}_{21}\boldsymbol{\Sigma}_1^{-1}\boldsymbol{\mu}_1 \end{bmatrix} \qquad [8.33]$$

In the absence of correlation between the acquired and missing measurements, that is, under the assumption that $\boldsymbol{\Sigma}_{21} = \boldsymbol{0}$, and when the measurements have zero means, namely for $\boldsymbol{\mu}_2 = \boldsymbol{0}$, equation [8.33] is then reduced to the simple expression for the pseudo-inverse given by equation [8.24].

In Figure 8.11, we compare, for some images, the pseudo-inverse solution, the one obtained by Bayesian completion, as well as the one obtained by learning the first layer $\boldsymbol{\omega}^1 = (\boldsymbol{W}^1, \boldsymbol{b}^1)$. In the latter case, the fully connected layer $\boldsymbol{\omega}^1$ is jointly learned with the downstream convolution layers $\boldsymbol{\omega}^\ell$, $2 \leq \ell \leq 4$. It should be pointed out that the first learned layer actually provides an approximate solution in the image domain. The PSNR is particularly low due to poor scaling; however, the objects existing on the original image are easily recognizable for the three reconstructed images. The pseudo-inverse solution improves the reconstruction quality very significantly, as well as the completed solution which offers the best reconstruction quality both visually and in terms of PSNR.

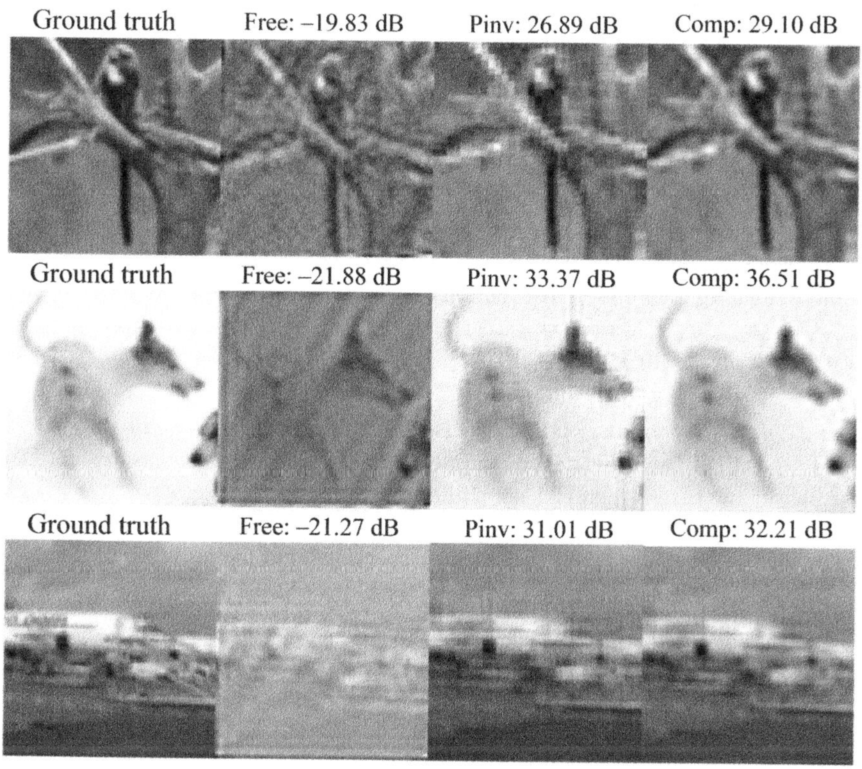

Figure 8.11. *Output from the first fully connected layer of a deep reconstruction network*

COMMENTS ON FIGURE 8.11.– *"Free" for free layer, that is, whose parameters are learned during training; "Pinv" for pseudo-inverse given by [8.24]; "Comp" for completion of missing measurements given by [8.33]. When training "free", the layers downstream of the first are the ones described in Figure 8.8. We include above each reconstructed image its PSNR expressed in decibels.*

8.4.6. *Taking noise into consideration*

We are now interested in the influence of measurement noise on reconstruction quality. In particular, we consider the Poisson noise intrinsic to any light signal measurement. The noisy measurements $\boldsymbol{y}^{\alpha}$ are given by:

$$\boldsymbol{y}^{\alpha} \sim \frac{1}{\alpha}\mathcal{P}(\alpha \boldsymbol{y}) \qquad [8.34]$$

where α is a multiplicative factor that drives the noise level and $\mathcal{P}$ represents the Poisson distribution. The larger α is, the larger the number of photons collected and the better the signal-to-noise ratio measurement. The division by α simply aims at bringing the data into the same range of variation, independently of the noise level. By approximating the Poisson distribution by a normal distribution, we have:

$$\boldsymbol{y}^{\alpha} \sim \boldsymbol{y} + \mathcal{N}(\boldsymbol{0}, \boldsymbol{\Sigma}_{\alpha}) \qquad [8.35]$$

where $\mathcal{N}(\boldsymbol{\mu}, \boldsymbol{\Sigma})$ represents the normal distribution of mean $\boldsymbol{\mu}$ and with variance $\boldsymbol{\Sigma}$ and $\boldsymbol{\Sigma}_{\alpha} \in \mathbb{R}^{M \times M}$ is a covariance matrix, which depends on the measurement. The noise considered here is therefore not additive.

The idea of Bayesian completion can be generalized in the presence of noise. To this end, the raw measurements $\boldsymbol{y}$ in equation [8.27] need to be replaced by a denoised version $\tilde{\boldsymbol{y}}_1$ of these measurements, thus leading to:

$$\tilde{\boldsymbol{x}} = \boldsymbol{H}^{\top}\tilde{\boldsymbol{y}} \quad \text{with} \quad \tilde{\boldsymbol{y}} = \begin{bmatrix} \tilde{\boldsymbol{y}}_1 \\ \tilde{\boldsymbol{y}}_2 \end{bmatrix} \qquad [8.36]$$

The denoised and completed measurements are given by (Lorente Mur et al. 2021):

$$\tilde{\boldsymbol{y}}_1 = \boldsymbol{\mu}_1 + \boldsymbol{\Sigma}_1[\boldsymbol{\Sigma}_1 + \boldsymbol{\Sigma}_{\alpha}]^{-1}(\boldsymbol{y}^{\alpha} - \boldsymbol{\mu}_1) \qquad [8.37a]$$

$$\tilde{\boldsymbol{y}}_2 = \boldsymbol{\mu}_2 + \boldsymbol{\Sigma}_{21}\boldsymbol{\Sigma}_1^{-1}[\tilde{\boldsymbol{y}}_1 - \boldsymbol{\mu}_1] \qquad [8.37b]$$

where equation [8.37a] corresponds to the denoising of acquired measurements, whereas equation [8.37b] corresponds to the completion of missing measurements. Comparing equations [8.37b] and [8.28], it can be noted that the completion steps with and without noise are identical (addition and subtraction of the averages and multiplication by $\boldsymbol{\Sigma}_{21}\boldsymbol{\Sigma}_1^{-1}$). Only the data to which these operations are applied change: raw measurements $\boldsymbol{y}$ in one case, denoised measurements $\tilde{\boldsymbol{y}}$ in the other. This solution is the one with the minimum mean squared error (MMSE) that can be obtained by a linear estimator.

By identification between [8.23], [8.36] and [8.37], we can choose the parameters of the first layer of the network, making it possible to compute the linear MMSE solution. These are given by:

$$\boldsymbol{W}^1_{\text{mmse}} = \boldsymbol{H}^\top \begin{bmatrix} \boldsymbol{\Sigma}_1[\boldsymbol{\Sigma}_1 + \boldsymbol{\Sigma}_\alpha]^{-1} \\ \boldsymbol{\Sigma}_{21}\boldsymbol{\Sigma}_1^{-1} \end{bmatrix} \tag{8.38a}$$

$$\boldsymbol{b}^1_{\text{mmse}} = \boldsymbol{H}^\top \begin{bmatrix} \boldsymbol{\mu}_1 - \boldsymbol{\Sigma}_1[\boldsymbol{\Sigma}_1 + \boldsymbol{\Sigma}_\alpha]^{-1}\boldsymbol{\mu}_1 \\ \boldsymbol{\mu}_2 - \boldsymbol{\Sigma}_{21}\boldsymbol{\Sigma}_1^{-1}\boldsymbol{\mu}_1 \end{bmatrix} \tag{8.38b}$$

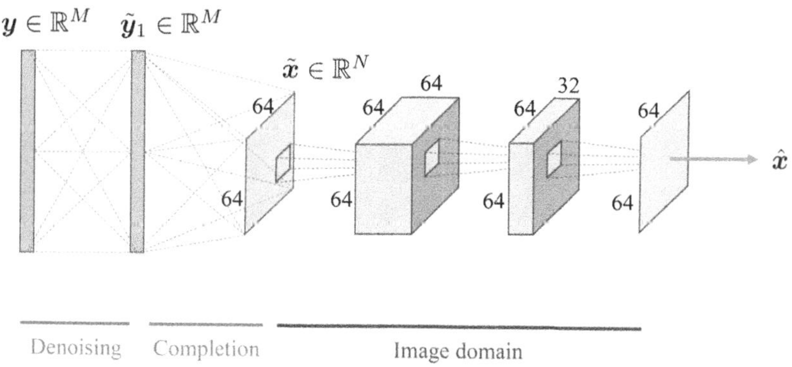

Figure 8.12. *Denoised completion network (DC-Net). For a color version of this figure, see www.iste.co.uk/fournier/unconventional.zip*

COMMENTS ON FIGURE 8.12.– *The first layer is a fully connected layer that computes the lowest mean squared error image using the analytical formula shown in equation [8.37]. As with the network introduced in Figure 8.8, the approximate solution $\tilde{x}$ is corrected by cascaded convolution layers, which has the effect of correcting residual artifacts in the image domain.*

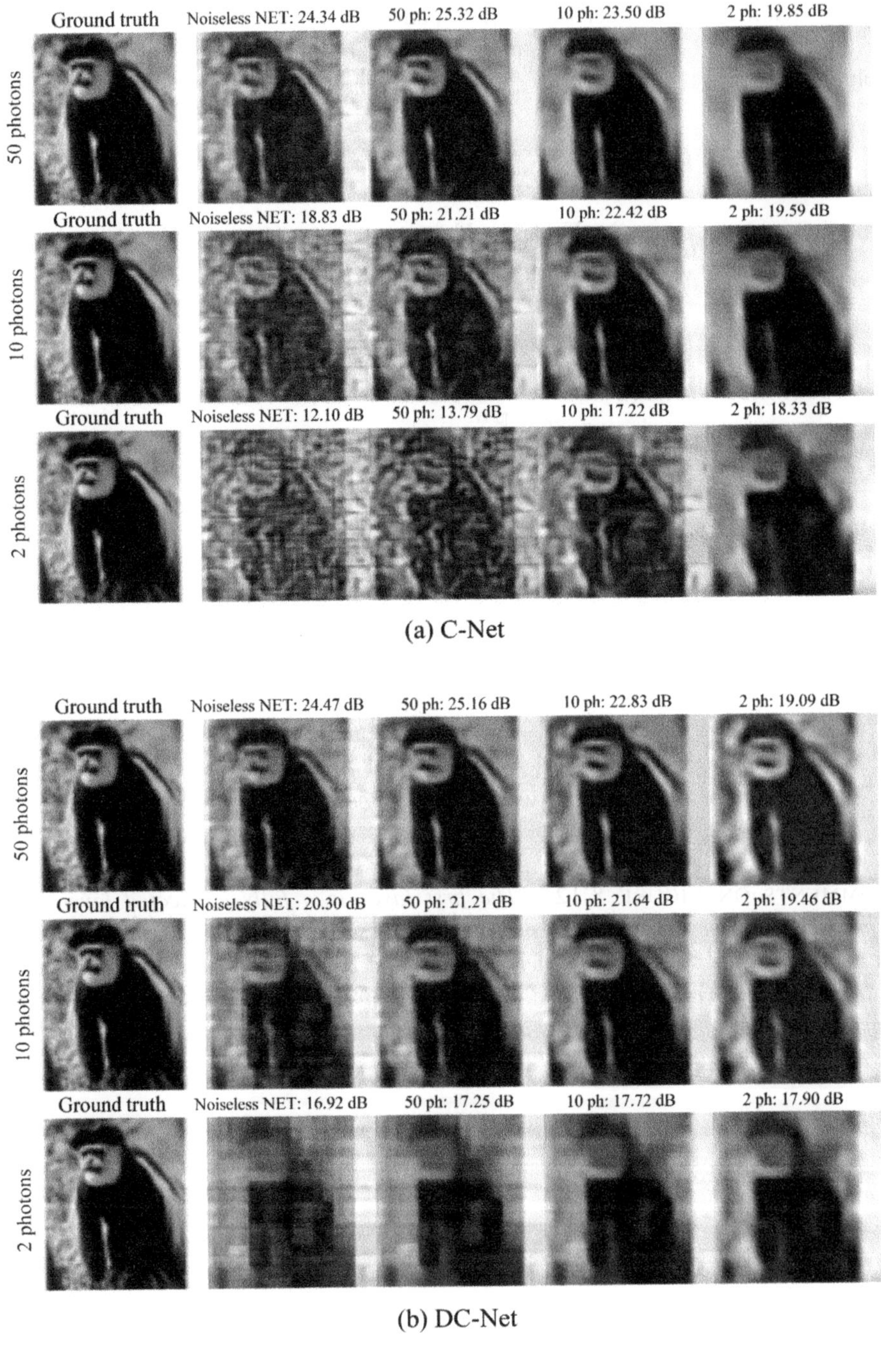

Figure 8.13. *Influence of noise level for two network architectures*

COMMENTS ON FIGURE 8.13.– *(a) C-Net defined by equation [8.33]. (b) DC-Net defined by equation* [8.38]. *Each of the figures (a) and (b) gathers reconstructions obtained with different levels of measurement and training noise. Each line corresponds to a measurement noise level. The signal-to-noise ratio increases from top to bottom:* $\alpha = 50$ *photons for the first line,* $\alpha = 10$ *photons for the second and* $\alpha = 2$ *photons for the third. Each column shows the reconstructions obtained by networks trained at increasing signal-to-noise ratios from left to right: no noise,* $\alpha = 50$ *photons,* $\alpha = 10$ *photons and* $\alpha = 2$ *photons.*

In Figure 8.13, we study the influence of measurement noise on reconstruction quality. We observe that a noiselessly trained reconstruction network will see its performances quickly decrease in the presence of noisy measurements (second column of Figure 8.13). For $\alpha = 2$ photons, the object in the scene is hardly discernible, which illustrates the need to train the network in the presence of noise. For a given measurement noise level, the best performing network is the one trained for the same noise level. As an example, for measurements with $\alpha = 10$ photons, the best network is the one trained at 10 photons (PSNR equal to 22.42 dB), while those trained with 50 and two photons lead to reduced PSNR of 21.21 and 19.59 dB, respectively. Visually, a network trained with too low a noise level leads to many artifacts, while a network trained with too high a noise level excessively smoothes the reconstruction.

8.5. Conclusion

This chapter provides a brief overview of single-pixel imaging from Hadamard transform optics to recent deep learning-based approaches. Hadamard transform optics was the first to have proposed acquiring an image by combining the signals from different pixels of the scene on a single-point detector. Under the assumption of additive Gaussian noise, this approach leads to significantly improving the signal-to-noise ratio of the acquired image, compared to a naive scanning approach. The compressed sensing theory then offered an elegant solution to reconstruct an image from a small number of measurements, which greatly reduces the number of measurements and therefore the acquisition time. More recently, learning approaches have contributed to considerably reduce the reconstruction time while improving the quality of the obtained images.

As we have strived to demonstrate, there are close links existing between classical and more recent learning-based reconstruction methods. The first layer of a reconstruction network in particular can be chosen to implement conventional solutions to inverse problems, such as the pseudo-inverse solution or the linear MMSE solution. The downstream layers can then be learned in order to correct the residual artifacts.

Reconstruction networks are currently the best performing, both visually and in terms of signal-to-noise ratios. When the photon noise becomes significant, typically below 50 photons per pixel, the network must be trained with noise. The level of training noise must be comparable to that of the measurements, otherwise performance will be significantly affected. Network robustness against an unknown noise level is currently part of the research themes of various groups. It is an extensive field of study, which would require its own chapter. The methods that should be mentioned include those that interpret classical iterative algorithms as successive network layers. Then, during the learning phase the hyperparameters are set, a regularization term or its gradient determined, or a proximal operator approximated. For more information about the subject, the reader can refer to the review by Arridge et al. (2019).

8.6. Acknowledgments

I would like to thank Corinne Fournier, Antonio Lorente Mur, Laurent Mahieu Williame as well as Françoise Peyrin for their kind and careful proofreading.

8.7. References

Adcock, B., Hansen, A.C., Poon, C., Roman, B. (eds) (2017). Breaking the coherence barrier: A new theory for compressed sensing. *Forum of Mathematics*, 5(e4), 84.

Arridge, S., Maass, P., Öktem, O., Schönlieb, C.-B. (2019). Solving inverse problems using data-driven models. *Acta Numerica*, 28, 1–174.

Baldassarre, L., Li, Y.-H., Scarlett, J., Gözcü, B., Bogunovic, I., Cevher, V. (2016). Learning-based compressive subsampling. *IEEE Journal of Selected Topics in Signal Processing*, 10(4), 809–822.

Barbastathis, G., Ozcan, A., Situ, G. (2019). On the use of deep learning for computational imaging. *Optica*, 6(8), 921–943.

Candes, E.J. and Wakin, M.B. (2008). An introduction to compressive sampling. *IEEE Signal Processing Magazine*, 25(2), 21–30.

Chan, W.L., Charan, K., Takhar, D., Kelly, K.F., Baraniuk, R.G., Mittleman, D.M. (2008). A single-pixel terahertz imaging system based on compressed sensing. *Applied Physics Letters*, 93(12), 121105.

Donoho, D.L. (2006). Compressed sensing. *IEEE Transactions on Information Theory*, 52, 1289–1306.

Duarte, M., Davenport, M., Takhar, D., Laska, J., Sun, T., Kelly, K., Baraniuk, R. (2008). Single-pixel imaging via compressive sampling. *Signal Processing Magazine, IEEE*, 25(2), 83–91.

Ducros, N., Lorente Mur, A., Peyrin, F. (2020). A completion network for reconstruction from compressed acquisition. *Proceedings of the IEEE 17th International Symposium on Biomedical Imaging (ISBI)*. IEEE, Iowa City, IA.

Edgar, M.P., Gibson, G.M., Padgett, M.J. (2019). Principles and prospects for single-pixel imaging. *Nature Photonics*, 13(1), 13–20.

Goodfellow, I., Bengio, Y., Courville, A. (2016). *Deep Learning*. MIT Press, Cambridge, MA.

Higham, C.F., Murray-Smith, R., Padgett, M.J., Edgar, M.P. (2018). Deep learning for real-time single-pixel video. *Scientific Reports*, 8(1), 2369.

Lorente Mur, A., Lorente Mur, A., Leclerc, P., Peyrin, F., Ducros, N., Ducros, N. (2021). Single-pixel image reconstruction from experimental data using neural networks. *Optics Express*, 29(11), 17097–17110.

Nelson, E.D. and Fredman, M.L. (1970). Hadamard spectroscopy. *JOSA*, 60(12), 1664–1669.

Ochoa, M., Pian, Q., Yao, R., Ducros, N., Intes, X. (2018). Assessing patterns for compressive fluorescence lifetime imaging. *Optics Letters*, 43(18), 4370–4373.

Openspyrit/Spyrit (2021). Openspyrit [Online]. Available at: https://github.com/openspyrit/spyrit.

Pian, Q., Yao, R., Sinsuebphon, N., Intes, X. (2017). Compressive hyperspectral time-resolved wide-field fluorescence lifetime imaging. *Nature Photonics*, 11, 411–414.

Radwell, N., Mitchell, K.J., Gibson, G.M., Edgar, M.P., Bowman, R., Padgett, M.J. (2014). Single-pixel infrared and visible microscope. *Optica*, 1(5), 285–289.

Rousset, F., Ducros, N., Peyrin, F., Valentini, G., D'Andrea, C., Farina, A. (2018). Time-resolved multispectral imaging based on an adaptive single-pixel camera. *Optics Express*, 26(8), 10550–10558.

Sloane, N.J.A. and Harwit, M. (1976). Masks for Hadamard transform optics, and weighing designs. *Applied Optics*, 15(1), 107–114.

Studer, V., Bobin, J., Chahid, M., Mousavi, H.S., Candes, E., Dahan, M. (2012). Compressive fluorescence microscopy for biological and hyperspectral imaging. *Proceedings of the National Academy of Sciences of the United States of America*, 109(26), E1679–E1687.

Vaz, P.G., Amaral, D., Ferreira, L.F.R., Morgado, M., Morgado, M., Cardoso, J. (2020). Image quality of compressive single-pixel imaging using different Hadamard orderings. *Optics Express*, 28(8), 11666–11681.

Glossary

Aperture synthesis: an interferometric process based on merging in amplitude and phase the data captured by a set of sensors in order to produce an image of better resolution. In optical or radio astronomy, a pupil synthesis of data from several distant (radio)telescopes is performed, which yields the same final angular resolution as would have been obtained with a (radio)telescope whose size would be the maximum distance between the individual sensors. In holographic microscopy, the principle is the same but angular aperture synthesis is performed on the illumination, which yields the same spatial resolution as if a condenser of large numerical aperture had been used.

Born approximation: in optics, the (first-order) Born approximation consists of considering that the interaction between the impinging illumination field and the investigated sample results in a single scattering event. Under this assumption, the influence of the diffracted field in the source term of the diffraction integral is neglected, and the total field detected in the sensor plane can be approximated by the illumination field plus a diffracted field, which is of much lower amplitude than the illumination field.

Cell dry mass: the mass of everything that composes a biological cell, except water (which represents 70% of the total mass). Somewhat surprisingly, this important parameter is directly proportional to the integral of the optical path difference on the surface of the cell (with a constant and known proportionality coefficient).

Coherence scanning interferometry: a technique that utilizes the limited coherence of white light fringes in incoherent light in interference microscopy by scanning over the whole depth of the structure to be measured. It is used to measure

Unconventional Optical Imaging for Biology,
coordinated by Corinne FOURNIER and Olivier HAEBERLÉ. © ISTE Ltd 2024.

large roughness and surface structures typically over a few micrometers to a few tens of micrometers (or even hundreds).

Convolution (convolution product): a mathematical operation between two functions. It models the filtering by a translation-invariant linear system. One of the functions corresponds to the input signal of the system i(x) and the other to the filter f(x). The result of the convolution corresponds to the system output $o(X)=\int e(X-x).f(x)dx$. The *Fourier transform* of a convolution product is obtained by multiplying the Fourier transforms of the input functions.

Deep learning: a set of machine learning methods that make use of deep neural networks (see *neural network*). The adjective "deep" is conventionally used for networks comprising at least four layers but this number is often higher (up to several hundred).

Digital holographic microscopy: the application of holography at the microscopic scale. As in traditional holography (at the macroscopic scale), the wavefront resulting from the interaction of the observed specimen is digitally recorded as a hologram, after modulation by a reference wave; a numerical reconstruction of this wavefront (demodulation) makes it possible to rebuild an image of this specimen by taking advantage of the strong magnification allowed by a microscope.

Digital micromirror device (DMD): an electromechanical microsystem comprising several hundred thousand micromirrors capable of rotating in two different positions. DMDs make it possible to spatially modulate light by reflection, at rates of several kilohertz.

(Dis)similarity measure: a mathematical relation for objectively quantifying the (non)similarity of two given sets (images, surfaces, textures, etc.).

Epoch: an iteration during which all signals/images in a database have been processed once during a learning phase (see *learning phase*). This terminology typically applies to stochastic gradient descent algorithms used for training a neural network (see *deep learning* and *neural network*).

Ewald sphere: a geometric construction used in the description of the diffraction phenomenon under elastic conditions. In the elastic scattering regime, the ends of the wave vectors describe a sphere centered at the origin of the spatial frequencies.

Fluorescence (light-induced): the property of certain molecules and biomolecules to spontaneously emit photons of wavelength $\lambda_{\text{emission}}$ (fluorescence light) as a result of electronic excitation caused by the absorption of photons of wavelength $\lambda_{excitation} < \lambda_{emission}$ (excitation light).

Fluorescence labeling: specific labeling using fluorophores, which are fluorescent molecules. The three main advantages of fluorescence are as follows: the very high contrast of the resulting images (dark background), making it possible to detect even a single molecule; the possibility of working on living cells; the huge variety of markers available and their functional specificity. It should be noted that all recent techniques of fluorescence super-resolution microscopy (resolution better than the diffraction limit) employ the nonlinear properties of fluorescence emission.

Forward model/direct model (in imaging): a numerical model of image formation. This model is used to compute image simulations. The problem of defining a forward model is called a forward problem.

Full-field optical coherence tomography: an imaging technique based on the principle of coherence scanning interferometry for observing structures in transparent and turbid media. The zero step difference makes it possible to detect only the ballistic photons that have been backscattered by an interface in the sample (e.g. an organic tissue) and to reconstruct its volumetric information, typically over a few hundred micrometers in depth. This technique is similar to ultrasound echography.

Hadamard transform: an orthogonal transform that can be seen as a discrete 2^m dimension Fourier transform. The Hadamard transform of a signal of length $n = 2^m$ can be obtained by a fast algorithm that requires only $n \log n$ additions or subtractions.

Homologous points: these are projections of a point of the scenic three-dimensional reference frame onto the two-dimensional reference frames of images acquired from at least two different points of view.

Image reconstruction: the estimation of physical and/or geometric quantities of imaged objects from one or more images (indirect measurements).

Image registration: a superposition technique of the regions of two images containing homologous points in the same scene.

Immersion medium: the medium between the microscope slide and the entrance lens of a microscope objective. The most common objectives are air, or dry objectives, the index of air being $n_{air} = 1$, water immersion ($n_{water} = 1.33$) objectives and oil immersion (n_{oil} = 1.515) objectives, but there are also immersion objectives using silicone oils ($n_{silicon}$ = 1.4).

In-line holography: a holography configuration where, unlike off-axis holography, the sample illumination wave is also the reference wave.

Interference microscopy: an optical microscopy method used for the three-dimensional measurement of microscopic structures on the surface and inside transparent or turbid media by interferometry and different types of signal/image processing.

Inverse problem: a problem whose objective is to find the parameters of interest from measurements and the associated forward model (see *forward model*). An inverse problem is generally solved by finding the parameters of interest minimizing a criterion that combines a data-fidelity term (see *likelihood*) and a regularization term (see *regularization*).

Köhler illumination: in optical microscopy, Köhler illumination is a sample illumination technique that ensures a homogeneous illumination, a high but adjustable illumination numerical aperture, and the limitation of the stray light entering the optical system.

Labeling: a targeted insertion of molecules used to highlight a set of target molecules in the sample (e.g. staining and fluorescence); the degree of specificity derives from the type of chemical bond between the labeling molecule and the target molecule (example of strong specificity: antibody labeling or immunolabeling).

Learning phase: the stage during which the parameters (bias, weights) of a neural network (see *neural network*) are adjusted in order to be able to perform a given task (such as classification, segmentation, image reconstruction, etc.).

Likelihood (term): a measure of how accurately a model fits to data. For finer results, this measure takes into account the uneven quality of data (via the data covariance matrix, for instance).

Linear model: a direct model (see *forward model*) that linearly depends on the parameters of interest (see *linear operator*). A discretized linear model can be represented by a matrix. The model is said to be nonlinear if it depends on the parameters of interest in a nonlinear way.

Linear operator: follows the principle of superposition. Applying it to a linear combination of (input) variables is equivalent to making a linear combination of the results of this operator on these same input variables.

Local spectroscopy: a technique based on coherence scanning interferometry for measurement of the local reflection spectrum of microscopic surfaces by using a Fourier transform applied to white fringe signals. It is used to measure the spectral distribution of a surface for colorimetry and to identify the different existing materials.

Mapping methods (or mosaicing): a set of methods based on registration techniques that insert all of the information seen in a set of images in a single frame of reference, thus leading to a global representation, expanded and without redundancy of the data of a scene.

Medical endoscopy: a method for visual exploration of the interior of the human body that uses a flexible or rigid optical tube a few millimeters in diameter (endoscope) to illuminate the internal tissues and acquire images thereof by means of a camera.

Microsphere-assisted microscopy: a super-resolution technique that employs a glass microsphere (in air) between the sample and the microscope objective to improve lateral resolution. Use in interferometric microscopy enables nanometrology to be performed.

Multi- and hyperspectral imaging: a set of methods for acquiring highly spatially and spectrally resolved images, that is, images formed in a large number of different spectral bands or wavelengths (typically a few dozen to several hundred); stacking these monochromatic images leads to a hyperspectral "cube" being constituted whose dimensions are those of the image (number of pixel columns x number of pixel rows) and the number of spectral bands acquired.

Neural network: a parametric model consisting of elementary units, called artificial neurons, connected to each other according to a model inspired by neural networks in biology. Forward propagation networks are composed of neurons organized in successive layers so that the information propagates in a single direction.

Noise (in imaging): undesirable and unpredictable signal that degrades image data quality. It can be statistically modeled for example to be taken into account in a reconstruction process.

Numerical aperture (NA): in microscopy, the numerical aperture is a quantity characterizing the objective, defined by the formula NA = n sinα. In this formula, n is the immersion medium refractive index, and α is the half-angle of the objective aperture, that is, the angle between the optical axis and the extremal ray entering the objective. It should be noted that if the index of the observed specimen is lower than the index of the immersion medium, the former limits the numerical aperture.

Off-axis holography: an interferometric setup with two waves. Here, the two waves interfere with a small angle on the sensor, generating a spatial modulation of the hologram. By demodulating the images thus acquired, the amplitude and the phase of the wave diffracted by the object can be reconstructed.

Optical etendue: a quantity characterizing the way in which light "spreads" in terms of area and angle. It corresponds to the product of the source area by the solid angle formed by the entrance pupil of the optical system seen from the source.

Optical flow: a field of vectors whose origin and end correspond to pairs of homologous points in two images.

Optical path difference (OPD): used to measure an optical thickness (see *thickness or optical path*) with respect to a reference thickness. Typically, this reference corresponds to the path of the wave through a homogeneous medium (air or water most of the time). Consequently, a measurement of the OPD gives information on what, in the sample, deviates from the reference medium.

Optical super-resolution: in recent years, several methods have been developed to improve the resolution of optical systems. The most spectacular results have been obtained in fluorescence microscopy, with the development of techniques such as PALM, STORM, F-PALM, STED, SSIM, SAX, MINFLUX and MINSTED through which it has been possible, by skilfully employing the characteristics of the fluorescence phenomenon, to "break" the Abbe limit, and usually reach resolutions of a few tens of nanometers, and in some particular cases, to reach a few nanometers.

Optimization methods: numerical techniques that can iteratively approximate an exact solution (a vector of parameters to be estimated) by automatically adjusting, from an initial solution, a set of values that allows for converging toward the final solution in the parameter space.

Phase mask or phase-shift mask: a (static) optical system that shifts the phase of light according to a spatial distribution that can be arbitrary (also called diffractive optical elements), which can be used in reflection or transmission and that allows wavefronts with known characteristics to be generated. They can be found for example in optical lithography, for generating Airy beams, or extending the depth of field of imaging systems. Their total transparency is their main advantage.

Phase modulator: an electro-optical device for dynamically creating a phase mask (as opposed to static phase masks). These devices can be discrete (e.g. liquid crystal modulator) or continuous (e.g. deformable mirror). There are a number of existing variants in transmission and reflection.

Phase retrieval: in interferometric imaging, this consists of reconstructing the phase information based on intensity measurements.

Phase shift (of a plane/an object): a negative or positive phase shift corresponds to how a wave is delayed or advanced when traveling through an object. This phase shift is classically expressed in radians. It can be expressed by a time unit by dividing it by $2\pi\nu$, ν being the wave frequency in the medium.

Phase-shifting: a method consisting of combining holograms for which the reference wave is shifted by a known quantity. The sequence thus acquired considers phase shifts of the reference wave ranging from 0 to 2 pi. For example, to carry out an acquisition in *phase-shifting* with four images, the reference phase will be shifted by pi/2 between each acquisition. By digitally processing these images, the wave phase can be estimated from intensity measurements.

Phase-shifting microscopy: a mathematical technique used to quantify interference fringes in monochromatic or quasi-monochromatic light in interference microscopy by introducing several phase shifts (typically 3–7) between the two interferometer arms to measure small roughnesses, usually below half the wavelength.

Pinhole model: a geometric camera model for which all the light rays reaching the image plane travel through a single point (the pinhole) and whose parameters are related to the optics (focal length, pixel size and projection of the optical center onto the image).

Pixel super-resolution: refers to the process that involves improving the digital spatial resolution of an image (by virtually decreasing the sampling step). Usually, super-resolution algorithms use a stack of images acquired with slight transverse shifts to compute an image with better resolution.

Point spread function (PSF): describes the response of an imaging system as the image of a single-point source through this system. Because of the limited system bandwidth, the image of a point is not a point but a blurry spot. Impulse response is a more general term, where PSF is the impulse response of an optical system.

Poisson noise (shot-noise): a type of noise (see *noise (in imaging)*) intrinsic to light measurements, which originates from the discrete nature of particles, namely photons and their conversion to photoelectrons. It is characterized by a variance equal to an expected value: the mean.

Regularization: "regularity" constraint (smoothness, sparsity, positivity, etc.) introducing a priori knowledge (independently of the data) on the parameters of interest when solving an inverse problem (see *inverse problem*). Such constraints offset the loss of information due to the instrument and prevent noise amplification.

Spatial coherence: a measure of the cross-correlation of information from two points on the same wavefront. A source is spatially coherent as long as the cross-correlation is not zero. A plane wave or a wave originating from a point source are perfect coherent waves.

Spatial resolution: the typical size of the smallest structure of the object of interest visible in measurements. For example, in astronomy (focusing to infinity), $1.22\lambda/D$ is the commonly used resolution criterion (Rayleigh criterion) for the angular resolution (in radians), with the observation wavelength λ, of a diffraction-limited imaging system, where D is the pupil diameter. In microscopy, the Abbe criterion gives for the resolution $d = \lambda/(2NA)$, with NA the objective numerical aperture (see *numerical aperture*). There are several variants of these criteria, depending on the configurations being considered (Sparrow criterion, Schuster criterion), and many techniques have been developed to measure them, which explains the wide variety of resolution test patterns depending on the measurement considered (USAF-1951 test pattern, Siemens test pattern, IEEE test pattern, Ronchi test pattern, etc.).

Temporal coherence: related to the width of the emission spectrum of a source and characterizes the ability of a source to generate interferences. The finer the spectrum, the easier it will be to record interference.

Thickness or optical path: the product of the geometrical thickness by the refractive index of the medium through which light travels. It should be noted that the index may not be homogeneous across the thickness traveled through.

Tomographic diffractive microscopy: a transmission microscopy technique, based on aperture synthesis, through which 3D imaging of unlabeled microscopic specimens is obtained. This technique is known by various names: diffractive optical microscopy, aperture synthesis microscopy, phase tomography, holotomography, scanning holographic microscopy, phase tomographic microscopy, etc.

Transmittance (of a plane/object): the ratio between the radiant energy of the light wave that has traveled through a plane and the radiant energy of the incident light wave. For the ratio between complex amplitudes, it is usually referred to as complex transmittance.

Twin or virtual image: an artifact ensuing from the reconstruction due to the backpropagation of an in-line hologram (from which only the intensity is recorded). It corresponds to the image the sensor would have recorded if the virtual object was at a distance –z therefrom (the real object being located at distance z).

Wavefront: a surface with the same phase as a wave field. For example, for a collimated laser source, wavefronts are plane and perpendicular to the optical axis. For a single-point source, wavefronts are spherical. There are continuous transformations for representing any wavefront as a sum of plane waves, or spherical waves depending on the configuration being considered.

Wavefront sensor: a device that allows direct analysis of the shape of the wavefront, without using holography. Many techniques have been developed, initially for astronomy, but have since been adapted to the specific characteristics of microscopy or to the analysis of laser beams.

List of Authors

Walter BLONDEL
CRAN
CNRS
Université de Lorraine
Vandœuvre-lès-Nancy
France

Pierre BON
Université de Limoges
CNRS
XLIM
France

Rémy CLAVEAU
ICube
CNRS
Université de Strasbourg
Illkirch
France

Christian DAUL
CRAN
CNRS
Université de Lorraine
Vandœuvre-lès-Nancy
France

Matthieu DEBAILLEUL
IRIMAS
Université de Haute-Alsace
Mulhouse
France

Nicolas DUCROS
CREATIS
INSA Lyon
and
Institut Universitaire de France (IUF)
Paris
France

Manuel FLURY
ICube
CNRS
Université de Strasbourg
Illkirch
France

Corinne FOURNIER
Laboratoire Hubert Curien
CNRS
IOGS
Télécom Saint-Étienne
Université Jean Monnet
Saint-Etienne
France

Michel GROSS
L2C
CNRS
Université de Montpellier
France

Olivier HAEBERLÉ
IRIMAS
Université de Haute-Alsace
Mulhouse
France

Sébastien MARBACH
ICube
CNRS
Université de Strasbourg
Illkirch
France

Fabien MOMEY
Laboratoire Hubert Curien
CNRS
IOGS
IUT de Saint-Étienne
Université Jean Monnet
Saint-Étienne
France

Serge MONNERET
Aix-Marseille Université
CNRS
Centrale Marseille
Institut Fresnel
France

Paul MONTGOMERY
ICube
CNRS
Université de Strasbourg
Illkirch
France

Amir NAHAS
ICube
CNRS
Université de Strasbourg
Illkirch
France

Thomas OLIVIER
Laboratoire Hubert Curien
CNRS
IOGS
Faculté des sciences et techniques
Université Jean Monnet
Saint-Étienne
France

Stéphane PERRIN
ICube
CNRS
Université de Strasbourg
Illkirch
France

Julien SAVATIER
Aix-Marseille Université
CNRS
Centrale Marseille
Institut Fresnel
Marseille
France

Bertrand SIMON
LP2N
CNRS
IOGS
Université de Bordeaux
Talence
France

Ferréol SOULEZ
Université de Lyon
Université Lyon 1
ENS de Lyon
CNRS
Centre de recherche
astrophysique de Lyon
Saint-Genis-Laval
France

Éric THIÉBAUT
Université de Lyon
Université Lyon 1
ENS de Lyon
CNRS
Centre de recherche
astrophysique de Lyon
Saint-Genis-Laval
France

Nicolas VERRIER
IRIMAS
Université de Haute-Alsace
Mulhouse
France

Index

A, B, C

D, E, F

G, H, I

L, M, N

O, P

R, S, T

U, V, W, Z

Printed and bound by CPI Group (UK) Ltd, Croydon, CR0 4YY
13/09/2026
14960999-0003